Dana Carpender's

KETO
FAT GRAM
COUNTER

The Quick-Reference
Guide to Balancing Your
MACROS and CALORIES

Dana Carpender

Author of the best-selling *500 Ketogenic Recipes*

FAIR WINDS

Brimming with creative inspiration, how-to projects, and useful information to enrich your everyday life, Quarto Knows is a favorite destination for those pursuing their interests and passions. Visit our site and dig deeper with our books into your area of interest: Quarto Creates, Quarto Cooks, Quarto Homes, Quarto Lives, Quarto Drives, Quarto Explores, Quarto Gifts, or Quarto Kids.

© 2020 Quarto Publishing Group USA Inc.
Text © 2020 Dana Carpender

First Published in 2020 by Fair Winds Press, an imprint of The Quarto Group, 100 Cummings Center, Suite 265-D, Beverly, MA 01915, USA.
T (978) 282-9590 F (978) 283-2742 QuartoKnows.com

Fair Winds Press titles are also available at discount for retail, wholesale, promotional, and bulk purchase. For details, contact the Special Sales Manager by email at specialsales@quarto.com or by mail at The Quarto Group, Attn: Special Sales Manager, 100 Cummings Center, Suite 265-D, Beverly, MA 01915, USA.

24 23 22 21 20   1 2 3 4 5

ISBN: 978-1-59233-908-2

Digital edition published in 2020

Library of Congress Cataloging-in-Publication Data available

Cover Design and Page Layout: Sporto

Printed in China

The information in this book is for educational purposes only. It is not intended to replace the advice of a physician or medical practitioner. Please see your health-care provider before beginning any new health program.

All product and company names are trademarks™ or registered® trademarks of their respective holders. Use of them does not imply any affiliation with or endorsement by them.

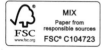

CONTENTS

Introduction

Welcome to the wonderful world of keto! I've been running my body on fat and ketones for almost twenty-four years now, and I have never considered going back to the mood and energy swings that came from running a glucose-based metabolism. You know those ads about "that three o'clock feeling," the ones that assume that everybody's energy crashes a few hours after lunch? Or the ones about how you just *have* to have a snack halfway through the afternoon or you'll fall over? Yeah, no. Haven't had a blood sugar crash in years.

Snacks just aren't a big thing for me anymore. Once I've had a cheese and avocado omelet fried in bacon grease for breakfast, I'm not hungry again for... well, quite a while. I have long since fallen into a pattern of eating two meals a day, rather than three. I'm just not hungry enough for three meals a day. When I think back on the years when I ate a Low fat diet centered on whole grains and other "good" carbs, and how ravenous I constantly felt, it's nightmarish. Yes, my life still centers on food to a large degree, since I write about it for a living. But that desperate "OMG, I have to eat something *right now* or I'll collapse!" feeling? Nope.

Though my body has adapted to running on fat and ketones—which took just a few days for me—my energy level still fluctuates, sure, depending on how much sleep I've had, my stress level, the weather. But my actual fuel supply has been steady, constant, and reliable. When I burn through the fuel from my last meal, I shift smoothly over to burning body fat with no energy drop. Just the way the body evolved to work.

Are you ready for limitless energy? Are you ready to teach your body to burn fat for fuel? Are you ready to finally not be hungry all the time?

WHAT ARE KETONES?

So what is a ketone, anyway? Ketones are a by-product of burning fat for fuel and are themselves a valuable fuel source. You may have heard that coal can be partially burned, yielding coke—not the soft drink, but a secondary fuel that burns hotter and cleaner than coal. Think of ketones as the coke that is derived from the burning of fat.

Most of your body's tissues will run just fine on free fatty acids. But there are some tissues, most notably the brain, that cannot burn fat. The vast majority of tissues that will not burn fat, *especially* the brain, will happily run on ketones.

Indeed, a ketogenic diet was first devised to treat epilepsy, a purpose for which it is still used today.

There are a few—a very few—tissues that require glucose, and a healthy person will have roughly a teaspoon of glucose in their blood while fasting. The liver can easily keep up with that demand through gluconeogenesis, the creation of glucose from protein and, to a lesser degree, from fat. There is no biochemical need for dietary carbohydrate.

WHAT IS A KETOGENIC DIET?

A ketogenic diet is a diet that forces the body to turn to fat and ketones for fuel. This is done by strictly limiting carbohydrates. I repeat: *This is done by strictly limiting carbohydrates.* I stress this because so much emphasis is being put on increasing fat intake that limiting carbs can get lost in the static. To be in dietary ketosis, most people need to cut carbohydrate intake to 50 grams or less per day, and many need to stay below 20 grams per day.

You can, of course, determine if and to what degree you are in ketosis through urine test strips, a blood ketone meter, or a breath meter (my choice). These can tell you whether you are creating ketones and, therefore, whether you are running a fat-based metabolism. What they cannot tell you is *where that fat is coming from*. Just because you are in ketosis does not mean you are losing weight. You may be burning body fat, sure. But you might be burning dietary fat, instead of body fat.

So let's be clear: Yes, I am in favor of a high-fat diet. I am a fan of rib-eye steaks, pork shoulder, eggs scrambled in bacon grease, plenty of olive oil on salads, pecans, walnuts, macadamia nuts, butter-dipped asparagus, plenty of mayo in my tuna salad (made with olive-oil-packed tuna), and yes, bacon-bacon-bacon, all that stuff. But adding fat to your diet without slashing the carb count to the bone will not get you into ketosis.

On the other hand, if you cut carbs back to 20 grams per day, you will very likely go into ketosis even without deliberately adding fat to your diet. And unless you're doing something bizarre, like eating nothing but water-packed tuna and grilled skinless chicken breast,* you will be eating a relatively high-fat diet.

Whether you need to deliberately strive to increase your fat intake depends on your purpose for eating a ketogenic diet. If you are shooting for a therapeutic degree of ketosis—for, say, seizure control or to improve cognitive function—then

---

*Need I say, this is not recommended?

adding fats, especially coconut oil and MCT oil, is a good way to get there. Similarly, if you are using ketones to fuel endurance exercise, fat bombs and butter-and-coconut-oil–laced coffee are great tools.

But if you are eating a ketogenic diet to lose and control your weight, some of the fat you burn must come from your body's fat stores. In other words, butter on your broccoli and asparagus, sautéed mushrooms on your steak, coleslaw made with mayo and sour cream? Good. Five or six cups of butter-and-oil–laced coffee or a dozen fat bombs a day? You may be overshooting the mark. I find this sort of thing (for me, it's likely super-low-carb shirataki noodles with butter and Parmesan) is best used in place of a meal, not *in addition to* them.

You're not adding fat to your usual caloric intake. You're substituting it for the carbs you used to eat. And since fat has 9 calories per gram to carbohydrate's 4 calories per gram, the volume doesn't need to be as great.

WHAT ARE MACROS?

"Macros" is short for macronutrients, aka stuff that yields calories. These would be protein, carbohydrate, and fat. One very popular form of the ketogenic diet involves eating to hit specific macronutrient ratios: commonly somewhere between 10 and 20 percent of calories from protein, 75 to 85 percent of calories from fat, and the remaining 5 to 10 percent from carbohydrate. This is why, in particular, this book lists the percentage of calories from fat for each entry. If you pay attention to the percentage of fat you're getting—a little more from one food, a little less from another—and make sure you stay under your carb count, your macros should be good.

In calculating macros, it is helpful to know that fats have 9 calories per gram, while both protein and carbohydrate have 4 calories per gram. Still, if you're being strict about macros, you'll probably want an app to help you track them. (I'd recommend one, but I don't have one. A search in the app store for "track your macros" turns up tons of 'em.)

How Much Protein?

Since protein is more readily converted to glucose than fat is, some keto dieters limit it pretty strictly. If, for instance, you are eating 85 percent fat, 10 percent protein, and 5 percent carbohydrate, on 2,000 calories per day, that would allow 200 calories of protein, or 50 grams. Since meat generally runs about 7 grams of protein per ounce (the rest being fat and water), that would be about

7 ounces of meat per day. Eggs have about 6 grams of protein apiece, so this plan would allow 8 eggs instead of the meat, or some combination of the two.

However, many people eat more protein than this and stay in ketosis. Again, your meter is your friend. You might also get a glucometer (blood sugar meter) and check your fasting blood sugar when you wake up. If it's above 100 when you know you've been eating very low carb, you're likely among those whose bodies are a little too good at converting protein to glucose.

The general recommendation is 1 gram of protein per kilogram of healthy body weight, which, for those of us still mired in pounds and ounces, means about a gram per every 2 pounds of healthy body weight. If your healthy weight (*not* your super-model-skinny weight!) would be, say, 130 pounds, that means that 65 grams of protein per day is a reasonable number to shoot for. I can't recommend dropping below 50 grams per day except for short fasts and the like.

If you find you do need to limit your protein, consider combining it with fat and perhaps some very-low-carb veggies: a 6-ounce steak with mushrooms sautéed in garlic butter; tuna salad with celery, a little onion, sugar-free bread-and-butter pickles, and plenty of mayo; shrimp sautéed in olive oil and garlic, tossed with shirataki noodles, sliced olives, capers, and pine nuts; an omelet cooked in bacon grease and filled with cheese and guacamole. Any of these will be delicious meals with satisfying portions that will help you stay within your macros.

The Other Source of Calories

There is one other source of calories: alcohol, at 7 calories per gram. It is possible to drink some alcohol on a keto diet, but it will skew your macros.

- Unsweetened, basic hard liquors—vodka, gin, whisky, Scotch, rum, tequila—are zero carb and, therefore, your best bet. Avoid the trendy, sweetened, flavored liquors, and, of course, be careful about your mixers.

- Dry wines run 1 - 4 grams carbohydrate per glass. No sweet wine!

- Most beers are way too high carb, but you can squeeze in a Michelob Ultra, Miller Lite, or Corona Premier now and then.

Two more thoughts on alcohol: One, like carbohydrate, alcohol stops fat burning until you burn through it. It is a luxury, to be sure. And two, some breath ketone meters pick up alcohol as ketones and will give you a false reading if you test after drinking.

HOW STRICT DO I HAVE TO BE?

That will depend on two things: your body and your definition of "strict."

I wish I could give credit where credit is due, but I've lost the original post. I saw a meme on Facebook that defined the three kinds of keto dieters: The super-strict kind, who track all their macros, eat only "clean" foods, shun everything processed or artificial—for whom the diet works. The semi-strict kind, who pay attention to macros and eat mostly real, unprocessed foods—for whom the diet also works. And the kind who just slash the carbs out of their diet, shun starches and sugars, and eat mostly animal foods and low-carb vegetables—for whom the diet works as well. The point is, there's no one precise way to follow a keto diet.

I have seen opinions kicking around the internet, people stating that keto is "like Atkins, but you only eat *clean* foods, organic vegetables, grass-fed meat, no artificial sweeteners." I have no problem with any of those ideas, but none of them is essential to a ketogenic diet. In fact, Atkins (properly *Dr. Atkins' Diet Revolution* and *Dr. Atkins' New Diet Revolution*) was and is a ketogenic diet. It was the world's big introduction to the concept, all the way back in 1972. I know: I tried it, peeing on Ketostix and all. I invented my first low-carb dessert by whipping heavy cream with cocoa powder and saccharin. I lost weight! It's just that, at thirteen, the concept of "permanent lifestyle change" was not on my radar.

When I went low carb in 1995, I didn't pick a particular diet. I'd been a nutrition buff for long enough to know which foods were high carb and which were not. I just dropped the starches and sugars and ate grocery-store meat, cheese, eggs, and produce. I lost weight and gained all the other benefits of ketosis: high energy, low appetite, clear head, great mood. When I finally got around to buying a bottle of Ketostix, sure enough, I was in ketosis.

No matter what else I ate, I was shunning starches and sugars almost entirely. *The thing to be strictest about is that carb intake.* (I do know people who have had to quit dairy and/or nuts to get the weight loss they wanted, and it's entirely possible I'd lose another fifteen pounds if I quit them, too. Honestly, it's not worth it to me. I'd also probably lose weight if I gave up wine in the evenings—but again, not worth it to me. If you're having trouble losing, these are worthwhile things to try.)

If you're the sort who loves going whole-hog on something, who will get satisfaction from seeing that neat pie chart every day of your 80 percent fat/15 percent protein/5 percent carbs, do it! And if you're the type who would rather just fry your eggs in butter every morning, order the bunless fast food burger for lunch, have sugar-free coffee syrup along with heavy cream in your coffee, and have a grocery-store rotisserie chicken along with whatever looks good at the salad bar for dinner, go for it. So long as your meter says you're in ketosis, it's all good.

TOTAL VERSUS NET CARBS

Some people count total carbs; others count net carbs. "Total carbs" is an easy concept: all of the carbohydrate in a serving, regardless of kind. "Net carbs," however, can get fuzzy.

Originally introduced as the "effective carb count" by Drs. Michael and Mary Dan Eades in their 1996 book *Protein Power*, the idea was simple: Since the human gut cannot digest or absorb fiber, which is a carbohydrate, they subtracted fiber from the total carb count of any food to get the number of grams of carbohydrate that would actually raise blood sugar and stimulate an insulin release. This allowed the dieter to eat more vegetables, low-sugar fruits, and nuts.

Then in the early 2000s, low-carbohydrate and, yes, ketogenic diets caught on in a big way. Cue the food-processing industry. All of a sudden, the market was flooded with foods making dubious claims about their "net carb" counts. Instead of allowing the consumption of nutritious real foods, the net carbs concept was used to push highly processed "treats." Along with fiber, companies subtracted sugar alcohols, "low glycemic monosaccharide" (aka fructose), glycerine, and resistant starches from the carb count for the consumer, largely in service of being able to offer highly processed, low-carb junk food.

Still, 20 to 50 grams of carbs per day add up quickly. Even many herbs and spices will add a gram or two to a dish, and a couple of green leafy salads, half an avocado, or some sautéed mushrooms and onions in a day will get you up to 20 grams total carbs. Which foods will bring more interest and variety, not to mention vitamins and minerals, to your diet: these vegetables, or a low-carb cookie? Make your choices with your eyes open.

As to what can legitimately be subtracted from total carbs to get an honest net-carb count, I'm going with two things, and two things only: fiber, which we've discussed, and erythritol. Let me explain that second one.

Sugar Alcohols

Sugar alcohols, aka polyols, are long-chain carbohydrates that are slowly and incompletely absorbed by the human body. They are widely used in commercial sugar-free sweets because (unlike artificial sweeteners, or stevia or monk fruit) they have the bulk of sugar, and also produce a lot of the textural effects of sugar. Food processors routinely subtract them from carbohydrate counts to get the lowest net-carb count possible.

Not so fast! According to the International Food Information Council Foundation, most sugar alcohols are absorbed to some degree, from roughly half of maltitol, the most-used of the bunch, to 65 percent of sorbitol. (Xylitol, quite popular, is in between those two at 60 percent absorption.) This means you cannot discount these sugar alcohols completely. When I eat, say, a sugar-free mini Reese's cup, I count half the maltitol carbs. So should you.

However, there is one sugar alcohol that is virtually unabsorbed, passing through the body unchanged in urine and feces: erythritol. This has made erythritol and erythritol blends (such as Swerve, Natural Mate, Virtue, and Truvia) the up-and-coming sugar-free sweeteners. I reach for them often.

Erythritol is the only sugar alcohol I consider valid to subtract entirely from your carb count when calculating net carbs. Since the food processors will inevitably subtract all of any sugar alcohol from their net-carb counts, it is up to you to read the labels and see which, if any, sugar alcohol is used. If it's erythritol, consider the net carb number valid. If it is any of the other sugar alcohols—maltitol, xylitol, sorbitol, etc.—add half of the "sugar alcohols" number back to that net carb count for a closer approximation. In this book, we've subtracted erythritol, if that's the only sugar alcohol used.

And if you've had an embarrassing experience with sugar-free candy in the past, it's good to know that erythritol also does not cause gastric distress.

Other Sweeteners

The Sweetener Wars rage on. I remain largely neutral. I have only a couple of points to make on the subject.

Artificial sweeteners are not inimical to ketosis. Indeed, when ketogenic diets were first used for seizure control nearly a hundred years ago, they included saccharin. Many people have done just fine on a ketogenic diet that included artificial sweeteners. I dislike saccharin (Sweet'N Low) and aspartame (Equal), but I still keep sucralose (Splenda) on hand, though I reach for flavored liquid stevia and monk fruit more and more. When I need a granular sweetener, I generally grab an erythritol-stevia or an erythritol-monk fruit blend. The point is, if you like sucralose, don't buy the hype that says it's not okay on a keto diet.

Do, however, use liquid sucralose, rather than granular, whenever possible. The granular stuff is bulked with maltodextrin, a carbohydrate, to make it measure like sugar. The "zero carb" claim on the label is an artifact of federal labeling law combined with a small serving size: the government allows anything with less than 0.5 gram of carbohydrate per serving to claim zero grams, and a "serving" of granular Splenda or its knock-offs is 1 teaspoon. When calculating nutritional stats for recipes, I assume granular sucralose to have 0.5 gram of carb per teaspoon, which adds up to 24 grams per cup—far less than sugar, but enough to pay attention to.

Allulose

Recently, a new sweetener, allulose, has hit the market. It is being touted as low carbohydrate. I do not yet have enough information to come to any kind of conclusion. I do know it is a form of fructose, a sugar that has a low glycemic impact but is very hard on the body. At this writing, I am not willing to use it.

Agave Nectar Is Sugar

Agave nectar has an undeserved reputation of being safe for keto dieters and low carbers. I consider this the greatest fraud perpetrated on the nutrition-conscious public since I became interested in nutrition forty years ago. Agave nectar is a processed food, made similarly to high fructose corn syrup, and even higher in fructose. Don't fall for it.

Regarding Sweeteners in General

I think it's important to limit your consumption of sweet things in general, whether they are sweetened with artificial sweeteners, stevia, monk fruit, or erythritol. I learned from Mary Vernon, MD, a diabetologist and bariatric physician, that we have taste buds in our small intestines, identical to those on our tongues. When they taste anything sweet, whether it's sugary or not, they trigger an insulin release to deal with the expected rise in blood sugar. If that sugar rush doesn't come, there shouldn't be a big insulin rush, but even a modest rise in insulin will slow the release of fat from storage and increase the risk of insulin resistance—and dampen ketone production.

ABOUT FATS

When you're deliberately eating a high-fat diet, it is vital that you pay attention to the quality of those fats. Unfortunately, officialdom has misinformed us about "healthy fats" for a good thirty years now. We were told to drastically limit "artery clogging saturated fats" and substitute unsaturated vegetable oils. This led to the current disastrous imbalance of unsaturated fatty acids in the American diet; the optimal 1:1 ratio of omega-3 and omega-6 fatty acids has been skewed to an average of 1:15.

You think sugar intake has increased? According to the *American Journal of Clinical Nutrition*, "The estimated per capita consumption of soybean oil increased >1000-fold from 1909 to 1999." The result is a harvest of all kinds of inflammatory illnesses, including cardiovascular disease, cancer, and auto-immune illnesses.

The demonizing of traditional animal fats was to a great degree driven by the burgeoning vegetable oil industry. Are you old enough to remember ads crowing about how polyunsaturated this-or-that vegetable oil was? Have you noticed that those ads have passed quietly from our midst? Margarine ads have been radically reduced, as well. You know why? Because it turns out that swapping in highly processed vegetable oils for traditional animal fats like butter, lard, tallow, and chicken fat is terrible for you, increasing the risk of everything from heart disease to cancer. Oops.

I trust you know, too, that substituting trans-fat-rich hydrogenated vegetable shortening for naturally saturated fats has turned out to be a disaster.

On a keto diet, natural fats are considered healthful, period. There are, however, a few fats that are most useful.

Coconut Oil

Coconut oil is a favorite of keto dieters, and with good reason: Coconut oil is very healthful stuff. It is highly saturated, far more so than lard, beef fat, or butter. It turns out this is a good thing. Saturated fats barely oxidize, you see, eliminating the risk of rancidity. Even at room temperature, coconut oil will keep for as long as a year.

Coconut oil raises your HDL cholesterol levels (the good stuff), increases immunity, improves insulin sensitivity, and stimulates the thyroid gland. Most of the saturated fat in coconut oil is in the form of medium chain triglycerides (MCTs), a fat that can be used directly by the muscles for fuel—it's true energy food. MCTs are also profoundly ketogenic; they are readily absorbed by the gut with no extra processing needed, providing a source of quick energy without the spike-and-crash that sugar creates.

Coconut oil is great for frying, sautéing, and baking when used in place of nasty hydrogenated shortening. (Solid at room temperature, coconut oil doesn't work for salad dressing or mayonnaise.) It is also great blended into coffee along with unsalted, grass-fed butter for a huge, hunger-killing, energy-boosting, ketone-and-caffeine rush.

Medium Chain Triglyceride Oil

Derived from coconut oil, MCT oil has been popular with athletes for a while because it can be burned directly by the muscles, offering a quick burst of energy without the crash that sugar would bring. It is also used by people who need concentrated nutrition; it can be particularly useful in cancer patients, for instance. And because MCTs are highly ketogenic, the oil is a great choice for keto dieters.

Because it is concentrated, MCT oil is even more ketogenic than coconut oil. Unlike coconut oil, MCT oil is liquid at room temperature, making it useful for salad dressings and the like. It has become my oil of choice for making mayonnaise.

Butter

The con-job from the margarine industry convinced twentieth-century Americans that butter was a ticket to a heart attack. Hah. Butter is health food!

Butter is a good source of vitamin A—true, preformed vitamin A, rather than the "provitamin A" you get from plant sources. It's also a source of vitamin E, a powerful antioxidant, and vitamin K, essential for calcium absorption to create strong bones and teeth. This is especially true if the butter is from grass-fed cows. Butter is also a source of selenium and iodine, the main constituents of thyroid hormone.

Butter is rich in saturated fats, it's true—about 60 percent of the fatty acids in butter is saturated. Interestingly, quite a lot of that is in the form of lauric acid. More than any other fat, lauric acid raises HDL ("good") cholesterol, which is thought to lower heart disease risk. There is some feeling that lauric acid has other benefits, ranging from antimicrobial and antifungal activity to stimulating the thyroid gland, thus increasing metabolism.

Then there's conjugated linoleic acid (CLA), a naturally occurring trans fat in butter that is not only harmless, but beneficial. When CLA was first identified in the 1980s, it was shown to help prevent and even treat cancer; there were gleeful headlines about how Velveeta was a cancer cure. Exaggerated, of course, but the benefits of CLA are real. Further testing has shown an effect on body composition, reducing fat and increasing muscle mass.

Grass-fed raw butter is higher in nutrients than the standard grocery-store stuff, and worth the extra money. That said, standard grocery-store butter is still a healthful fat. If you are lactose intolerant, you may well still be able to eat ghee, or clarified butter. Consult your doctor.

Lard

Yes, lard. Until Americans were sold a bill of goods about vegetable oils and hydrogenated shortening, lard was the most-used fat in the American diet, not only for frying and sautéing, but also as shortening in baked goods. Yet lard has been so defamed that it has become symbolic of "artery clogging saturated fat," though, ironically, it has slightly more unsaturated than saturated fat—about 57 percent. Most of that unsaturated fat in lard is in the form of monounsaturates, the same sort of fat that is considered healthful when found in olive oil.

Unfortunately, most of the lard in grocery stores cannot be considered a good fat. It comes from animals raised on the cheapest, nastiest feed, and much of it is hydrogenated, because lard is unsaturated enough to be soft at room temperature. Seek out a local small farm that produces pasture-raised pork, and buy a bucket of unprocessed lard. This is glorious stuff, bland yet rich, wonderful for all kinds of cooking and baking. Because lard is rich in monounsaturates, it will go rancid eventually. Scoop enough for a week or so, put it in a clean jar, and freeze the rest.

Bacon Grease

Think of it as lard with a salty, smoky, amazing flavor, but any way you look at it, bacon grease is pure culinary gold. If you shell out the money for good, small-farm bacon from pastured hogs, then throw out the grease, I will personally come to your house and dope-slap you. Around here, we keep the stuff from cheap grocery-store bacon, too. I pour it into an old salsa jar, keep it by the stove, and use it for all sorts of things, from frying eggs to roasting vegetables. I'd refrigerate it, but I use it up too fast for it to go bad.

Olive Oil

It's hard to get a handle on olive oil. The common wisdom is that it's the healthiest possible fat, but the paleo faction disputes that, especially if used for cooking, rather than in uncooked applications like salad dressings. I'm of the opinion that olive oil has been around long enough to be considered pretty safe, and the flavor is essential to Mediterranean and Middle Eastern cuisines, of which I am seriously fond. I use it for salad dressings and in cooking, where the flavor is essential to the dish.

Other Fats to Consider

Chicken Fat: Also known as *schmaltz*, rendered chicken fat is a staple of Jewish cuisine. Whether you can find it in local stores may depend upon whether you live where there is a substantial Jewish population. Good specialty butchers should have it, too. Properly rendered, chicken fat is a bland, neutral fat that can be used in a wide variety of foods—my mother claimed her mother used it as shortening in brownies! Again, the quality of chicken fat will depend on how the chicken was raised. No hormones, antibiotics, or soy feed will make for more healthful schmaltz.

Duck Fat: If you roast a duck, do not—I repeat, DO NOT—throw away the fat. Use it for sautéing and roasting vegetables. Amazing. And ducks have a lot of fat!

Tallow: Remember how good McDonald's fries were when you were a kid? You know why? They were fried in tallow, also known as beef fat. In the 1980s, the OMG-Saturated-Fat-Is-Eeeevul Squad bullied them into switching to vegetable oil, which not only made the fries less tasty, but filled them with trans fats, too. It's an excellent cooking fat, especially if you can get it from grass-fed beef. Indeed, make it a rule never to discard fat from properly raised meat.

EAT SALT!

Because lower insulin levels improve your kidneys' ability to excrete sodium, it is not uncommon for keto dieters to become sodium deficient. Despite scare tactics, salt is an essential nutrient. If you're feeling washed out, tired, achy, and/or head-achy, with no obvious reason, the first thing to try is salt. Heavily salted broth or bouillon is a good choice, as are pickles. Or just pour a little salt into your palm, lick it, and drink some water.

EXOGENOUS KETONES

As understanding of the benefits of dietary ketosis has spread, there has naturally been a proliferation of products to serve the market. One class of products is exogenous ketones, or ketones you take as a supplement. Do you need these?

Once again, it depends on why you are eating a ketogenic diet. If your aim is to treat cognitive impairment or seizures, or any other condition for which the ketones serve as a therapy, exogenous ketones may well be a godsend. If this is the case, you'll have to do your own research. I've never read the labels on 'em, since I make my own ketones by burning fat.

If, on the other hand, you are eating a keto diet to lose weight or for general health, exogenous ketones are simply another fuel source. Remember, testing positive for ketosis only shows you that you have ketones in your blood, breath, or urine. It does not tell you whether those ketones came from burning dietary fat or body fat. If you also swallow exogenous ketones, your deep state of ketosis *really* doesn't tell you if you're burning body fat—or burning much fat at all.

Be aware that some of the exogenous ketones are being sold through network marketing, with pressure to buy into the "business opportunity." I have seen good nutritional products sold by network marketing companies, but they have almost invariably been overpriced. If you're in it for weight loss, save your money and make your own ketones.

TIPS FOR DINING OUT

There is a myth that it's hard to eat keto if you frequently eat at restaurants. This is an excuse. It is a rare restaurant that doesn't offer *anything* we can eat. It is simply up to us to choose it.

This means getting over your own personal mythology. I knew a woman—morbidly obese—who said she "had" to have Curly Fries every time she went to Arby's. She said this with conviction, as if it had the same force as, say, the laws of kosher for an observant Jew, or skipping meat on Fridays during Lent for Catholics. If there is a restaurant you "can't go to" without ordering something carby, steer clear, at least until you're so comfortable with this Way of Eating that ordering, say, fettuccini Alfredo is unthinkable.

If you know ahead of time where you'll be eating, it's a good idea to peruse the menu; most restaurants now have their menus available online. This can save you from the odd eatery where there really is nothing low carb on the menu—a few places are truly hopeless.

In this book, we've given you as much information as we could find for the most popular restaurants in America, but some only give numbers for a whole meal, not allowing for holding sweet sauces or substituting for carby sides. For those restaurants where we couldn't calculate accurate, "safe" meals or menu items, we note "Insufficient information." This is not to say that these restaurants have no suitable items; it's just that we couldn't get accurate nutritional information on them.

Should you find yourself in a restaurant that doesn't give complete information, here are some tips:

- Restaurants are in the service industry. Substitutions within reason—steamed vegetables instead of the potato, the meat and cheese of a sandwich on a bed of lettuce instead of bread, lemon butter or tartar sauce instead of cocktail sauce with your shrimp—should be cheerfully granted. If not, take your money elsewhere. If they go above and beyond for you, tip heavily and write a great review online!

- It's hard to go wrong with a steak and a salad, with steamed broccoli or grilled asparagus, well buttered. Ditto grilled or steamed fish or seafood with lemon butter, or a grilled chicken breast, though that's pretty darned lean. Do they have a rich sauce you can top it with?

- Even if the numbers are not available, most fast food burgers will be okay. You will need to ask them to hold the bun, of course, but also ketchup, barbecue sauce, fried onion rings or "straws," and anything else that is carb laden. Cheese is safe, though cheese sauce may contain starchy thickeners. Bacon is awesome, of course, so order the bacon cheeseburger. Your basic lettuce, tomato, and pickle should be fine, as should sautéed mushrooms.

- Restaurants centering on animal foods of one kind or another are a good bet; steak houses, seafood restaurants, and chicken wing places all should have some kind of meat that hasn't been gooped up. Two possible exceptions are fried chicken restaurants, where all the chicken may be breaded, and rib joints, though often you can get them with only dry rub, not the sugary sauce.

- "Clean" food is currently trendy. This is not synonymous with "low carb" or "keto." Most restaurants will use ingredients you would not use at home, whether it's soy oil in the salad dressing or cornstarch in the sauce.

- Beware the main-dish salad. The health-conscious have been trained to choose the main-dish salad, but read the descriptions carefully. Croutons? Tortilla strips? Chow mein noodles? Yeah, no. Also appearing in many main-dish salads are things like grapes, apples, and raisins. Add those to the carbs in the lettuce, tomato, and all that, and you may well be over 20 grams of carbs for the meal. Throw in a sugary dressing, and it climbs even higher. The chicken or shrimp Caesar salad, sans croutons, is usually safe. (If they bring the croutons by mistake, pick them out and build things with them. Yes, I have done this. More than once.) Oh! And grilled chicken, not crispy!

- In general, Caesar, blue cheese, and full-fat ranch are the most keto friendly dressings. Vinaigrettes vary, as some are sweetened. If you're a fan, get the vinaigrette on the side. Or ask for olive oil, vinegar, and a wedge of lemon. These, with a little salt and pepper, are a real favorite of mine. And for the love of all that's keto, skip the Low fat dressings, and anything obviously sweet: honey mustard, poppy seed, raspberry vinaigrette, and the like.

- Sadly, Chinese restaurants are one of the hardest for us. Yes, you can skip the rice or noodles, but the combination of plenty of vegetables with cornstarch and often sugar in sauces pushes the limits.

- You can always get a keto meal at a restaurant that serves breakfast all day!

- While more and more restaurants offer gluten-free options, be aware that "gluten free" does not necessarily mean "low carb." Be aware, too, that IHOP adds pancake batter to the eggs for their omelets. Request they make yours with unadulterated eggs.

- If all that's at hand is a mini-mart, consider pork rinds, almonds, or a hot dog eaten without the bun. Some mini-marts also have hard-boiled eggs, which can be a lifesaver, as can string cheese sticks.

- In a desperate situation, do what you can. Pick the breading off the fried mozzarella sticks. Peel the toppings off the pizza and toss the crust. Use that hot dog bun as a holder, sliding the hot dog out a bite at a time. Thanks to keto, you'll be so much less hungry that desperate situations will be infrequent.

WHAT'S NEW ABOUT THIS BOOK?

If you've seen my *Carb Gram Counter*, you may wonder how this book is different. There are a few differences: We've included fat grams and fat percentages, to help you hit your macros. This is also more specifically geared toward people eating a ketogenic diet, rather than to all forms of carbohydrate restriction. And we've added more than 1,500 new entries, including dishes from popular restaurants and the plethora of keto-geared food and beverage products flooding onto the market. Indeed, those products are proliferating so rapidly that new ones have hit the market since I wrote this—I guarantee there will be products on the market that we missed, for just this reason. Need I warn you? READ THE LABELS!

HOW TO USE THIS BOOK

This book is designed to help you count calories, carbohydrates, and nutrients accurately, quickly, and easily. Alphabetical listings make locating your foods simple. To improve clarity and speed in locating food choices, this book is divided into three sections:

> Beverages
> Foods
> Dining Out

Abbreviation and Symbol Key

&	and
>	greater than
<	less than
appx	approximately
as prep	prepared as instructed on package, usual method
avg	average size
bev	beverage
cal	calorie
dia	diameter
ea	each
fl oz	fluid ounce
g	gram(s)
"	inch(es)
lb	pound
lg	large
med	medium
misc	miscellaneous
oz	ounce
pc	piece

pkg	package
pkt	packet
prep	prepared
reg	regular
sm	small
svg	serving
sq	square
Tbsp	tablespoon
Tr	trace—less than 1 g
tsp	teaspoon
w/	with
w/o	without
xl	extra-large

Be Aware

Working with online restaurant nutrition charts, we occasionally found the numbers didn't quite "work." For example, Cracker Barrel's online menu notes that their pork chops have 0 g total carbs and 2 g fiber; this would mean they have "-2 g" net carbs, which is impossible. It is possible that they subtracted the fiber from the carb count in advance; we can't know. But the pork chops should be fine. Too, some products' fat percentages worked out to greater than 100 percent, a mathematical impossibility. We've changed those to 100 percent.

Please Note

- All listings are medium- or average-portion size, unless specified.

- "Cooked" means the food is cooked without added fats, sauces, or sugars. This includes boiling, steaming, and heating in a microwave oven.

- "Baked" and "broiled" describe the normal methods of baking and broiling, without oil, or minimal cooking oil for a non-stick surface. No other fats, sauces, or sugars have been added.

- Names in *italics* signify registered trademarks.

- Net carbs are calculated by subtracting fiber (and in some cases, erythritol) from total carbs. Net carbs are rounded to whole numbers.

- The data is accurate at the time of publication. However, food manufacturers may change their ingredients at any time without notice. Food nutrition labels should also be checked.

- Keep your eyes open for new low-carb products!

References

- The United States Department of Agriculture (USDA), National Nutrient Database for Standard Reference, Release 21, (2008) and Nutritional analysis from The Food Processor® Nutrition and Fitness Software (version 11.6), © 2018 ESHA Research, Inc.

- Food manufacturers' nutrient labels (2009 and 2019).

- Restaurants' printed nutritional data (2009) and online nutritional data (2019).

BEVERAGES

	Serving Size	Calories	Fat (g)	Calories from Fat (%)	Total Carbs (g)	Fiber (g)	Net Carbs (g)	Protein (g)
Almond Milk								
Almond Breeze original	8 fl oz	60	3	45	1	0	1	1
Chocolate	8 fl oz	120	3	23	2	0	2	2
Chocolate, unsweetened	8 fl oz	51	4	71	2	0	2	2
Unsweetened	8 fl oz	39	3	69	2	0	2	2
Vanilla	8 fl oz	93	3	29	1	0	1	1
Vanilla, unsweetened	8 fl oz	37	3	73	1	0	1	1
Apple Juice, canned or bottled	8 fl oz	120	Tr	0	28	Tr	28	Tr
Apple Juice, frozen concentrate (prepared)	8 fl oz	110	Tr	0	28	Tr	28	Tr
Apple-Cranberry Juice	8 fl oz	120	Tr	0	29	Tr	29	Tr
Apple-Grape Juice	8 fl oz	130	Tr	0	31	Tr	31	Tr
Apricot Nectar	8 fl oz	140	Tr	0	36	2	34	Tr
Beer	***	***	*	*	*	*	*	*
Light Beer	12 fl oz	100	0	0	6	0	6	Tr
Light, Low Carb Beer	12 fl oz	96	0	0	3	0	3	Tr
Low Carb Beer	12 fl oz	97	0	0	3	0	3	Tr
Regular Beer	12 fl oz	150	0	0	13	0	13	2
Bourbon - see Distilled Spirits	***	***	*	*	*	*	*	*
Brandy - see Distilled Spirits	***	***	*	*	*	*	*	*
Capri Sun **juice drink**	8 fl oz	120	0	0	29	Tr	29	Tr
Carbonated Beverages - see Soda	***	***	*	*	*	*	*	*
Carrot Juice	8 fl oz	90	Tr	0	22	2	20	2
Cashew Milk	***	***	*	*	*	*	*	*
Original/plain	8 fl oz	78	5	58	8	0	8	2
Unsweetened	8 fl oz	38	3	71	2	0	2	1
Vanilla, *Pacific Natural*	8 fl oz	70	4	51	8	0	8	2
Vanilla, unsweetened, *Pacific Natural*	8 fl oz	50	4	72	2	0	2	1
Club Soda - see Soda	***	***	*	*	*	*	*	*

	Serving Size	Calories	Fat (g)	Calories from Fat (%)	Total Carbs (g)	Fiber (g)	Net Carbs (g)	Protein (g)
Cocoa/Chocolate Beverage, Hot	***	***	*	*	*	*	*	*
Regular, as prep	6 fl oz	110	1	8	24	1	23	2
Diet or sugar free, as prep	6 fl oz	60	Tr	0	11	1	10	2
Nestlé Rich Chocolate Hot Cocoa Mix	1 envelope	80	3	34	15	Tr	15	Tr
Nestlé Rich Chocolate Hot Cocoa Mix, w/ marshmallows	1 envelope	80	3	34	15	Tr	15	Tr
Ovaltine Sugar-Free Hot Cocoa	6 fl oz	40	Tr	0	7	Tr	7	3
Coconut Milk Beverage - see also Coconut Milk, canned	***	***	*	*	*	*	*	*
So Delicious, chocolate	8 fl oz	90	5	50	12	0	12	1
So Delicious, original	8 fl oz	70	4.5	58	8	0	8	0
So Delicious, unsweetened	8 fl oz	45	4.5	90	2	0	2	0
So Delicious, vanilla	8 fl oz	80	4.5	51	10	0	10	0
Coconut Water, *Zico*, original	11.2 fl oz	60	0	0	15	0	15	0
Coconut Water, *Zico*, original	16.9 fl oz	90	0	0	22	0	22	0
Coffee - see also specific restaurants	***	***	*	*	*	*	*	*
Brewed coffee, regular or decaf	6 fl oz	0	0	0	0	0	0	Tr
Instant coffee, regular or decaf	6 fl oz	0	0	0	Tr	0	Tr	Tr
Cappuccino, made w/ 4 oz milk	***	***	*	*	*	*	*	*
w/ whole milk (3.25)	6 fl oz	80	4	45	6	0	6	4
w/ reduced fat milk (2)	6 fl oz	60	2	30	6	0	6	4
w/ low fat milk (1)	6 fl oz	50	1	18	6	0	6	4
w/ nonfat milk	6 fl oz	45	Tr	0	6	0	6	4
Espresso	2 fl oz	0	Tr	0	0	0	0	Tr
Instant powder	***	***	*	*	*	*	*	*
Cappuccino flavor	4 tsp	50	Tr	0	11	Tr	11	Tr
French flavor	4 tsp	60	3	45	9	0	9	Tr
Mocha flavor	2 Tbsp	60	2	30	10	Tr	10	Tr
Latte, made w/ 10 oz milk	***	***	*	*	*	*	*	*
w/ whole milk (3.25)	12 fl oz	180	10	50	14	0	14	10
w/ reduced fat milk (2)	12 fl oz	150	6	36	14	0	14	10

	Serving Size	Calories	Fat (g)	Calories from Fat (%)	Total Carbs (g)	Fiber (g)	Net Carbs (g)	Protein (g)
w/ lowfat milk (1)	12 fl oz	130	3	21	15	0	15	10
w/ nonfat milk	12 fl oz	100	Tr	0	15	0	15	10
Coffee Cream - see Creamer	***	***	*	*	*	*	*	*
Coffee Liqueur, 53 proof	1.5 fl oz	170	Tr	0	24	0	24	Tr
Coke - see Soda	***	***	*	*	*	*	*	*
Cola - see Soda	***	***	*	*	*	*	*	*
Cranberry-Apple Juice Drink	8 fl oz	150	Tr	0	39	0	39	0
Cranberry-Apricot Juice Drink	8 fl oz	160	0	0	40	Tr	40	Tr
Cranberry-Grape Drink	8 fl oz	140	Tr	0	34	Tr	34	Tr
Cranberry Juice Cocktail, bottled	8 fl oz	140	Tr	0	34	0	34	0
Cranberry Juice Cocktail, frozen concentrate, as prep	8 fl oz	110	0	0	28	0	28	0
Cream Soda - see Soda	***	***	*	*	*	*	*	*
Creamer	***	***	*	*	*	*	*	*
Coffee-Mate, Original liquid creamer	1 Tbsp	20	1	45	2	0	2	0
Coffee-Mate, Original powdered creamer	1 tsp	10	Tr	0	1	0	1	0
Half & half (cream & milk)	1 Tbsp	20	2	90	Tr	0	Tr	Tr
Half & half (cream & milk)	1 cup	320	28	79	10	0	10	7
Half & half, fat free	1 Tbsp	10	Tr	0	1	0	1	Tr
Liquid creamer	1 container	20	2	90	2	0	2	Tr
Liquid creamer, flavored	1 Tbsp	40	2	45	5	Tr	5	Tr
Liquid creamer, light	1 Tbsp	10	Fat	0	1	0	1	Tr
Powdered creamer	1 tsp	10	Tr	0	1	0	1	Tr
Powdered creamer, flavored	1 tsp	10	Tr	0	2	0	2	0
Powdered creamer, light	1 pkt	15	Tr	0	2	0	2	Tr
Silk Original Creamer	1 Tbsp	15	1	60	1	0	1	0
So Delicious Almond Milk Creamer, original	1 Tbsp	5	0	0	1	0	1	0
So Delicious Coconut Milk Creamer, original	1 Tbsp	10	0	0	1	0	1	0
Crème de Menthe	1.5 fl oz	190	Tr	0	21	0	21	?
Crystal Light, all flavors	8 fl oz	5	0	0	0	0	0	0
Daiquiri	2 fl oz	110	Tr	0	4	Tr	4	Tr

	Serving Size	Calories	Fat (g)	Calories from Fat (%)	Total Carbs (g)	Fiber (g)	Net Carbs (g)	Protein (g)
Diet Cola - see Soda	***	***	*	*	*	*	*	*
Diet Soda - see Soda	***	***	*	*	*	*	*	*
Distilled Spirits	***	***	*	*	*	*	*	*
80 proof	1.5 fl oz	100	0	0	0	0	0	0
86 proof	1.5 fl oz	110	0	0	Tr	0	Tr	0
90 proof	1.5 fl oz	110	0	0	0	0	0	0
Eggnog, light	1 cup	189	8	38	17	0	17	12
Eggnog, plain	1 cup	340	19	50	34	0	34	10
Eggnog, *Silk* (soy), original	½ cup	80	1.5	17	13	1	12	3
Fruit Juice Drink, citrus, frozen concentrate, as prep	8 fl oz	110	Tr	0	28	Tr	28	Tr
Fruit Juice Drink, frozen concentrate, as prep	8 fl oz	110	0	0	29	Tr	29	Tr
Fruit Punch Juice Drink, frozen concentrate, as prep	8 fl oz	100	Tr	0	24	0	24	Tr
Fruit-Flavored Drink Mix, powdered, low calorie	1 tsp	5	0	0	2	0	2	0
Fruit-Flavored Drink Mix, powdered, unsweetened	2 tsp	60	0	0	23	0	23	0
Gatorade	8 fl oz	50	0	0	14	0	14	0
Gin - see Distilled Spirits	***	***	*	*	*	*	*	*
Goat Milk	8 fl oz	168	10	54	11	0	11	9
Grape Juice, canned or bottled, unsweetened	8 fl oz	150	Tr	0	37	Tr	37	Tr
Grape Juice Cocktail, frozen concentrate, as prep	8 fl oz	130	Tr	0	32	Tr	32	Tr
Grapefruit Juice	***	***	*	*	*	*	*	*
Canned, unsweetened	8 fl oz	90	Tr	0	22	Tr	22	1
Canned, sugar sweetened	8 fl oz	120	Tr	0	28	Tr	28	2
Fresh squeezed	8 fl oz	100	Tr	0	23	Tr	23	1
Frozen concentrate, unsweetened, as prep	8 fl oz	100	Tr	0	24	Tr	24	1
Half & Half - see Creamer	***	***	*	*	*	*	*	*
Hawaiian Punch	***	***	*	*	*	*	*	*
Regular	8 fl oz	120	0	0	30	Tr	30	0
Light	8 fl oz	45	0	0	11	0	11	0
Hemp Milk	***	***	*	*	*	*	*	*

	Serving Size	Calories	Fat (g)	Calories from Fat (%)	Total Carbs (g)	Fiber (g)	Net Carbs (g)	Protein (g)
Pacific Natural, chocolate	8 fl oz	200	5	23	35	0	35	3
Pacific Natural, original	8 fl oz	140	5	32	20	0	20	3
Pacific Natural, unsweetened	8 fl oz	60	4.5	68	0	0	0	3
Pacific Natural, vanilla	8 fl oz	160	5	28	24	0	24	3
Pacific Natural, vanilla unsweetened	8 fl oz	60	4.5	68	0	0	0	3
Hot Cocoa/Chocolate - see Cocoa	***	***	*	*	*	*	*	*
Iced Tea - see Tea, Iced	***	***	*	*	*	*	*	*
Juice - see specific listings	***	***	*	*	*	*	*	*
Kefir	***	***	*	*	*	*	*	*
Plain	1 cup	127	2	14	18	0	18	9
Plain, low fat	1 cup	110	2	16	12	0	12	10
Kool Aid	***	***	*	*	*	*	*	*
Sugar free, as prep	8 fl oz	5	0	0	0	0	0	0
Sugar sweetened, as prep	8 fl oz	60	0	0	16	Tr	16	0
Unsweetened packet	1 pkt	0	0	0	0	0	0	0
Lemon Juice	***	***	*	*	*	*	*	*
Canned or bottled, unsweetened	1 Tbsp	0	Tr	0	Tr	Tr	Tr	Tr
Canned or bottled, unsweetened	1 cup	50	Tr	0	16	1	15	Tr
Fresh squeezed	1 Tbsp	0	0	0	1	Tr	1	Tr
Fresh squeezed	1 cup	60	0	0	21	1	20	Tr
Lemonade	***	***	*	*	*	*	*	*
Frozen concentrate, as prep (white or pink)	8 fl oz	100	Tr	0	26	Tr	26	Tr
Powdered, as prep	8 fl oz	100	0	0	26	0	26	0
Powdered, sugar free, as prep	8 fl oz	5	0	0	2	0	2	Tr
Lemonade, *Minute Maid* Light	12 fl oz	5	0	0	2	0	2	0
Lemonade, *Minute Maid* Light	16 fl oz	10	0	0	3	0	3	0
Lemonade, *Minute Maid* Light	32 fl oz	15	0	0	5	0	5	0
Lemon-Flavored Drink	***	***	*	*	*	*	*	*
Powdered, as prep	8 fl oz	70	0	0	17	0	17	Tr
Lime Juice	***	***	*	*	*	*	*	*

	Serving Size	Calories	Fat (g)	Calories from Fat (%)	Total Carbs (g)	Fiber (g)	Net Carbs (g)	Protein (g)
Canned or bottled, unsweetened	1 Tbsp	0	Tr	0	1	Tr	1	Tr
Canned or bottled, unsweetened	1 cup	50	Tr	0	17	1	16	Tr
Fresh squeezed	1 Tbsp	0	Tr	0	1	Tr	1	Tr
Fresh squeezed	1 cup	60	Tr	0	20	1	19	1
Limeade	***	***	*	*	*	*	*	*
Frozen concentrate, as prep	8 fl oz	130	0	0	34	0	34	0
Liqueur, 53 proof	1.5 fl oz	170	Tr	0	24	0	24	Tr
Liqueur, 63 proof	1.5 fl oz	160	Tr	0	17	0	17	Tr
Macadamia Nut Milk, *Milkadamia*	***	***	*	*	*	*	*	*
Original	8 fl oz	70	5	64	7	1	6	1
Unsweetened	8 fl oz	50	5	90	1	1	0	1
Unsweetened Vanilla	8 fl oz	50	5	90	1	1	0	1
Mai Tai	5 fl oz	280	0	0	28	1	27	0
Margarita	5 fl oz	150	0	0	10	Tr	10	0
Martini, plain	2.5 fl oz	155	0	0	0	0	0	0
Milk, chocolate	***	***	*	*	*	*	*	*
Whole	8 fl oz	210	9	39	26	2	24	8
Reduced fat	8 fl oz	190	5	24	30	2	28	7
Low fat	8 fl oz	154	2	12	24	1	23	9
Milk, white	***	***	*	*	*	*	*	*
Whole, 3.25 fat	8 fl oz	150	8	48	11	0	11	8
Reduced fat, 2 fat	8 fl oz	120	5	38	11	0	11	8
Low fat, 1 fat	8 fl oz	100	2	18	12	0	12	8
Nonfat (skim)	8 fl oz	90	Tr	0	12	0	12	8
Nonfat instant, as prep	8 fl oz	80	Tr	0	12	0	12	8
Nonfat instant, dry powder only	1 cup	240	Tr	0	36	0	36	24
Milk, misc products	***	***	*	*	*	*	*	*
Almond - see Almond Milk	***	***	*	*	*	*	*	*
Buttermilk, low fat	1 cup	100	2	18	12	0	12	8
Buttermilk, powdered (dried)	1 Tbsp	25	Tr	0	3	0	3	2
Cashew - see Cashew Milk	***	***	*	*	*	*	*	*

	Serving Size	Calories	Fat (g)	Calories from Fat (%)	Total Carbs (g)	Fiber (g)	Net Carbs (g)	Protein (g)
Coconut - see Coconut Milk Beverage	***	***	*	*	*	*	*	*
Condensed, sweetened	1 cup	980	27	25	167	0	167	24
Evaporated, skim	1 cup	200	Tr	0	29	0	29	19
Evaporated, whole	1 cup	340	19	50	25	0	25	17
Goat - see Goat Milk	***	***	*	*	*	*	*	*
Hemp - see Hemp Milk	***	***	*	*	*	*	*	*
Macadamia Nut - see Macadamia Nut Milk	***	***	*	*	*	*	*	*
Malted, chocolate	1 cup	225	9	36	30	1	29	9
Malted, natural	1 cup	230	10	39	27	Tr	27	10
Oat Milk - see Oat Milk	***	***	*	*	*	*	*	*
Rice - see Rice Milk	***	***	*	*	*	*	*	*
Saco Cultured Buttermilk Blend, powdered	4 Tbsp	80	Tr	0	13	0	13	5
Soy - see Soy Milk	***	***	*	*	*	*	*	*
Milk Shake - see Shake	***	***	*	*	*	*	*	*
Nesquik	***	***	*	*	*	*	*	*
Chocolate syrup	1 Tbsp	70	0	0	16	0	16	0
Chocolate syrup, ⅓ less sugar	1 Tbsp	50	0	0	10	0	10	0
Strawberry, ⅓ less sugar	1 Tbsp	50	0	0	11	1	10	0
Vanilla, ⅓ less sugar	1 Tbsp	50	0	0	12	0	12	0
Oat Milk, *Elmhurst*	8 fl oz	100	1.5	14	18	2	16	4
Orange Juice	***	***	*	*	*	*	*	*
Canned, unsweetened	8 fl oz	120	Tr	0	27	Tr	27	2
Chilled, from concentrate	8 fl oz	110	Tr	0	25	Tr	25	2
Fresh squeezed	8 fl oz	110	Tr	0	26	Tr	26	2
Frozen concentrate, as prep	8 fl oz	110	Tr	0	27	Tr	27	2
Peach Nectar	8 fl oz	130	Tr	0	35	2	33	Tr
Pear Nectar	8 fl oz	150	Tr	0	39	2	37	Tr
Pepsi - see Soda	***	***	*	*	*	*	*	*
Pina Colada	4.5 fl oz	250	3	11	32	Tr	32	Tr
Pineapple Grapefruit Juice	8 fl oz	120	Tr	0	29	Tr	29	Tr
Pineapple Juice	***	***	*	*	*	*	*	*

	Serving Size	Calories	Fat (g)	Calories from Fat (%)	Total Carbs (g)	Fiber (g)	Net Carbs (g)	Protein (g)
Canned, unsweetened	8 fl oz	130	Tr	0	32	Tr	32	Tr
Frozen concentrate, as prep	8 fl oz	130	Tr	0	32	Tr	32	1
Pineapple Orange Juice	8 fl oz	125	0	0	30	Tr	30	3
Powerade, lemon-lime flavored	8 fl oz	80	Tr	0	19	0	19	0
Powerade Zero, any flavor, any size	***	0	0	0	1	0	1	0
Propel Fitness Water, fruit flavored	8 fl oz	10	0	0	3	0	3	0
Prune Juice	8 fl oz	180	Tr	0	45	3	42	2
Red Bull Energy Drink	***	***	*	*	*	*	*	*
Regular	12 fl oz	157	0	0	40	0	40	1
Sugar free	12 fl oz	14	0	0	4	0	4	1
Total Zero	12 fl oz	0	0	0	0	0	0	1
Rice Milk	***	***	*	*	*	*	*	*
Chocolate, *Rice Dream*	8 fl oz	160	3	17	34	0	34	1
Original	8 fl oz	120	2.5	19	23	0	23	1
Unsweetened	8 fl oz	113	2	16	22	0	22	1
Vanilla, *Rice Dream*	8 fl oz	130	2.5	17	26	0	26	1
Root Beer - see Soda	***	***	*	*	*	*	*	*
Rum - see Distilled Spirits	***	***	*	*	*	*	*	*
Sake (rice wine)	1 fl oz	40	0	0	2	0	2	Tr
Scotch - see Distilled Spirits	***	***	*	*	*	*	*	*
Screwdriver	7 fl oz	160	Tr	0	17	1	16	Tr
Shake	***	***	*	*	*	*	*	*
Chocolate, regular milk shake	11 oz	370	8	19	66	Tr	66	10
Vanilla, regular milk shake	11 oz	350	10	26	56	0	56	12
Atkins Advantage low carb shake	***	***	*	*	*	*	*	*
Café Caramel	11 oz	160	9	51	3	2	1	15
Chocolate Royale	11 oz	160	9	51	5	4	1	15
Milk Chocolate Delight	11 oz	160	9	51	4	3	1	15
Mocha Latte	11 oz	160	9	51	5	3	2	15
Strawberry	11 oz	150	9	54	2	2	0	15
Vanilla	11 oz	150	9	54	2	2	0	15

	Serving Size	Calories	Fat (g)	Calories from Fat (%)	Total Carbs (g)	Fiber (g)	Net Carbs (g)	Protein (g)
Soda/Cola/Soft Drink (Carbonated Beverages)	***	***	*	*	*	*	*	*
Barq's Root Beer	12 fl oz	170	0	0	45	0	45	0
Barq's Root Beer, diet	12 fl oz	0	0	0	Tr	0	Tr	0
Cherry Coke	12 fl oz	160	0	0	42	0	42	0
Cherry Coke, diet	12 fl oz	0	0	0	Tr	0	Tr	0
Cherry Coke, Cherry Zero, any size	***	0	0	0	0	0	0	0
Club Soda	12 fl oz	0	0	0	0	0	0	0
Coca-Cola Classic	12 fl oz	150	0	0	41	0	41	0
Coke, diet, caffeine free, any size	***	0	0	0	0	0	0	0
Coke, diet	< 30 fl oz	0	0	0	0	0	0	0
Coke, diet	> 30 fl oz	0	0	0	Tr	0	Tr	0
Coke, diet, flavored	12 fl oz	0	0	0	0	0	0	0
Coke Zero Sugar, original or orange vanilla, any size	***	0	0	0	0	0	0	0
Cola	12 fl oz	140	Tr	0	35	0	35	Tr
Cola, no caffeine	12 fl oz	150	0	0	39	0	39	0
Cream Soda	12 fl oz	190	0	0	49	0	49	0
Diet Cola, w/ aspartame	12 fl oz	5	Tr	0	1	0	1	Tr
Diet Cola, w/ sodium saccharin	12 fl oz	0	0	0	Tr	0	Tr	0
Dr Pepper	12 fl oz	150	0	0	41	0	41	0
Dr Pepper, diet	12 fl oz	0	0	0	0	0	0	0
Fanta Zero Sugar, orange flavored, any size	***	0	0	0	1	0	1	0
Fresca	12 fl oz	0	0	0	Tr	0	Tr	0
Ginger Ale	12 fl oz	120	0	0	32	0	32	0
Ginger Ale, diet	12 fl oz	0	0	0	0	0	0	0
Grape Soda	12 fl oz	160	0	0	42	0	42	0
Lemon Lime Soda	12 fl oz	150	0	0	39	0	39	Tr
Mello Yello Zero	12 fl oz	0	0	0	0	0	0	0
Mountain Dew	12 fl oz	170	0	0	46	0	46	0
Mountain Dew, diet	12 fl oz	0	0	0	0	0	0	0
Mug Cream Soda	12 fl oz	180	0	0	47	0	47	0
Mug Cream Soda, diet	12 fl oz	0	0	0	0	0	0	0

	Serving Size	Calories	Fat (g)	Calories from Fat (%)	Total Carbs (g)	Fiber (g)	Net Carbs (g)	Protein (g)
Mug Root Beer	12 fl oz	160	0	0	43	0	43	0
Mug Root Beer, diet	12 fl oz	0	0	0	0	0	0	0
Orange Soda	12 fl oz	180	0	0	46	0	46	0
Pepsi, regular & caffeine free	12 fl oz	150	0	0	41	0	41	0
Pepsi, diet	12 fl oz	0	0	0	0	0	0	0
Pepsi, diet, caffeine free	12 fl oz	0	0	0	0	0	0	0
Pepsi Max	12 fl oz	0	0	0	0	0	0	0
Pepsi One	12 fl oz	0	0	0	0	0	0	0
Pepsi Zero Sugar, original and wild cherry	12 fl oz	0	0	0	0	0	0	0
Pibb Xtra	12 fl oz	150	0	0	39	0	39	0
Pibb Zero	12 fl oz	0	0	0	Tr	0	Tr	0
RC Cola	12 fl oz	160	0	0	43	0	43	0
RC Cola, diet	12 fl oz	0	0	0	0	0	0	0
Root Beer	12 fl oz	150	0	0	39	0	39	0
Seltzer Water, sparkling	12 fl oz	0	0	0	0	0	0	0
Seven Up	12 fl oz	150	0	0	39	0	39	0
Seven Up, diet	12 fl oz	0	0	0	0	0	0	0
Sierra Mist	12 fl oz	140	0	0	39	0	39	0
Sierra Mist, diet	12 fl oz	0	0	0	0	0	0	0
Sprite	12 fl oz	150	0	0	37	0	37	0
Sprite Zero	12 fl oz	0	0	0	0	0	0	0
Stewart's Root Beer	12 fl oz	150	0	0	38	0	38	0
Stewart's Root Beer, diet	12 fl oz	0	0	0	0	0	0	0
Tab	12 fl oz	0	0	0	Tr	0	Tr	0
Tonic Water	12 fl oz	120	0	0	32	0	32	0
Tonic Water, diet	12 fl oz	0	0	0	1	0	1	0
Soft Drinks - see Soda	***	***	*	*	*	*	*	*
Soy Milk	***	***	*	*	*	*	*	*
Chocolate	1 cup	150	4	24	24	1	23	6
Unsweetened	1 cup	80	4	45	4	1	3	7
Vanilla	1 cup	100	4	36	12	Tr	12	6

	Serving Size	Calories	Fat (g)	Calories from Fat (%)	Total Carbs (g)	Fiber (g)	Net Carbs (g)	Protein (g)
SILK, chocolate	1 cup	140	4	26	23	2	21	5
SILK, unsweetened	1 cup	80	4	45	4	1	3	7
SILK, vanilla	1 cup	100	4	36	10	1	9	6
Vitasoy Organic Classic Original	1 cup	45	2	40	5	Tr	5	3
Vitasoy Light Vanilla	1 cup	70	2	26	10	Tr	10	4
Sport Drinks - see specific listings	***	***	*	*	*	*	*	*
Sugar Free Beverage - see specific listings	***	***	*	*	*	*	*	*
SunnyD	***	***	*	*	*	*	*	*
Fruit Punch	8 fl oz	80	0	0	21	Tr	21	0
Mango	8 fl oz	90	0	0	22	Tr	22	0
Smooth Style	8 fl oz	90	0	0	22	Tr	22	0
Tangy Original Style	8 fl oz	90	0	0	22	Tr	22	0
***SunnyD* with calcium**	8 fl oz	140	0	0	35	Tr	35	0
***SunnyD* Reduced Sugar**	8 fl oz	60	0	0	15	Tr	15	0
Tang	***	***	*	*	*	*	*	*
Regular	8 fl oz	115	0	0	29	Tr	29	0
Sugar free	8 fl oz	5	0	0	0	0	0	0
Tangerine Juice, fresh squeezed	8 fl oz	110	Tr	0	25	Tr	25	1
Tea, Hot	***	***	*	*	*	*	*	*
Regular, Decaf, or Herbal	***	***	*	*	*	*	*	*
sweetened w/ 1 tsp sugar	8 fl oz	20	0	0	5	0	5	0
sweetened w/ 1 pkt aspartame	8 fl oz	5	0	0	2	0	2	Tr
unsweetened	8 fl oz	0	0	0	Tr	0	Tr	0
Instant	***	***	*	*	*	*	*	*
sweetened w/ sodium saccharin, lemon flavored	8 fl oz	5	0	0	1	0	1	Tr
sweetened w/ sugar, lemon flavored	8 fl oz	90	Tr	0	22	Tr	22	Tr
unsweetened	8 fl oz	0	0	0	Tr	0	Tr	Tr

	Serving Size	Calories	Fat (g)	Calories from Fat (%)	Total Carbs (g)	Fiber (g)	Net Carbs (g)	Protein (g)
Tea, Iced	***	***	*	*	*	*	*	*
Arizona iced tea, lemon flavor	8 fl oz	90	0	0	22	0	22	0
Fuze, diet iced tea, lemon, any size	***	0	0	0	0	0	0	0
Fuze, unsweetened brewed iced tea, any size	***	0	0	0	0	0	0	0
Gold Peak, diet tea, original or green	18.5 fl oz	0	0	0	0	0	0	0
Gold Peak, unsweetened tea, original or raspberry	18.5 fl oz	0	0	0	0	0	0	0
Gold Peak, unsweetened lemon tea	18.5 fl oz	0	0	0	2	0	2	0
Honest Tea, unsweetened, lemon, mint, or peach ginger	16.9 fl oz	0	0	0	0	0	0	0
Lipton Brisk iced tea, lemon flavor	8 fl oz	90	0	0	22	0	22	0
Nestle Cool Nestea iced tea, lemon flavor	8 fl oz	90	0	0	22	0	22	0
Tequila	1.5 fl oz	100	0	0	0	0	0	0
Tequila Sunrise	5.5 fl oz	190	Tr	0	19	0	19	Tr
Tomato Juice, canned	8 fl oz	40	Tr	0	10	1	9	2
Tomato & Clam Juice, canned	8 fl oz	120	Tr	0	27	1	26	2
Tonic Water - see Soda	***	***	*	*	*	*	*	*
V8 SPLASH **Juice Drinks**	***	***	*	*	*	*	*	*
Berry Blend, Orange Pineapple, Strawberry Banana, Strawberry Kiwi, Tropical Blend	8 fl oz	70	0	0	18	0	18	0
Fruit Medley, Guava Passion Fruit, Orchard Blend	8 fl oz	80	0	0	19	0	19	0
Mango Peach	8 fl oz	80	0	0	20	0	20	0
V8 SPLASH **Juice Drinks,** all diet blends	8 fl oz	10	0	0	3	0	3	0

	Serving Size	Calories	Fat (g)	Calories from Fat (%)	Total Carbs (g)	Fiber (g)	Net Carbs (g)	Protein (g)
V8 SPLASH Smoothies	***	***	*	*	*	*	*	*
Peach Mango	8 fl oz	90	0	0	19	0	19	3
Strawberry Banana	8 fl oz	90	0	0	20	0	20	3
Tropical Colada	8 fl oz	100	0	0	21	1	20	3
V8 Vegetable Juice	8 fl oz	50	0	0	10	2	8	2
Vodka - see Distilled Spirits	***	***	*	*	*	*	*	*
Water	8 fl oz	0	0	0	0	0	0	0
Water, Bottled, any size	***	0	0	0	0	0	0	0
Whisky/Whiskey - see Distilled Spirits	***	***	*	*	*	*	*	*
Wine	***	***	*	*	*	*	*	*
Cooking Wine	1 fl oz	15	0	0	2	0	2	Tr
Dessert Wine, dry	3.5 fl oz	150	0	0	12	0	12	Tr
Dessert Wine, sweet	3.2 fl oz	170	0	0	14	0	14	Tr
Non-alcoholic Wine	5 fl oz	10	0	0	2	0	2	Tr
Red Wine (table wine)	5 fl oz	130	0	0	4	0	4	Tr
Rice Wine - see Sake	***	***	*	*	*	*	*	*
Rosé Wine	5 fl oz	120	0	0	4	0		Tr
Sparkling Wine, Champagne	5 fl oz	123	0	0	4	0	4	Tr
White Wine (table wine)	5 fl oz	120	0	0	4	0		Tr
White Zinfandel	5 fl oz	120	0	0	4	0		Tr

FOODS

	Serving Size	Calories	Fat (g)	Calories from Fat (%)	Total Carbs (g)	Fiber (g)	Net Carbs (g)	Protein (g)	Sugar Alcohol (g)
Alfalfa Sprouts, fresh	1 cup	10	Tr	0	Tr	Tr	Tr	1	0
Almonds - see Nuts	***	***	*	*	*	*	*	*	*
Anchovy - see Fish/ Seafood	***	***	*	*	*	*	*	*	*
Anise Seed	1 Tbsp	25	1	36	3	1	2	1	0
Apple	***	***	*	*	*	*	*	*	*
Dried	5 rings	80	Tr	0	21	3	18	Tr	0
Fresh, peeled, sliced	1 cup	50	Tr	0	14	1	13	Tr	0
Fresh, unpeeled, sm 2¾" dia	1	80	Tr	0	21	4	17	Tr	0
Fresh, unpeeled, med 3" dia	1	100	Tr	0	25	4	21	Tr	0
Apple Butter	1 Tbsp	30	Tr	0	7	Tr	7	Tr	0
Apple Pie Filling, 1 portion	2⅔ oz	80	Tr	0	20	Tr	20	Tr	0
Applesauce	***	***	*	*	*	*	*	*	*
Sweetened	½ cup	100	Tr	0	25	2	23	Tr	0
Unsweetened	½ cup	50	Tr	0	14	2	12	Tr	0
Apricot	***	***	*	*	*	*	*	*	*
Canned halves, in heavy syrup	1 cup	220	Tr	0	55	4	51	1	0
Canned halves, in juice	1 cup	120	Tr	0	30	4	26	2	0
Dried, halves	10	90	Tr	0	22	3	19	1	0
Fresh, med, 1.3 oz	1	15	Tr	0	4	1	3	Tr	0
Artichoke, globe or French	***	***	*	*	*	*	*	*	*
Fresh, cooked med whole	1	60	Tr	0	14	10	4	4	0
Fresh, cooked hearts, drained	½ cup	45	Tr	0	10	7	3	2	0
Frozen, thawed and cooked	½ cup	40	Tr	0	8	4	4	3	0
Artichoke, Jerusalem, raw, sliced	1 cup	110	Tr	0	26	2	24	3	0

	Serving Size	Calories	Fat (g)	Calories from Fat (%)	Total Carbs (g)	Fiber (g)	Net Carbs (g)	Protein (g)	Sugar Alcohol (g)
Arugula, fresh	½ cup	0	Tr	0	Tr	Tr	Tr	Tr	0
Asparagus, cooked	***	***	*	*	*	*	*	*	0
Canned, 5" spears	4	15	Tr	0	2	1	1	2	0
Canned, chopped pieces	1 cup	45	2	40	6	4	2	5	0
Fresh, med spears	4	15	Tr	0	3	1	2	1	0
Fresh, chopped pieces	½ cup	20	Tr	0	4	2	2	2	0
Frozen, spears	4	10	Tr	0	1	1	0	2	0
Frozen, chopped pieces	1 cup	30	Tr	0	4	3	1	5	0
Aspartame Sweetener (Equal)	1 pkt	0	0	0	Tr	0	Tr	Tr	0
Aspartame Sweetener (Equal)	1 tsp	15	0	0	3	0	3	Tr	0
Avocado	***	***	*	*	*	*	*	*	0
California, ⅕ of whole	1 oz	45	4	80	3	2	1	Tr	0
Florida, ⅒ of whole	1 oz	35	3	77	2	2	0	Tr	0
Bacon - see Pork	***	***	*	*	*	*	*	*	*
Bacon Bits	1 Tbsp	35	2	51	2	Tr	1	2	0
Bagel, regular, med, 3¾ oz	***	***	*	*	*	*	*	*	*
Blueberry	1	270	1	3	54	3	51	9	0
Cinnamon raisin	1	290	2	6	58	2	56	10	0
Egg	1	290	2	6	56	2	54	11	0
Everything	1	310	3.5	10	59	4	55	12	0
Oat bran	1	270	1	3	56	4	52	11	0
Onion	1	290	2	6	56	2	54	11	0
Plain	1	290	2	6	56	2	54	11	0
Poppyseed	1	290	2	6	56	2	54	11	0
Sesame	1	290	2	6	56	2	54	11	0
Whole wheat	1	240	2	8	49	7	42	10	0
Bagel, Low Carb	***	***	*	*	*	*	*	*	*
ThinSlim Foods Love-the-Taste Zero-Carb bagels (all flavors)	1	90	4	40	14	14	0	14	0

	Serving Size	Calories	Fat (g)	Calories from Fat (%)	Total Carbs (g)	Fiber (g)	Net Carbs (g)	Protein (g)	Sugar Alcohol (g)
ThinSlim Foods Love-Your-Waist bagels (all flavors)	1	35	0	0	9	8	1	8	0
Baking Powder	1 tsp	0	0	0	1	0	1	0	0
Baking Soda	1 tsp	0	0	0	0	0	0	0	0
Bamboo Shoots, canned, drained	1 cup	25	Tr	0	4	2	2	2	0
Banana	***	***	*	*	*	*	*	*	*
Fresh, 7" long	1	110	Tr	0	27	3	24	1	0
Fresh, sliced	1 cup	130	Tr	0	34	4	30	2	0
Barley, pearled, cooked	1 cup	190	Tr	0	44	6	38	4	0
Bars, Keto, Low Carb, Protein	***	***	*	*	*	*	*	*	*
(See also Energy Bar)	***	***	*	*	*	*	*	*	*
Adapt Your Life Low Carb Protein Bars (all flavors)	1	170	6	32	15	10	1	19	4
Adapt Your Life Mini Keto Bars (all flavors)	1	100	9	81	2	1	1	5	0
Atkins Harvest Trail Bars	***	***	*	*	*	*	*	*	*
Coconut Almond	1	160	11	62	16	10	6	8	0
Dark Chocolate Peanut Butter	1	170	13	69	13	9	4	8	0
Dark Chocolate Sea Salt Caramel	1	180	14	70	13	9	4	8	0
Atkins Protein-Rich Meal Bars	***	***	*	*	*	*	*	*	*
Almond Coconut	1	200	11	50	16	10	6	15	3
Blueberry Greek Yogurt	1	200	9	41	21	9	12	14	8
Chocolate Almond Caramel	1	190	9	43	17	11	6	15	4
Chocolate Chip Cookie Dough	1	220	10	41	32	14	18	13	15
Chocolate Chip Granola	1	200	9	41	18	7	11	17	8
Chocolate Peanut Butter	1	250	14	50	23	12	11	16	8

	Serving Size	Calories	Fat (g)	Calories from Fat (%)	Total Carbs (g)	Fiber (g)	Net Carbs (g)	Protein (g)	Sugar Alcohol (g)
Chocolate Peanut Butter Pretzel	1	200	9	41	18	7	11	16	7
Cookies n' Crème	1	200	11	50	22	9	13	14	9
Peanut Butter Granola	1	210	11	47	16	8	8	16	6
Peanut Fudge Granola	1	220	11	45	18	6	12	16	8
Vanilla Pecan Crisp	1	200	10	45	17	11	6	16	3
Atkins Snacks	***	***	*	*	*	*	*	*	*
Caramel Chocolate Peanut Nougat Bar	1	170	11	58	20	11	9	9	7
Caramel Double Chocolate Crunch Bar	1	160	9	51	20	14	6	10	2
Cashew Trail Mix Bar	1	170	11	58	19	6	13	7	7
Cranberry Almond Bar	1	1	140	5	32	16	6	10	10
Chocolate Chip Crisp Bar	1	140	6	39	16	7	9	10	5
Chocolate Hazelnut Bar	1	180	14	70	18	7	11	6	8
Coconut Almond Delight Bar	1	200	15	68	18	6	12	7	9
Dark Chocolate Almond Coconut Crunch Bar	1	170	13	69	15	10	5	7	1
Dark Chocolate Decadence Bar	1	160	9	51	22	11	11	9	8
Lemon Bar	1	160	7	39	15	9	6	13	3
Peanut Butter Fudge Crisp Bar	1	150	8	48	13	7	6	11	4
Triple Chocolate Bar	1	160	8	45	15	8	7	13	3
White Chocolate Macadamia Nut Bar	1	170	8	42	15	8	7	12	3
Caramel Chocolate Nut Roll	1	190	13	62	19	6	13	7	10
Sweet & Salty Trail Mix	1 pkt	190	14	66	15	3	12	7	8

	Serving Size	Calories	Fat (g)	Calories from Fat (%)	Total Carbs (g)	Fiber (g)	Net Carbs (g)	Protein (g)	Sugar Alcohol (g)
Chocolate Mint Protein Wafer Crisps	1	190	14	66	10	5	5	10	1
Lemon Vanilla Protein Wafer Crisps	1	200	15	68	8	4	4	11	1
Peanut Butter Protein Wafer Crisps	1	190	14	66	9	5	4	11	1
Julian Bakery	***	***	*	*	*	*	*	*	*
InstaKetones Protein Bar, Orange Burst	1	140	8	51	18	14	4	15	0
PaleoThin Protein Bars	***	***	*	*	*	*	*	*	*
Almond Fudge	1	170	8	42	24	23	1	20	0
Blueberry Tart	1	210	10	43	23	21	2	20	0
Chocolate Brownie	1	170	8	42	25	24	1	20	0
Chocolate Mint	1	190	10	47	24	22	2	20	0
Cinnamon Roll	1	190	5	24	25	19	6	20	0
Coconut Cream	1	190	5	24	24	19	5	20	0
Espresso	1	170	5	26	28	26	2	20	0
Glazed Donut	1	190	5	24	24	19	5	20	0
Sunflower Butter	1	150	7	42	25	24	1	20	0
Vanilla Cake	1	180	4	20	25	21	4	20	0
Vanilla Pudding	1	170	6	32	23	22	1	20	0
PeganThin Protein Bars	***	***	*	*	*	*	*	*	*
Chocolate Lava	1	190	9	43	27	26	1	20	0
Ginger Snap Cookie	1	170	6	32	28	27	1	20	0
Sweet Sunflower	1	187	11	53	26	24	2	20	0
Vanilla Cinnamon Twist	1	150	6	36	26	23	3	20	0
PrimalThin Whey Protein Bar, Sweet Cream	1	130	5	35	19	18	1	20	0
StayThin Protein Bars	***	***	*	*	*	*	*	*	*

	Serving Size	Calories	Fat (g)	Calories from Fat (%)	Total Carbs (g)	Fiber (g)	Net Carbs (g)	Protein (g)	Sugar Alcohol (g)
Peanut Butter Grass-Fed Whey Protein	1	160	7	39	24	22	2	20	0
Peanut Butter Egg-White Protein	1	170	7	37	29	26	3	20	0
Kiss My Keto Keto Bars	***	***	*	*	*	*	*	*	*
Chocolate Coconut	1	240	20	75	16	10	4	9	2
Chocolate Cookie Dough	1	230	19	74	16	12	2	10	2
Chocolate Peanut Butter	1	240	20	75	16	11	3	10	2
Perfect Keto Keto Bar, Almond Butter Brownie	1	230	19	74	12	9	3	10	0
Quest Protein Bars	***	***	*	*	*	*	*	*	*
Apple Pie	1	190	6	28	24	16	6	20	2
Birthday Cake	1	180	6	30	24	14	4	21	6
Blueberry Muffin	1	200	8	36	21	15	4	21	2
Chocolate Brownie	1	180	6	30	23	17	4	20	2
Chocolate Chip Cookie Dough	1	200	9	41	21	14	4	21	3
Chocolate Hazelnut	1	190	8	38	23	14	4	20	5
Chocolate Peanut Butter	1	210	10	43	22	13	5	20	4
Cinnamon Roll	1	180	6	30	24	16	4	20	4
Coconut Cashew	1	190	7	33	23	15	4	20	4
Cookies & Cream	1	200	8	36	21	15	4	21	2
Double Chocolate Chunk	1	180	7	35	24	14	4	20	6
Maple Waffle	1	190	6	28	24	16	5	20	3
Mint Chocolate Chunk	1	200	8	36	22	16	4	20	2
Mocha Chocolate Chip	1	180	6	30	24	14	4	20	6
Oatmeal Chocolate Chip	1	190	7	33	23	16	5	20	2
Peanut Butter Brownie Smash	1	190	7	33	24	14	6	20	4

	Serving Size	Calories	Fat (g)	Calories from Fat (%)	Total Carbs (g)	Fiber (g)	Net Carbs (g)	Protein (g)	Sugar Alcohol (g)
Peanut Butter Supreme	1	200	8	36	22	15	5	20	2
Rocky Road	1	210	9	39	21	14	5	20	2
S'mores	1	190	7	33	22	14	4	21	4
Strawberry Cheesecake	1	180	5	25	25	15	5	20	5
Vanilla Almond Crunch	1	200	9	41	21	15	4	20	2
White Chocolate Raspberry	1	200	8	36	22	15	5	20	2
Quest Hero Protein Bars	***	***	*	*	*	*	*	*	*
Blueberry Cobbler	1	170	7	37	30	10	20	17	4
Chocolate Caramel Pecan	1	200	11	50	27	11	16	15	1
Vanilla Caramel	1	180	9	45	29	10	19	16	4
SlimFast Keto Meal Bar, Whipped Peanut Butter Chocolate	1	190	14	66	15	9	4	7	2
SlimFast Keto Meal Bar, Whipped Triple Chocolate	1	190	14	66	15	9	4	7	2
Stoka Bar, Coco Almond	1	260	23	80	18	6	4	9	8
Stoka Bar, Vanilla Almond	1	260	23	80	17	6	4	9	7
Zenwise Health Keto-Crave Energy Bar, Cacao Almond	1	210	16	69	13	8	5	9	0
Zenwise Health Keto-Crave Energy Bar, Choc Chip Cookie Dough	1	210	16	69	10	7	3	12	0
Bars, Sweet - see Sweets, Low Carb	***	***	*	*	*	*	*	*	*
Basil	***	***	*	0	*	*	*	*	*
Dried spiced	1 tsp	0	Tr	0	Tr	Tr	Tr	Tr	0
Fresh, chopped pieces	2 Tbsp	0	Tr	0	Tr	Tr	Tr	Tr	0
Fresh, whole leaves	¼ cup	0	Tr	0	Tr	Tr	Tr	Tr	0

	Serving Size	Calories	Fat (g)	Calories from Fat (%)	Total Carbs (g)	Fiber (g)	Net Carbs (g)	Protein (g)	Sugar Alcohol (g)
Bean Sprouts (mung)	***	***	*	*	*	*	*	*	*
Cooked, boiled	1 cup	25	Tr	0	5	1	4	3	0
Cooked, stir-fried	1 cup	60	Tr	0	13	2	11	5	0
Fresh	1 cup	30	Tr	0	6	2	4	3	0
BEANS	***	***	*	*	*	*	*	*	*
Dried Beans, cooked w/o fats	***	***	*	*	*	*	*	*	*
Adzuki	½ cup	150	Tr	0	29	8	21	9	0
Black	½ cup	110	Tr	0	20	8	12	8	0
Black-eyed peas	½ cup	80	Tr	0	17	4	13	3	0
Cranberry (roman)	½ cup	120	Tr	0	22	9	13	8	0
Fava (broad beans)	½ cup	90	Tr	0	17	5	12	7	0
Garbanzo (chickpeas)	½ cup	130	2	14	23	6	17	7	0
Great Northern	½ cup	100	Tr	0	19	6	13	7	0
Kidney (dark or light red)	½ cup	110	Tr	0	20	7	13	8	0
Lima, baby	½ cup	120	Tr	0	21	7	14	7	0
Lima, large	½ cup	110	Tr	0	20	7	13	7	0
Navy	½ cup	130	Tr	0	24	10	14	8	0
Pinto	½ cup	120	Tr	0	22	8	14	8	0
Soy	½ cup	150	8	48	9	5	4	14	0
White	½ cup	120	Tr	0	23	6	17	9	0
Snap Beans (string beans), cooked w/o fats	***	***	*	*	*	*	*	*	*
Canned, drained	1 cup	25	Tr	0	6	3	3	2	0
Frozen, cooked	1 cup	40	Tr	0	9	4	5	2	0
Green beans, fresh	1 cup	45	Tr	0	10	4	6	2	0
Yellow (wax) beans, fresh	1 cup	45	Tr	0	10	4	6	2	0
Bean Dishes, misc., as prep	***	***	*	*	*	*	*	*	*
Baked beans, plain or vegetarian	½ cup	120	Tr	0	27	5	22	6	0
Baked beans w/ frankfurters	½ cup	180	9	45	20	9	11	9	0

	Serving Size	Calories	Fat (g)	Calories from Fat (%)	Total Carbs (g)	Fiber (g)	Net Carbs (g)	Protein (g)	Sugar Alcohol (g)
Baked beans w/ pork	½ cup	130	2	14	25	7	18	7	0
Baked beans w/ pork & tomato sauce	½ cup	120	1	8	23	5	18	6	0
Baked beans w/ pork & sweet sauce	½ cup	140	2	13	27	5	22	7	0
Campbell's Brown Sugar and Bacon flavored beans	½ cup	160	3	17	30	8	22	5	0
Campbell's Pork and Beans	½ cup	140	2	13	25	7	18	6	0
Refried beans	½ cup	110	1	8	18	6	12	6	0
Refried beans, fat free	½ cup	90	Tr	0	16	5	11	6	0
Refried beans, vegetarian	½ cup	100	1	9	16	6	10	6	0
Refried red beans	½ cup	170	8	42	18	6	12	6	0
BEEF	***	***	*	*	*	*	*	*	*
(Weights for meat w/o bones)	***	***	*	*	*	*	*	*	*
(Meats trimmed to 0 fat, unless otherwise noted)	***	***	*	*	*	*	*	*	*
Bottom Round, braised	***	***	*	*	*	*	*	*	*
lean & fat	3 oz	190	8	38	0	0	0	29	0
lean only	3 oz	189	7	33	0	0	0	29	0
Brisket, braised	***	***	*	*	*	*	*	*	*
flat half, lean & fat	3 oz	180	7	35	0	0	0	28	0
flat half, lean only	3 oz	170	6	32	0	0	0	28	0
point half, lean & fat	3 oz	300	24	72	0	0	0	20	0
point half, lean only	3 oz	210	12	51	0	0	0	24	0
whole, lean & fat	3 oz	250	17	61	0	0	0	23	0
whole, lean only	3 oz	190	9	43	0	0	0	25	0
Chuck Blade, Blade Roast, braised	***	***	*	*	*	*	*	*	*
lean & fat	3 oz	300	22	66	0	0	0	23	0

	Serving Size	Calories	Fat (g)	Calories from Fat (%)	Total Carbs (g)	Fiber (g)	Net Carbs (g)	Protein (g)	Sugar Alcohol (g)
lean only	3 oz	220	11	45	0	0	0	26	0
Chuck, Top Blade, broiled	***	***	*	*	*	*	*	*	*
lean & fat	3 oz	180	10	50	0	0	0	22	0
lean only	3 oz	170	9	48	0	0	0	22	0
Corned Beef	3 oz	210	13	56	0	0	0	23	0
Dried Beef, chipped	1 oz	45	Tr	0	Tr	0	Tr	9	0
Eye of Round, roasted	***	***	*	*	*	*	*	*	*
lean & fat	3 oz	140	4	26	0	0	0	25	0
lean only	3 oz	140	4	26	0	0	0	25	0
Flank Steak, broiled	***	***	*	*	*	*	*	*	*
lean & fat	3 oz	160	7	39	0	0	0	24	0
lean only	3 oz	160	6	34	0	0	0	24	0
Ground Beef/ Hamburger Meat, broiled	***	***	*	*	*	*	*	*	*
75 lean	3 oz	240	16	60	0	0	0	22	0
80 lean	3 oz	230	15	59	0	0	0	22	0
85 lean	3 oz	210	13	56	0	0	0	22	0
90 lean	3 oz	180	10	50	0	0	0	22	0
95 lean	3 oz	164	6	33	0	0	0	25	0
Liver, fried	3 oz	150	4	24	4	0	4	23	0
Pastrami	2 oz	80	3	34	0	0	0	12	0
Porterhouse Steak, broiled	***	***	*	*	*	*	*	*	*
lean & fat	3 oz	240	16	60	0	0	0	20	0
lean only	3 oz	180	10	50	0	0	0	22	0
Pot Roast, Chuck, braised	***	***	*	*	*	*	*	*	*
lean & fat	3 oz	250	16	58	0	0	0	25	0
lean only	3 oz	170	5	26	0	0	0	28	0
Prime Rib (trimmed to ⅛" fat), broiled	3 oz	330	28	76	0	0	0	19	0
Rib Roast (trimmed to ⅛" fat), roasted	3 oz	300	24	72	0	0	0	19	0

	Serving Size	Calories	Fat (g)	Calories from Fat (%)	Total Carbs (g)	Fiber (g)	Net Carbs (g)	Protein (g)	Sugar Alcohol (g)
Roast Beef, sliced deli meat	2 oz	70	2	26	2	0	2	10	0
Short Ribs, braised	***	***	*	*	*	*	*	*	*
lean & fat	3 oz	400	36	81	0	0	0	18	0
lean only	3 oz	250	15	54	0	0	0	26	0
Top Sirloin, broiled	***	***	*	*	*	*	*	*	*
lean & fat	3 oz	180	8	40	0	0	0	25	0
lean only	3 oz	160	5	28	0	0	0	26	0
T-bone Steak, broiled	***	***	*	*	*	*	*	*	*
lean & fat	3 oz	210	14	60	0	0	0	21	0
lean only	3 oz	160	7	39	0	0	0	22	0
Tenderloin Steak, broiled	***	***	*	*	*	*	*	*	*
lean & fat	3 oz	190	10	47	0	0	0	23	0
lean only	3 oz	160	7	39	0	0	0	24	0
Top Round, braised	***	***	*	*	*	*	*	*	*
lean & fat	3 oz	180	6	30	0	0	0	30	0
lean only	3 oz	170	4	21	0	0	0	31	0
Tri-tip Steak, broiled	***	***	*	*	*	*	*	*	*
lean & fat	3 oz	230	13	51	0	0	0	26	0
lean only	3 oz	210	11	47	0	0	0	26	0
(Other Beef Products, see:	***	***	*	*	*	*	*	*	*
Bologna, Hot Dog, Salami, Sausage & specific entrées)	***	***	*	*	*	*	*	*	*
Beef Jerky	1 piece	80	5	56	2	Tr	2	7	0
Beef Macaroni, frozen entrée	8.5 oz	210	2	9	34	5	29	14	0
Beef Stew, *Dinty Moore,* canned	1 cup	220	13	53	16	3	13	11	0
Beet Greens, chopped, cooked	½ cup	20	Tr	0	4	2	2	2	0
Beets	***	***	*	*	*	*	*	*	*

	Serving Size	Calories	Fat (g)	Calories from Fat (%)	Total Carbs (g)	Fiber (g)	Net Carbs (g)	Protein (g)	Sugar Alcohol (g)
Canned, drained, slices	½ cup	25	Tr	0	6	2	4	Tr	0
Canned, drained, whole	1 cup	50	Tr	0	12	3	9	2	0
Canned, pickled, slices w/ liquid	½ cup	70	Tr	0	19	3	16	Tr	0
Fresh, cooked, slices	½ cup	35	Tr	0	9	2	7	Tr	0
Fresh, cooked, whole, 2" dia	2	45	Tr	0	10	2	8	2	0
Biscuit, Low Carb	***	***	*	*	*	*	*	*	*
Linda's Diet Delites Low Carb Biscuits	1	70	4.5	58	12	10	2	4	0
Biscuit, plain or buttermilk	***	***	*	*	*	*	*	*	*
Prep from recipe, 2½" dia	1	210	10	43	27	1	26	4	0
Prep from recipe, 4" dia	1	360	17	43	45	2	43	7	0
Refrigerated dough, baked	***	***	*	*	*	*	*	*	*
regular 2½" dia	1	100	4	36	13	Tr	13	2	0
reduced fat, 2¼" dia	1	60	1	15	12	Tr	12	2	0
Blackberries	***	***	*	*	*	*	*	*	*
Fresh	1 cup	60	Tr	0	14	8	6	2	0
Frozen, unthawed	1 cup	100	Tr	0	24	8	16	2	0
Blueberries	***	***	*	*	*	*	*	*	*
Fresh	1 cup	80	Tr	0	22	4	18	1	0
Frozen, sweetened, thawed	1 cup	190	Tr	0	51	5	46	Tr	0
Frozen, unsweetened, unthawed	1 cup	80	Tr	0	19	4	15	Tr	0
Frozen, wild, unthawed	1 cup	70	Tr	0	19	6	13	0	0
Bok Choy - see Cabbage	***	***	*	*	*	*	*	*	*
Bologna	***	***	*	*	*	*	*	*	*

	Serving Size	Calories	Fat (g)	Calories from Fat (%)	Total Carbs (g)	Fiber (g)	Net Carbs (g)	Protein (g)	Sugar Alcohol (g)
Beef	1 slice	90	8	80	1	0	1	3	0
Beef, low fat	1 slice	60	4	60	2	0	2	3	0
Beef & pork	1 slice	90	7	70	2	0	2	4	0
Beef & pork, low fat	1 slice	60	5	75	Tr	0	Tr	3	0
Boars Head, beef & pork	2 oz	150	13	78	1	0	1	7	0
Louis Rich, turkey bologna	1 slice	50	4	72	1	0	1	3	0
Oscar Mayer, beef light	1 slice	60	4	60	2	0	2	3	0
Oscar Mayer, bologna	1 slice	90	8	80	Tr	0	Tr	3	0
Oscar Mayer, bologna, fat free	1 slice	20	Tr	0	2	0	2	4	0
Turkey	1 slice	60	5	75	1	Tr	1	3	0
Bouillon - see Soup	***	***	*	*	*	*	*	*	*
Bratwurst, *Boars Head*	1	300	25	75	0	0	0	19	0
Braunschweiger, *Oscar Mayer*, 1 slice	1 oz	90	8	80	Tr	Tr	Tr	4	0
BREAD/BREAD PRODUCTS	***	***	*	*	*	*	*	*	*
(avg ½" thick slice, unless noted)	***	***	*	*	*	*	*	*	*
(See also Bagel & Biscuit)	***	***	*	*	*	*	*	*	*
Boston brown, canned	1 slice	90	Tr	0	20	2	18	2	0
Cornbread, 3" x 2"	1 pc	190	6	28	29	1	28	4	0
Cracked wheat	1 slice	80	1	11	15	2	13	3	0
Croissant	1 med	230	12	47	26	2	24	5	0
Croissant, apple	1 med	150	5	30	21	1	20	4	0
Croissant, cheese	1 med	240	12	45	27	2	25	5	0
Croissant, chocolate	1 med	240	13	49	28	2	26	4	0
Egg bread	1 slice	110	2	16	19	Tr	19	4	0
English muffin, traditional	***	***	*	*	*	*	*	*	*
cinnamon raisin	1 whole	140	1	6	27	2	25	5	0

	Serving Size	Calories	Fat (g)	Calories from Fat (%)	Total Carbs (g)	Fiber (g)	Net Carbs (g)	Protein (g)	Sugar Alcohol (g)
light, multigrain, *Thomas'*	1 whole	100	1	9	25	8	13	5	0
multigrain	1 whole	160	1	6	31	2	29	6	0
oat bran (gluten free)	1 whole	137	2.5	16	23	3	20	6	0
regular	1 whole	130	Tr	0	25	2	23	5	0
whole wheat	1 whole	130	1	7	27	4	23	6	0
English muffin, low carb, *Mikey's Paleo*	½ ea	86	6	63	4	2	2	4	0
French bread	1 slice	90	Tr	0	18	Tr	18	4	0
Garlic bread, *Pepperidge Farm*, frozen	1 slice	170	7	37	24	2	22	4	0
Irish soda bread	1 oz	80	1	11	16	Tr	16	2	0
Italian bread	1 slice	50	Tr	0	10	Tr	10	2	0
Low carb	***	***	*	*	*	*	*	*	*
Cali'flour Foods, Flatbreads, 5" low carb	1	50	2.5	45	4	1	3	5	0
Julian Bakery PaleoThin Bread	***	***	*	*	*	*	*	*	*
Almond	1 slice	60	3	45	6	5	1	7	0
Coconut	1 slice	35	1	26	6	5	1	5	0
Sandwich (gluten-free, grain-free)	1 slice	90	6	60	7	4	3	6	0
Seed Medley	1 slice	65	5	69	8	6	2	6	0
Outer Aisle Gourmet Cauliflower Sandwich Thins	1 pc	50	2.5	45	2	1	1	4	0
ThinSlim Foods, Love-the-Taste Zero-Carb Bread, all flavors	1 slice	45	2	40	7	7	0	7	0
Plain, Thin Sliced	2 slices	45	2	40	7	7	0	7	0
ThinSlim Foods, Love-the-Taste Zero-Carb rolls & buns	***	***	*	*	*	*	*	*	*

	Serving Size	Calories	Fat (g)	Calories from Fat (%)	Total Carbs (g)	Fiber (g)	Net Carbs (g)	Protein (g)	Sugar Alcohol (g)
Hamburger buns	1	90	4	40	14	14	0	14	0
Hot dog buns	1	90	4	40	14	14	0	14	0
Olive & garlic rolls	1	120	6	45	14	14	0	14	0
Onion pockets	1	90	4	40	14	14	0	14	0
ThinSlim Foods, Gluten-Free Zero-Carb rolls & buns (all flavors)	1	50	3	54	11	10	0	4.5	1
Multigrain bread	1 slice	70	1	13	11	2	9	4	0
Oat bread	1 slice	70	1	13	12	1	11	3	0
Oatmeal bread	1 slice	70	1	13	13	1	12	2	0
Pita bread, 4"	1 whole	80	Tr	0	16	Tr	16	3	0
Pita bread, 6½"	1 whole	170	Tr	0	33	1	32	5	0
Pita bread, whole-wheat, 4"	1 whole	70	Tr	0	15	2	13	3	0
Pita bread, whole-wheat, 6½"	1 whole	170	2	11	35	5	30	6	0
Pumpernickel bread	1 slice	80	1	11	15	2	13	3	0
Raisin bread	1 slice	90	1	10	17	1	16	3	0
Reduced calorie bread, white	1 slice	50	Tr	0	10	2	8	2	0
Ricebran bread	1 slice	70	1	13	12	1	11	2	0
Roll	***	***	*	*	*	*	*	*	*
dinner (egg)	1	110	2	16	18	1	17	3	0
French	1	110	2	16	19	1	18	3	0
hard or kaiser	1	170	3	16	30	1	29	6	0
hamburger or hot dog	1	120	2	15	21	Tr	21	4	0
hamburger or hot dog, multigrain	1	110	3	25	19	2	17	4	0
hamburger or hot dog, low cal	1	80	Tr	0	18	3	15	4	0
whole wheat	1	100	2	18	18	3	15	3	0
Rye bread	1 slice	80	1	11	16	2	14	3	0
Sourdough bread	1 slice	90	Tr	0	18	Tr	18	4	0

	Serving Size	Calories	Fat (g)	Calories from Fat (%)	Total Carbs (g)	Fiber (g)	Net Carbs (g)	Protein (g)	Sugar Alcohol (g)
Vienna bread	1 slice	90	Tr	0	18	Tr	18	4	0
Wheat bread	1 slice	70	Tr	0	12	Tr	12	3	0
White bread	1 slice	70	Tr	0	13	Tr	13	2	0
Whole-wheat bread	1 slice	79	Tr	0	12	2	10	4	0
Bread Crumbs	***	***	*	*	*	*	*	*	*
Dry, grated	1 cup	430	6	13	78	5	73	14	0
Dry, seasoned, grated	1 cup	460	7	14	82	6	76	17	0
Low Carb, Plain, *ThinSlim Foods* Love-the-Taste	4 Tbsp	45	2	40	7	7	0	7	0
Panko Bread Crumbs, *Ian's*	¼ cup	70	0	0	15	Tr	15	2	0
Panko Japanese Style, *Dynasty*	½ cup	110	1	8	20	1	19	4	0
Soft crumbs	1 cup	120	2	15	23	1	22	3	0
Bread Stick, med	1	40	Tr	0	7	Tr	7	1	0
Bread Stuffing - see Stuffing	***	***	*	*	*	*	*	*	*
Breakfast Bar, w/ oats, raisins & coconut	1	200	8	36	29	1	28	4	0
Breakfasts	***	***	*	*	*	*	*	*	*
Atkins Frozen Foodie Meal Kits	***	***	*	*	*	*	*	*	*
Bacon Scramble	1	370	28	68	5	1	4	23	0
Farmhouse-Style Sausage Scramble	1	340	27	71	7	2	5	20	0
Ham & Cheese Omelet	1	210	15	64	4	0	4	16	0
Jimmy Dean Simple Scrambles	***	***	*	*	*	*	*	*	*
Bacon	1	310	23	67	2	0	2	23	0
Sausage	1	290	22	68	3	0	3	20	0
Meat Lovers	1	300	24	72	2	0	2	23	0
Three Cheese	1	180	11	55	3	0	3	18	0
Turkey Sausage	1	150	7	42	3	0	3	17	0

	Serving Size	Calories	Fat (g)	Calories from Fat (%)	Total Carbs (g)	Fiber (g)	Net Carbs (g)	Protein (g)	Sugar Alcohol (g)
Breakfast Sandwich	***	***	*	*	*	*	*	*	*
(See also specific restaurants)	***	***	*	*	*	*	*	*	*
Biscuit w/ egg	1	370	22	54	32	Tr	32	12	0
Biscuit w/ egg & bacon	1	460	31	61	29	Tr	29	17	0
Biscuit w/ egg, bacon & cheese	1	440	25	51	35	Tr	35	17	0
Biscuit w/ egg & sausage	1	510	34	60	34	Tr	34	18	0
Biscuit w/ ham	1	390	18	42	44	Tr	44	13	0
Biscuit w/ sausage	1	410	27	59	33	Tr	33	11	0
Croissant w/ egg & cheese	1	370	25	61	24	Tr	24	13	0
Croissant w/ egg, cheese & bacon	1	410	28	61	24	Tr	24	16	0
Croissant w/ egg, cheese & ham	1	470	34	65	24	Tr	24	19	0
Croissant w/ egg, cheese & sausage	1	520	38	66	25	Tr	25	20	0
English muffin w/ egg, cheese & Canadian bacon	1	310	13	38	30	Tr	30	19	0
English muffin w/ egg, cheese & sausage	1	470	30	57	29	Tr	29	22	0
Broccoli	***	***	*	*	*	*	*	*	*
Florets, fresh	1 cup	20	Tr	0	4	2	2	2	0
Fresh, raw, spear, 5" long	1	10	Tr	0	2	Tr	2	Tr	0
Fresh, raw, chopped	1 cup	30	Tr	0	6	2	4	3	0
Fresh, cooked, spear, 5" long	1	10	Tr	0	3	1	2	Tr	0
Fresh, cooked, chopped	½ cup	25	Tr	0	6	3	3	2	0
Frozen, spears, cooked	½ cup	25	Tr	0	5	3	2	3	0
Frozen, chopped, cooked	1 cup	50	Tr	0	10	6	4	6	0

	Serving Size	Calories	Fat (g)	Calories from Fat (%)	Total Carbs (g)	Fiber (g)	Net Carbs (g)	Protein (g)	Sugar Alcohol (g)
Broccoli, Chinese, cooked	1 cup	20	Tr	0	3	3	1	1	0
Broccoli Rabe	***	***	*	*	*	*	*	*	*
Cooked	3 oz	30	Tr	0	3	2	1	3	0
Raw, chopped	1 cup	10	Tr	0	1	1	0	1	0
Broth - see Soup	***	***	*	*	*	*	*	*	*
Brownie, 2" square	1	240	10	38	39	Tr	39	3	0
(See also Sweets, Low Carb)	***	***	*	*	*	*	*	*	*
Brussels Sprouts	***	***	*	*	*	*	*	*	*
Fresh, cooked	1 cup	60	Tr	0	11	4	7	4	0
Frozen, cooked	1 cup	70	Tr	0	13	6	7	6	0
Bulgur	***	***	*	*	*	*	*	*	*
Cooked	1 cup	150	Tr	0	34	8	26	6	0
Uncooked	1 cup	480	2	4	106	26	80	17	0
Bun - see Bread/Bread Products, Roll	***	***	*	*	*	*	*	*	*
Burrito	***	***	*	*	*	*	*	*	*
Bean & cheese	1	310	9	26	48	12	36	10	0
Beef & bean	1	350	14	36	45	8	37	10	0
Butter	***	***	*	*	*	*	*	*	*
(See also Margarine)	***	***	*	*	*	*	*	*	*
Regular, salted or unsalted, 1 stick	8 Tbsp	810	92	100	Tr	0	Tr	Tr	0
Regular, salted or unsalted	1 Tbsp	102	12	100	Tr	0	Tr	Tr	0
Regular, salted or unsalted	1 tsp	35	4	100	0	0	0	Tr	0
Cabbage	***	***	*	*	*	*	*	*	*
Chinese cabbage (bok choy), shredded, cooked	1 cup	20	Tr	0	3	2	1	3	0
Chinese cabbage (bok choy), shredded, raw	1 cup	10	Tr	0	2	Tr	2	1	0
Green, shredded, cooked	½ cup	15	Tr	0	4	1	3	Tr	0

	Serving Size	Calories	Fat (g)	Calories from Fat (%)	Total Carbs (g)	Fiber (g)	Net Carbs (g)	Protein (g)	Sugar Alcohol (g)
Green, shredded, raw	1 cup	15	Tr	0	4	2	2	Tr	0
Napa cabbage	1 cup	15	Tr	0	2	Tr	2	1	0
Red/purple cabbage, shredded, cooked	1 cup	45	Tr	0	10	4	6	2	0
Red/purple cabbage, shredded, raw	1 cup	20	Tr	0	5	2	3	1	0
Savoy cabbage, shredded, cooked	1 cup	35	Tr	0	8	4	4	3	0
Savoy cabbage, shredded, raw	1 cup	20	Tr	0	4	2	2	1	0
Cake	***	***	*	*	*	*	*	*	*
(See also Sweets, Low Carb)	***	***	*	*	*	*	*	*	*
(average size slice of single layer cake, ⅛ of 9", unless noted)	***	***	*	*	*	*	*	*	*
Angel food, ¹⁄₁₂ of 10" cake	1 slice	130	Tr	0	29	Tr	29	3	0
Boston cream, ⅛ of cake	1 slice	230	8	31	40	1	39	2	0
Cheesecake, plain, ⅙ of 17 oz cake	1 slice	260	18	62	20	Tr	20	4	0
Chocolate cake w/ chocolate frosting	1 slice	240	11	41	35	2	33	3	0
Fruitcake, small slice	1 slice	140	4	26	27	2	25	1	0
Gingerbread	1 slice	260	12	42	36	1	35	3	0
Pineapple upside down	1 slice	370	14	34	58	Tr	58	4	0
Pound w/o glaze, ¹⁄₁₀ of cake	1 slice	120	6	45	15	Tr	15	2	0
Pound, fat free, ¹⁄₁₀ of cake	1 slice	100	Tr	0	21	Tr	21	2	0
Sponge, ¹⁄₁₀ of 10" cake	1 slice	110	1	8	23	Tr	23	2	0
White, ¹⁄₁₂ of cake, w/ coconut frosting	1 slice	400	12	27	71	1	70	5	0
White, ¹⁄₁₂ of cake, w/o frosting	1 slice	260	9	31	42	Tr	42	4	0

	Serving Size	Calories	Fat (g)	Calories from Fat (%)	Total Carbs (g)	Fiber (g)	Net Carbs (g)	Protein (g)	Sugar Alcohol (g)
Yellow w/ chocolate frosting	1 slice	240	11	41	36	1	35	2	0
Yellow w/ vanilla frosting	1 slice	240	9	34	38	Tr	38	2	0
CANDY	***	***	*	*	*	*	*	*	*
(See also Sweets, Low Carb)	***	***	*	*	*	*	*	*	*
Almond Joy, 1.8 oz bar	1	240	13	49	29	3	26	2	0
Baby Ruth, 2.1 oz bar	1	280	13	42	40	1	39	3	0
Bit-O-Honey	6 pc	150	3	18	32	Tr	32	Tr	0
Butterfinger, 2.1 oz bar	1	280	11	35	44	1	43	3	0
Caramel	***	***	*	*	*	*	*	*	*
regular caramel, 0.3 oz	1 pc	40	Tr	0	8	0	8	Tr	0
regular caramel, 2.5 oz	1 pkg	270	6	20	55	0	55	3	0
chocolate caramel roll	1 pc	25	Tr	0	6	0	6	Tr	0
chocolate covered, w/ nuts	1 pc	70	3	39	9	Tr	9	1	0
Caramello, 1.6 oz bar	1	210	10	43	29	Tr	29	3	0
Carob	1 oz	150	9	54	16	1	15	2	0
Charms Blow Pop	1	60	0	0	17	0	17	0	0
Chewing gum - see Chewing Gum	***	***	*	*	*	*	*	*	*
Chocolate Bars	***	***	*	*	*	*	*	*	*
(See also Chocolate for Baking)	***	***	*	*	*	*	*	*	*
Hershey's Milk Chocolate, 1.5 oz, plain	1	210	13	56	26	1	25	3	0
Hershey's Milk Chocolate, 1.5 oz, w/ almonds	1	210	14	60	21	2	19	4	0

	Serving Size	Calories	Fat (g)	Calories from Fat (%)	Total Carbs (g)	Fiber (g)	Net Carbs (g)	Protein (g)	Sugar Alcohol (g)
Hershey's Special Dark, 1.5 oz	1	180	12	60	25	3	22	2	0
Hershey's Special Dark, miniature size	1	100	6	54	10	1	9	Tr	0
Hershey's Extra Creamy Chocolate & Caramel, 1.25 oz	1	180	9	45	22	Tr	22	2	0
Hershey's Miniatures, 1.5 oz	5 pc	210	13	56	25	2	23	3	0
Hershey's Mr. Goodbar, 1.75 oz	1	250	17	61	26	2	24	5	0
Chocolate coated peanuts	10	210	13	56	20	2	18	5	0
Chocolate coated raisins	10	40	2	45	7	Tr	7	Tr	0
Chocolate Kiss, *Hershey's*	9 pc	230	13	51	24	1	23	3	0
Fifth Avenue, 2 oz bar	1	270	13	43	35	2	33	5	0
Fruit leather, pieces, 1 pkt	¾ oz	80	Tr	0	17	0	17	Tr	0
Fruit leather, small roll	1	50	Tr	0	12	0	12	Tr	0
Fudge, 1 piece	***	***	*	*	*	*	*	*	*
chocolate	¾ oz	90	2	20	16	Tr	16	Tr	0
chocolate w/ marshmallow	¾ oz	100	4	36	15	Tr	15	Tr	0
chocolate w/ marshmallow & nuts	¾ oz	100	4	36	14	Tr	14	Tr	0
chocolate w/ nuts	¾ oz	100	4	36	14	Tr	14	Tr	0
peanut butter	¾ oz	80	1	11	16	Tr	16	Tr	0
vanilla	¾ oz	80	1	11	17	0	17	Tr	0
vanilla w/ nuts	¾ oz	90	3	30	16	Tr	16	Tr	0
Goobers, 1.4 oz pkg	1	200	13	59	21	4	17	4	0
Gumdrops ¾" dia	5	80	0	0	21	0	21	0	0
Gummy bears	10	90	0	0	22	0	22	0	0

	Serving Size	Calories	Fat (g)	Calories from Fat (%)	Total Carbs (g)	Fiber (g)	Net Carbs (g)	Protein (g)	Sugar Alcohol (g)
Gummy worms	10	290	0	0	73	Tr	73	0	0
Hardy Candy	***	***	*	*	*	*	*	*	*
butterscotch	2	40	Tr	0	10	0	10	0	0
regular	2	45	Tr	0	12	0	12	0	0
sugar free	2	25	0	0	6	0	6	0	0
Jelly beans, regular size	10	110	Tr	0	26	Tr	26	0	0
Jelly beans, small pieces	10	40	Tr	0	10	0	10	0	0
Junior Mints	16	170	3	16	35	1	34	1	0
Kit Kat, 1.5 oz bar	1	220	11	45	27	Tr	27	3	0
Krackel, 1.5 oz bar	1	210	11	47	26	Tr	26	3	0
Licorice, black or red	1	41	0	0	10	0	10	0	0
M&M's	***	***	*	*	*	*	*	*	*
dark chocolate	48 g	240	11	41	33	2	31	2	0
dark chocolate mint	43 g	210	10	43	29	2	27	2	0
dark chocolate peanut	43 g	220	12	49	25	2	23	4	0
peanut butter	46 g	240	13	49	26	1	25	4	0
plain	10	35	2	51	5	Tr	5	Tr	0
w/ almonds	10	170	9	48	20	2	18	3	0
w/ peanuts	10	100	5	45	12	1	12	2	0
w/ pretzels	32 g	150	4.5	27	24	1	23	2	0
Mars Almond, 1.75 oz bar	1	230	12	47	31	1	30	4	0
Marshmallow, avg size (¼ oz)	1	25	Tr	0	6	0	6	Tr	0
Mentos	1 pc	10	0	0	3	0	3	0	0
Milky Way, regular size, 2 oz	1	260	10	35	41	Tr	41	2	0
Milky Way, fun size	1	80	3	34	12	Tr	12	Tr	0
Milky Way Dark, 1¾ oz	1	220	8	33	36	1	35	1	0
Mounds, 1.9 oz bar	1	260	14	48	31	2	29	2	0

	Serving Size	Calories	Fat (g)	Calories from Fat (%)	Total Carbs (g)	Fiber (g)	Net Carbs (g)	Protein (g)	Sugar Alcohol (g)
Nestlé Crunch, 1.55 oz bar	1	220	11	45	30	Tr	30	2	0
Nestlé Crunch, fun size	1	50	3	54	7	Tr	7	Tr	0
Oh Henry!, 2 oz bar	1	260	13	45	37	1	36	4	0
Oh Henry!, fun size	1	120	6	45	17	Tr	17	2	0
Peanut brittle	1 oz	140	5	32	20	Tr	20	2	0
Peppermint Pattie, York, 1.5 oz	1	170	3	16	35	Tr	35	Tr	0
Raisinets, 1.6 oz	1 pkg	190	8	38	31	1	30	2	0
Reese's Bites	16 pc	200	12	54	22	1	21	4	0
Reese's Fast Break	1 bar	280	13	42	36	2	34	5	0
Reese's Nutrageous, 1.92 oz bar	1	280	17	55	29	2	27	6	0
Reese's Peanut Butter Cup, regular size	2 cups	230	14	55	25	2	23	5	0
Reese's Peanut Butter Cup, miniature size	2 cups	70	4	51	8	Tr	8	1	0
Reese's Pieces, 1.6 oz pkg	1 pkg	230	11	43	28	1	27	6	0
Reese's Sticks, 1.5 oz	1	220	13	53	23	1	22	4	0
Rolo caramels	7 pc	200	9	41	29	Tr	29	2	0
Skittles, original	10 pc	45	Tr	0	10	0	10	Tr	0
Skor toffee, 1.4 oz bar	1	210	13	56	24	Tr	24	1	0
Snickers, regular size, 2 oz	1	270	14	47	35	1	34	4	0
Snickers, fun size	1	70	4	51	9	Tr	9	1	0
Starburst Fruit Chews, 2 oz	1 pkg	240	5	19	49	0	49	Tr	0
Three Musketeers, 2.1 oz bar	1	260	8	28	46	Tr	46	2	0
Three Musketeers, fun size	1	60	2	30	11	Tr	11	Tr	0
Toffee	1 oz	160	9	51	18	0	18	Tr	0
Tootsie Roll	6 pc	160	1	6	35	0	35	Tr	0

	Serving Size	Calories	Fat (g)	Calories from Fat (%)	Total Carbs (g)	Fiber (g)	Net Carbs (g)	Protein (g)	Sugar Alcohol (g)
Twix, fun size	1	80	4	45	11	0	11	1	0
Twizzlers, strawberry, 2.5 oz pkg	1 pkg	250	2	7	28	0	28	2	0
Whatchamacallit, 1.7 oz bar	1 bar	240	11	41	30	Tr	30	4	0
Cantaloupe	***	***	*	*	*	*	*	*	*
Fresh, balls	1 cup	60	Tr	0	14	2	12	2	0
Fresh, cubed	1 cup	50	Tr	0	13	1	12	1	0
Fresh, medium 5" dia	1 melon	190	1	5	45	5	40	5	0
Fresh, wedge, ⅛ melon	1 wedge	25	Tr	0	6	Tr	6	Tr	0
Carambola (starfruit)	***	***	*	*	*	*	*	*	*
Fresh, sliced	1 cup	30	Tr	0	7	3	4	1	0
Fresh, 3⅝", whole	1	30	Tr	0	6	3	3	Tr	0
Caramels - see Candy	***	***	*	*	*	*	*	*	*
Carrot	***	***	*	*	*	*	*	*	*
Baby, fresh, 3 oz	8–9 pc	30	Tr	0	7	3	4	Tr	0
Canned, drained, slices, cooked	1 cup	35	Tr	0	8	2	6	Tr	0
Fresh, cooked, slices	1 cup	60	Tr	0	13	5	8	1	0
Fresh, raw, shredded	1 cup	45	Tr	0	11	3	8	1	0
Fresh, raw, whole, 7½" long	1	30	Tr	0	7	2	5	Tr	0
Frozen, cooked, slices	1 cup	50	Tr	0	11	5	7	Tr	0
Cashew - see Nuts	***	***	*	*	*	*	*	*	*
Catsup, regular (see also Ketchup)	1 Tbsp	15	Tr	0	4	0	4	Tr	0
Restaurant-size packet	1 pkt	5	Tr	0	2	0	2	Tr	0
Cauliflower	***	***	*	*	*	*	*	*	*
Fresh, cooked, flowerets	3	10	Tr	0	2	1	1	Tr	0
Fresh, cooked, chopped	1 cup	30	Tr	0	5	3	2	2	0
Fresh, raw, flowerets	3	10	Tr	0	2	1	1	Tr	0

	Serving Size	Calories	Fat (g)	Calories from Fat (%)	Total Carbs (g)	Fiber (g)	Net Carbs (g)	Protein (g)	Sugar Alcohol (g)
Fresh, raw, chopped or diced	1 cup	25	Tr	0	5	3	2	2	0
Frozen, chopped, cooked	1 cup	35	Tr	0	7	5	2	3	0
Frozen, mashed	***	***	*	*	*	*	*	*	*
Birds Eye Veggie Made	***	***	*	*	*	*	*	*	*
Original	½ cup	50	3	54	6	3	3	2	0
Roasted Garlic	½ cup	60	3	45	6	3	3	2	0
Sour Cream & Chives	½ cup	90	6	60	8	3	5	3	0
Green Giant	***	***	*	*	*	*	*	*	*
Broccoli & Cheese	½ cup	90	5	50	8	2	6	3	0
Cheddar & Bacon	½ cup	90	6	60	6	2	4	3	0
Garlic & Herb	½ cup	80	4.5	51	8	2	6	3	0
Original w/ Olive Oil & Sea Salt	½ cup	80	5	56	7	2	5	3	0
Caviar	1 Tbsp	40	3	68	Tr	0	Tr	4	0
Cayenne, dried spice	¼ tsp	0	Tr	0	Tr	Tr	Tr	Tr	0
Celery	***	***	*	*	*	*	*	*	*
Cooked, diced pieces	1 cup	25	Tr	0	6	2	4	1	0
Cooked, stalk, 7½" long	2	15	Tr	0	3	1	2	Tr	0
Fresh, raw, diced	1 cup	15	Tr	0	3	2	1	Tr	0
Fresh, raw, stalk, 7½" long	1	5	Tr	0	1	Tr	1	Tr	0
Fresh, sticks, 4" long	10 pc	6	0	0	1	Tr	1	0	0
Celery Seed	1 tsp	10	Tr	0	Tr	Tr	Tr	Tr	0
CEREAL	***	***	*	*	*	*	*	*	*
Low-Carb	***	***	*	*	*	*	*	*	*
Adapt Your Life, Choc Chip or Original	30 g	142	10	63	6	4	2	10	0

	Serving Size	Calories	Fat (g)	Calories from Fat (%)	Total Carbs (g)	Fiber (g)	Net Carbs (g)	Protein (g)	Sugar Alcohol (g)
Catalina Crunch, Cinnamon Toast or Dark Chocolate	½ cup	90	4	40	12	7	5	8	0
Keto and Co	***	***	*	*	*	*	*	*	*
Hot Breakfast, Maple Brown Sugar	2 Tbsp mix	50	2	36	13	8	5	3	0
Hot Breakfast, Plain	2 Tbsp mix	50	2	36	12	8	4	3	0
Regular	***	***	*	*	*	*	*	*	*
All-Bran	½ cup	80	2	23	23	9	14	4	0
Apple Jacks	1 cup	130	Tr	0	30	Tr	30	1	0
Cap'n Crunch	***	***	*	*	*	*	*	*	*
Crunchberries	¾ cup	110	2	16	22	Tr	22	1	0
original	¾ cup	110	2	16	23	Tr	23	1	0
Peanut Butter Crunch	¾ cup	110	3	25	21	Tr	21	2	0
Cheerios	***	***	*	*	*	*	*	*	*
Ancient Grains	¾ cup	110	2	16	22	2	20	3	0
Apple Cinnamon	¾ cup	120	2	15	25	1	24	2	0
Banana Nut	¾ cup	110	1.5	12	22	2	20	2	0
Chocolate	¾ cup	100	1.5	14	21	2	19	3	0
Chocolate Peanut Butter	¾ cup	120	4	30	21	2	19	3	0
Frosted	¾ cup	100	1.5	14	22	2	20	3	0
Honey Nut	¾ cup	110	2	16	22	2	20	3	0
Multigrain	1 cup	110	1.5	12	24	3	21	2	0
Oat Crunch, cinnamon	1 cup	200	4.5	20	40	4	36	3	0
original	1 cup	100	2	18	21	3	18	3	0
Protein, cinnamon almond	1¼ cups	220	4.5	18	40	3	37	7	0
Protein, oats & honey	1¼ cups	210	2.5	11	41	4	37	7	0
Very Berry	¾ cup	110	1.5	12	22	2	20	2	0

	Serving Size	Calories	Fat (g)	Calories from Fat (%)	Total Carbs (g)	Fiber (g)	Net Carbs (g)	Protein (g)	Sugar Alcohol (g)
Chex	***	***	*	*	*	*	*	*	*
Blueberry	¾ cup	130	2.5	17	24	1	23	1	0
Chocolate	¾ cup	130	2.5	17	26	1	25	2	0
Cinnamon	¾ cup	120	2.5	19	24	1	23	1	0
Corn	1 cup	110	Tr	0	26	1	25	2	0
Frosted	¾ cup	110	Tr	0	27	0	27	1	0
Honey Nut	¾ cup	130	Tr	0	28	Tr	28	2	0
Multi Bran	¾ cup	150	1	6	40	6	34	3	0
Rice	1 cup	100	Tr	0	23	Tr	23	3	0
Vanilla	¾ cup	120	2.5	19	24	1	23	1	0
Wheat	¾ cup	170	Tr	0	38	5	33	5	0
Cinnamon Toast Crunch	¾ cup	130	3	21	25	1	24	2	0
Cocoa Krispies	¾ cup	120	Tr	0	27	Tr	27	2	0
Cocoa Puffs	¾ cup	110	1	8	23	1	22	Tr	0
Corn Flakes	***	***	*	*	*	*	*	*	*
Kellogg's	1 cup	100	Tr	0	24	Tr	24	2	0
Total	1 cup	110	Tr	0	26	Tr	26	2	0
Corn Pops	1 cup	120	Tr	0	28	Tr	28	1	0
Cracklin' Oat Bran	¾ cup	200	7	32	34	6	28	4	0
Cream of Rice, as prep	1 cup	130	Tr	0	28	Tr	28	2	0
Cream of Wheat, as prep	1 cup	150	Tr	0	32	1	31	4	0
Crispix	1 cup	110	1	8	26	Tr	26	1	0
Crispix Cinnamon Crunch	¾ cup	120	1	8	26	1	26	1	0
Froot Loops	1 cup	120	1	8	26	1	26	1	0
Froot Loops, reduced sugar	1 ¼ cup	130	1	7	28	1	27	2	0
Frosted Flakes	¾ cup	110	Tr	0	27	Tr	27	1	0
Frosted Flakes, reduced sugar	1 cup	120	Tr	0	28	Tr	28	2	0
Frosted Mini Wheats	***	***	*	*	*	*	*	*	*
bite size	24 biscuits	200	Tr	0	48	6	42	6	0

	Serving Size	Calories	Fat (g)	Calories from Fat (%)	Total Carbs (g)	Fiber (g)	Net Carbs (g)	Protein (g)	Sugar Alcohol (g)
regular size	5 biscuits	180	Tr	0	42	5	37	5	0
Golden Grahams	¾ cup	120	1	8	26	1	25	1	0
Granola	***	***	*	*	*	*	*	*	*
Bear Naked	***	***	*	*	*	*	*	*	*
Cacao & Cashew Butter (gluten free)	½ cup	250	11	40	34	3	31	5	0
Fit, Toasted Coconut Almond	½ cup	210	5	21	40	6	34	6	0
Fit, Triple Berry	½ cup	220	3.5	14	45	6	39	7	0
Fit, V'nilla Almond	½ cup	210	5	21	40	5	35	6	0
Honey Almond	½ cup	290	15	47	29	5	24	11	0
Original Cinnamon	½ cup	260	12	42	31	5	26	11	0
Cascadian Farm Oats & Honey	⅔ cup	270	7	23	46	3	43	6	0
homemade	1 cup	600	29	44	65	11	54	18	0
Honey Bunches of Oats, Crunchy Honey Roasted	¼ cup	110	3	25	19	2	17	2	0
Kashi	***	***	*	*	*	*	*	*	*
Mountain Medley	½ cup	220	7	29	37	6	31	6	0
Orchard Spice	½ cup	220	7	29	37	6	31	6	0
Summer Berry	½ cup	220	6	25	37	7	31	7	0
Kellogg's	***	***	*	*	*	*	*	*	*
Low Fat w/ Raisins	½ cup	190	3	14	40	3	37	4	0
Low Fat w/ Raisins	⅔ cup	230	3	12	49	4	45	5	0
Special K Granola, Touch of Honey	½ cup	200	3	14	40	5	35	6	0
Nature Valley	***	***	*	*	*	*	*	*	*
Low Fat Fruit	⅔ cup	210	3	13	44	3	41	4	0
Protein, Cranberry Almond	½ cup	210	5	21	32	2	30	10	0
Protein, Oats 'n Dark Chocolate	½ cup	210	5	21	32	2	30	10	0
Purely Elizabeth	***	***	*	*	*	*	*	*	*

	Serving Size	Calories	Fat (g)	Calories from Fat (%)	Total Carbs (g)	Fiber (g)	Net Carbs (g)	Protein (g)	Sugar Alcohol (g)
Ancient Grain, Blueberry Hemp	⅓ cup	130	5	35	18	2	16	3	0
Ancient Grain, Cranberry Pecan	⅓ cup	140	7	45	18	2	16	3	0
Ancient Grain, original	⅓ cup	140	6	39	18	2	16	3	0
Ancient Grain, Pumpkin Cinnamon	⅓ cup	140	6	39	17	2	15	4	0
Chocolate Sea Salt + Peanut Butter	⅓ cup	130	5	35	17	2	15	3	0
Grain Free, Banana Nut Butter	⅓ cup	150	11	66	9	2	7	5	0
Grain Free, Coconut Cashew	⅓ cup	170	13	69	9	2	7	5	0
Maple + Almond Butter	⅓ cup	140	6	39	19	3	16	4	0
Superfood, Dark Chocolate Strawberry	⅓ cup	140	6	39	20	3	17	3	0
Superfood, Pumpkin Spice (grain free)	⅓ cup	160	12	68	10	2	8	5	0
Quaker	***	***	*	*	*	*	*	*	*
Low Fat w/ Raisins	⅔ cup	220	3	12	45	3	42	4	0
Oats & Honey	½ cup	210	6	26	35	3	32	5	0
Sun Country w/ Almonds	½ cup	270	10	33	38	3	35	7	0
Granola, Low Carb	***	***	*	*	*	*	*	*	*
Diabetic Kitchen Cinnamon Pecan Granola Cereal	⅓ cup	160	14	79	8	5	3	4	0
Julian Bakery ProGranola	***	***	*	*	*	*	*	*	*
Espresso	½ cup	92	3.5	34	17	14	3	12	0
Peanut Butter Cluster	½ cup	110	6	49	16	14	2	12	0
Vanilla Cinnamon	½ cup	97	4.5	42	14	12	2	12	0
Vanilla Cluster	½ cup	83	3	33	17	15	2	12	0
Honey Smacks	¾ cup	100	Tr	0	24	1	23	2	0

	Serving Size	Calories	Fat (g)	Calories from Fat (%)	Total Carbs (g)	Fiber (g)	Net Carbs (g)	Protein (g)	Sugar Alcohol (g)
Kashi, GOLEAN, Cinnamon Crisp	¾ cup	180	4	20	32	9	23	11	0
Kashi, GOLEAN, original	1¼ cups	180	2	10	40	13	27	12	0
Kix Berry Berry	¾ cup	100	1	9	23	Tr	23	Tr	0
Kix original	1¼ cup	100	1	9	25	3	22	2	0
Life Cinnamon	¾ cup	120	1	8	25	2	23	3	0
Life Honey Graham	¾ cup	120	1	8	25	2	23	3	0
Life original	¾ cup	120	1	8	25	2	23	3	0
Lucky Charms	¾ cup	110	Tr	0	22	1	21	2	0
Lucky Charms Chocolate	1 cup	120	1	8	26	1	25	1	0
Malt-O-Meal, as prep	1 cup	110	Tr	0	23	1	22	4	0
Malt-O-Meal, Chocolate, as prep	1 cup	120	Tr	0	25	1	24	3	0
Maltex, as prep	1 cup	190	1	5	39	2	37	6	0
Oatmeal, warm - see Oatmeal	***	***	*	*	*	*	*	*	*
Product 19	1 cup	100	Tr	0	25	1	24	2	0
Puffed rice	1 cup	60	Tr	0	13	Tr	13	Tr	0
Puffed rice, Quaker	1 cup	50	Tr	0	12	Tr	12	Tr	0
Puffed wheat	1 cup	45	Tr	0	10	Tr	10	2	0
Raisin Bran	***	***	*	*	*	*	*	*	*
General Mills Raisin Nut Bran	¾ cup	200	4	18	42	5	37	4	0
General Mills Total Raisin Bran	1 cup	170	1	5	42	5	37	3	0
General Mills Wheaties Raisin Bran	1 cup	180	Tr	0	45	5	37	4	0
Kellogg's Raisin Bran	1 cup	190	1	5	46	7	39	5	0
Kellogg's Raisin Bran Crunch	1 cup	190	1	5	45	4	41	3	0
Kraft Post Raisin Bran	1 cup	190	2	9	45	7	38	6	0
Malt-O-Meal Raisin Bran	1 cup	210	1	4	45	8	37	5	0

	Serving Size	Calories	Fat (g)	Calories from Fat (%)	Total Carbs (g)	Fiber (g)	Net Carbs (g)	Protein (g)	Sugar Alcohol (g)
Rice Chex, General Mills	1 cup	100	Tr	0	23	Tr	23	2	0
Rice Krispies, Kellogg's	***	***	*	*	*	*	*	*	*
Cocoa	¾ cup	120	1	8	27	0	27	1	0
Frosted	¾ cup	120	Tr	0	27	Tr	27	2	0
original	1 ¼ cup	130	Tr	0	28	Tr	28	2	0
Strawberry	1 cup	120	Tr	0	26	Tr	26	2	0
Shredded Wheat	***	***	*	*	*	*	*	*	*
Kashi Berry Fruitful	32 biscuits	190	1	5	47	6	41	7	0
Kashi Cinnamon Harvest	31 biscuits	200	1	5	48	7	41	7	0
Kashi Island Vanilla	29 biscuits	200	1	5	47	6	41	7	0
Kellogg's Miniatures	30 biscuits	100	Tr	0	24	4	20	3	0
large frosted biscuits	2 biscuits	160	1	6	36	6	30	5	0
Post Original Shredded Wheat, spoon size	1 cup	170	Tr	0	41	6	35	5	0
Post Frosted Shredded Wheat	1 cup	180	Tr	0	44	5	39	4	0
Special K	1 cup	120	Tr	0	22	Tr	22	7	0
Special K Low Carb	¾ cup	100	3	27	14	4	10	10	0
Total - see Corn Flakes & Raisin Bran	***	***	*	*	*	*	*	*	*
Total Whole Grain	¾ cup	100	Tr	0	23	3	20	2	0
Trix	1 cup	130	2	14	28	1	27	1	0
Wheaties	¾ cup	100	Tr	0	22	3	19	3	0
Cereal Bar	***	***	*	*	*	*	*	*	*
Kashi, fruit filled	1	130	3	21	25	3	22	2	0
Nutrigrain, fruit filled	1	140	3	19	27	Tr	27	2	0
Chalupa - see individual restaurant listings	***	***	*	*	*	*	*	*	*

	Serving Size	Calories	Fat (g)	Calories from Fat (%)	Total Carbs (g)	Fiber (g)	Net Carbs (g)	Protein (g)	Sugar Alcohol (g)
CHEESE	***	***	*	*	*	*	*	*	*
American, pasteurized cheese	***	***	*	*	*	*	*	*	*
fat free	1 slice	30	Tr	0	3	0	3	5	0
low fat	1 slice	40	2	45	Tr	0	Tr	5	0
regular	1 oz	110	9	74	Tr	0	Tr	6	0
Blue cheese	1 oz	100	8	72	Tr	0	Tr	6	0
crumbled	1 cup	477	39	74	3	0	3	29	0
Cheddar	***	***	*	*	*	*	*	*	*
1 slice, regular	1 oz	110	9	74	Tr	0	Tr	7	0
1" cube	1	70	6	77	Tr	0	Tr	4	0
low fat slice	1 oz	50	2	36	Tr	0	Tr	7	0
shredded	1 cup	460	38	74	2	0	2	28	0
Cheese food, pasteurized	1 oz	90	7	70	2	0	2	5	0
Cheese spread	***	***	*	*	*	*	*	*	*
cream cheese base	1 oz	80	8	90	Tr	0	Tr	2	0
pasteurized	1 oz	80	6	68	3	0	3	5	0
Velveeta	1 oz	90	6	60	3	0	3	5	0
Colby	1 oz	110	9	74	Tr	0	Tr	7	0
Colby, low fat	1 oz	50	2	36	Tr	0	Tr	7	0
Cottage cheese	***	***	*	*	*	*	*	*	*
regular, creamed, 4 fat	***	***	*	*	*	*	*	*	*
large curd	1 cup	210	9	39	7	0	7	23	0
small curb	1 cup	220	10	41	8	0	8	25	0
with fruit	1 cup	220	9	37	10	Tr	10	24	0
low fat, 2 fat	1 cup	190	6	28	8	0	8	27	0
low fat, 1 fat	1 cup	160	2	11	6	0	6	28	0
low fat, 1 fat w/ vegetables	1 cup	150	2	12	7	0	7	25	0
fat free	1 cup	100	Tr	0	10	0	10	15	0

	Serving Size	Calories	Fat (g)	Calories from Fat (%)	Total Carbs (g)	Fiber (g)	Net Carbs (g)	Protein (g)	Sugar Alcohol (g)
dry curd, uncreamed, nonfat	1 cup	100	Tr	0	10	0	10	15	0
Cream cheese	***	***	*	*	*	*	*	*	*
regular	1 oz	100	10	90	1	0	1	2	0
regular	1 Tbsp	50	5	90	Tr	0	Tr	Tr	0
regular, whipped	1 Tbsp	35	3	77	Tr	0	Tr	Tr	0
low fat/light	1 Tbsp	30	2	60	1	0	1	1	0
low fat, whipped	1 Tbsp	20	2	90	Tr	0	Tr	Tr	0
fat free	1 oz	30	Tr	0	2	0	2	4	0
strawberry flavor, *Philadelphia*	1 oz	71	5	63	4	0	4	1	0
vegetable flavor, *Philadelphia*	1 oz	73	6	74	2	0	2	2	0
Feta	1 oz	80	6	68	1	0	1	4	0
crumbled	1 cup	400	32	72	6	0	6	21	0
Fontina	1 oz	110	9	74	Tr	0	Tr	7	0
shredded	1 cup	420	34	73	2	0	2	28	0
Gruyère	1 oz	117	9	69	Tr	0	Tr	8	0
Goat cheese, soft	1 oz	80	6	68	Tr	0	Tr	5	0
Goat cheese, semisoft	1 oz	100	9	81	Tr	0	Tr	6	0
Goat cheese, hard	1 oz	130	10	69	Tr	0	Tr	9	0
Manchego	1 oz	120	10	75	0	0	0	7	0
Mascarpone	1 oz	122	13	96	0	0	0	2	0
Monterey	***	***	*	*	*	*	*	*	*
regular	1 oz	110	9	74	Tr	0	Tr	7	0
shredded	1 cup	420	34	73	Tr	0	Tr	28	0
low fat	1 oz	90	6	60	Tr	0	Tr	8	0
low fat shredded	1 cup	350	24	62	Tr	0	Tr	32	0
Mozzarella	***	***	*	*	*	*	*	*	*
burrata, *BelGioioso*	1 oz	71	7	89	0	0	0	5	0
fat free, shredded	1 cup	170	0	0	4	2	2	36	0
part skim, 1 slice	1 oz	70	5	64	Tr	0	Tr	7	0
part skim, shredded	1 cup	333	22	59	6	0	6	27	0

	Serving Size	Calories	Fat (g)	Calories from Fat (%)	Total Carbs (g)	Fiber (g)	Net Carbs (g)	Protein (g)	Sugar Alcohol (g)
whole milk, regular, 1 slice	1 oz	90	6	60	Tr	0	Tr	6	0
whole milk, regular, shredded	1 cup	340	25	66	3	0	3	25	0
Muenster	***	***	*	*	*	*	*	*	*
low fat, sliced	1 oz	80	5	56	Tr	0	Tr	7	0
regular, shredded	1 cup	420	34	73	1	0	1	27	0
regular, sliced	1 oz	100	9	81	Tr	0	Tr	7	0
Neufchatel	1 oz	701	7	9	1	0	1	3	0
Parmesan, grated	1 cup	430	29	61	4	0	4	39	0
Parmesan, grated	1 Tbsp	20	1	45	Tr	0	Tr	2	0
Processed (*Velveeta*)	1 oz	70	4	51	3	0	3	4	0
Provolone	***	***	*	*	*	*	*	*	*
regular	1 oz	100	8	72	Tr	0	Tr	7	0
reduced fat	1 oz	80	5	56	Tr	0	Tr	7	0
Ricotta	***	***	*	*	*	*	*	*	*
regular	1 cup	430	32	67	8	0	8	28	0
part skim	1 cup	340	20	53	13	0	13	28	0
Romano, grated	1 oz	110	8	65	1	0	1	9	0
Roquefort, sheep's milk	1 oz	110	9	74	Tr	0	Tr	6	0
Swiss	***	***	*	*	*	*	*	*	*
low fat, 1 slice	1 oz	50	1	18	Tr	0	Tr	8	0
low fat, shredded	1 cup	190	6	28	4	0	4	31	0
regular, 1 slice	1 oz	110	8	65	2	0	2	8	0
regular, shredded	1 cup	410	30	66	6	0	6	29	0
Cheese Puffs or Twists	1 oz	160	10	56	15	Tr	15	2	0
Cheeze Whiz	2 Tbsp	90	7	70	3	Tr	3	4	0
Cheeze Whiz **Light**	2 Tbsp	80	3	34	6	Tr	6	6	0
Cherries	***	***	*	*	*	*	*	*	*
Fresh, sweet	10	50	Tr	0	13	2	11	Tr	0
Sour, canned, water packed	1 cup	90	Tr	0	22	3	19	2	0
Sour, frozen, unsweetened	1 cup	70	Tr	0	17	3	14	1	0

	Serving Size	Calories	Fat (g)	Calories from Fat (%)	Total Carbs (g)	Fiber (g)	Net Carbs (g)	Protein (g)	Sugar Alcohol (g)
Sweet, canned, water packed	1 cup	110	Tr	0	29	4	25	2	0
Sweet dark, frozen, unsweetened	1 cup	90	0.5	5	22	3	19	2	0
Cherry Pie Filling, canned	3 oz	100	Tr	0	24	tr	24	Tr	0
Chestnut - see Nuts	***	***	*	*	*	*	*	*	*
Chewing Gum	***	***	*	*	*	*	*	*	*
Block	1	20	Tr	0	5	Tr	5	0	0
Bubble Yum, all regular flavors	1	25	0	0	6	0	6	0	0
Chiclets	10	40	Tr	0	11	Tr	11	0	0
Dentyne Ice, all regular flavors	2	5	0	0	2	0	2	0	0
Ice Breakers	1	10	0	0	2	0	2	0	0
Orbit	1	5	0	0	1	0	0	0	1
Orbit White	2	5	0	0	2	0	0	0	2
Pur	2	10	0	0	2	0	0	0	2
Stick	1	7	Tr	0	2	Tr	2	0	0
Sugarless	1 pc	5	Tr	0	2	0	2	0	0
Trident, all flavors, 1" sticks	1	5	0	0	1	0	1	0	0
Wrigley's	***	***	*	*	*	*	*	*	*
regular	1	10	0	0	2	0	2	0	0
Eclipse	2 pc	5	0	0	2	0	2	0	0
Extra, sugar free	1	5	0	0	2	0	2	0	0
Chex Mix, 1 oz	⅔ cup	120	3	23	21	1	20	3	0
CHICKEN	***	***	*	*	*	*	*	*	*
Giblets, simmered, chopped	1 cup	230	7	27	Tr	0	Tr	39	0
Fried Chicken, batter dipped	***	***	*	*	*	*	*	*	*
½ breast, bone removed	5 oz	360	19	48	13	Tr	13	35	0
drumstick, avg size	1	190	11	52	6	Tr	6	16	0
thigh, avg size	1	240	14	53	8	Tr	8	19	0

	Serving Size	Calories	Fat (g)	Calories from Fat (%)	Total Carbs (g)	Fiber (g)	Net Carbs (g)	Protein (g)	Sugar Alcohol (g)
wing, avg size	1	160	11	62	5	Tr	5	10	0
Fried Chicken, breaded, boneless pieces	6 pc	290	18	56	16	Tr	16	15	0
Liver, simmered	3 oz	140	6	39	Tr	0	Tr	21	0
Neck, simmered	1	90	7	70	0	0	0	8	0
Roast Chicken	***	***	*	*	*	*	*	*	*
½ breast, bone removed	3.5 oz	190	8	38	0	0	0	29	0
drumstick, avg size	1	110	6	49	0	0	0	14	0
thigh, avg size	1	150	10	60	0	0	0	16	0
wing, avg size	1	100	7	63	0	0	0	9	0
white meat, skinless, chopped	1 cup	210	6	26	0	0	0	38	0
dark meat, skinless, chopped	1 cup	250	13	47	0	0	0	33	0
light & dark meat, skinless, chopped	1 cup	230	9	35	0	0	0	35	0
canned, boneless	5 oz	230	10	39	0	0	0	32	0
Stewed Chicken	***	***	*	*	*	*	*	*	*
white meat (breast), skinless, chopped	1 cup	210	4	17	0	0	0	41	0
dark meat, skinless, chopped	1 cup	270	13	43	0	0	0	36	0
light & dark meat, skinless, chopped	1 cup	250	10	36	0	0	0	38	0
drumstick, skinless	1	80	3	34	0	0	0	13	0
thigh, skinless	1	110	5	41	0	0	0	14	0
(Other Chicken Products, see:	***	***	*	*	*	*	*	*	*
Bologna, Hot Dog, Salami, Sausage & specific entrées)	***	***	*	*	*	*	*	*	*
Chicken Nuggets	***	***	*	*	*	*	*	*	*
Frozen, cooked	3 oz	250	17	61	12	2	10	13	0
Chicken Roll, light meat	2 oz	60	2	30	3	0	3	10	0

	Serving Size	Calories	Fat (g)	Calories from Fat (%)	Total Carbs (g)	Fiber (g)	Net Carbs (g)	Protein (g)	Sugar Alcohol (g)
Chicken Wings	***	***	*	*	*	*	*	*	*
Perdue Buffalo-Style Glazed Jumbo Wings	3 oz	140	9	58	1	0	1	13	0
Perdue Chicken wings, Savory Herb w/ Roasted Garlic	4 oz	200	12	54	3	0	3	17	0
Tyson Any'Tizers Bone-In Hot Wings, Buffalo Style	3 oz	190	13	62	3	0	3	14	0
Chickpeas, cooked	½ cup	130	2	14	23	6	17	7	0
Chili Powder	1 tsp	10	Tr	0	1	Tr	1	Tr	0
Chili w/ Beans, *Hormel,* canned	1 cup	190	7	33	18	3	15	17	0
Chili Con Carne w/ Beans, canned	1 cup	300	13	39	28	10	18	17	0
Chimichanga - see individual restaurant listings	***	***	*	*	*	*	*	*	*
Chips - see Corn Chips, Potato Chips & other specific listings	***	***	*	*	*	*	*	*	*
Chives, raw, chopped	1 Tbsp	0	Tr	0	Tr	Tr	Tr	Tr	0
Chives, freeze-dried	1 Tbsp	0	Tr	0	Tr	Tr	Tr	Tr	0
Chocolate for Baking	***	***	*	*	*	*	*	*	*
(See also Candy for other chocolates)	***	***	*	*	*	*	*	*	*
Mexican baking chocolate	1 sq	90	3	30	16	Tr	16	Tr	0
Nestlé Milk Chocolate Morsels	1 Tbsp	70	3	39	9	0	9	Tr	0
Nestlé Semi-Sweet Chocolate Morsels	1 Tbsp	70	3	39	9	Tr	9	Tr	0
Nestlé Premiere White Chocolate Morsels	1 Tbsp	70	3	39	9	0	9	0	0
Unsweetened for baking, solid	1 sq	150	15	90	9	5	4	4	0
Unsweetened, liquid	1 oz	130	14	97	10	5	5	3	0

	Serving Size	Calories	Fat (g)	Calories from Fat (%)	Total Carbs (g)	Fiber (g)	Net Carbs (g)	Protein (g)	Sugar Alcohol (g)
Chocolate for Snacking - see Sweets, Low Carb	***	***	*	*	*	*	*	*	*
Cilantro, raw	¼ cup	0	Tr	0	Tr	Tr	Tr	Tr	0
Cilantro, dried (coriander)	1 tsp	0	Tr	0	Tr	Tr	Tr	Tr	0
Cinnamon, ground	1 tsp	5	Tr	0	2	1	1	Tr	0
Cinnamon Roll w/ icing, *Pillsbury*	1	150	5	30	23	Tr	23	2	0
Cinnamon Sweet Roll w/ raisins & glaze, 2 ¾"	1	220	10	41	31	1	30	4	0
Clam Chowder - see Soup	***	***	*	*	*	*	*	*	*
Clams - see Fish/ Seafood	***	***	*	*	*	*	*	*	*
Cloves, ground	1 tsp	5	Tr	0	1	Tr	1	Tr	0
Cocoa Mix - see Beverages, Cocoa/ Chocolate, and Mixes	***	***	*	*	*	*	*	*	*
Cocoa, unsweetened powder	1 Tbsp	10	Tr	0	3	2	1	1	0
Coconut	***	***	*	*	*	*	*	*	*
Chips/flakes, dried, unsweetened	1 cup	400	40	90	16	8	8	4	0
Dried, sweetened, shredded	1 cup	460	33	65	44	4	40	3	0
Dried, unsweetened, shredded	1 oz	190	18	85	7	5	2	2	0
Fresh piece, 2" x 2" x ½"	1 pc	160	15	84	7	4	3	2	0
Fresh, shredded, not packed	1 cup	280	27	87	12	7	5	3	0
Coconut Cream, canned, unsweetened	1 Tbsp	70	3	39	10	0	10	Tr	0
Coconut Milk, canned	***	***	*	*	*	*	*	*	*
Light/lite, *KA-ME*	1 cup	160	16	90	4	0	4	0	0
Regular	1 cup	450	48	96	6	0	6	5	0

	Serving Size	Calories	Fat (g)	Calories from Fat (%)	Total Carbs (g)	Fiber (g)	Net Carbs (g)	Protein (g)	Sugar Alcohol (g)
Coffee - see Beverages, Coffee	***	***	*	*	*	*	*	*	*
Coleslaw	½ cup	45	2	40	8	Tr	8	Tr	0
Collards	***	***	*	*	*	*	*	*	*
Fresh, chopped, cooked	1 cup	50	Tr	0	9	5	4	4	0
Frozen, chopped, cooked	1 cup	60	Tr	0	12	5	7	5	0
Condiments - see Sauce or specific listings	***	***	*	*	*	*	*	*	*
COOKIES, 2 ¼" dia, unless noted	***	***	*	*	*	*	*	*	*
(See also Sweets, Low Carb)	***	***	*	*	*	*	*	*	*
Animal Crackers, 1" dia, sm box	2 oz	250	8	29	42	Tr	42	4	0
Butter Cookie	1	25	Tr	0	4	0	4	Tr	0
Chocolate Chip, regular	1	80	5	56	9	Tr	9	Tr	0
Chocolate Chip, reduced fat	1	45	2	40	7	Tr	7	Tr	0
Coconut Cookie, 2"	1	100	3	27	17	Tr	17	Tr	0
Fig Bar	1	60	1	15	11	Tr	11	Tr	0
Molasses cookie	1	70	2	26	11	Tr	11	Tr	0
Oatmeal, plain, 2⅝"	1	70	3	39	10	Tr	10	1	0
Oatmeal w/ raisins, 2⅝"	1	70	2	26	10	Tr	10	Tr	0
Peanut Butter, plain, 3"	1	100	5	45	12	Tr	12	2	0
Pecan Shortbread, 2"	1	80	5	56	8	Tr	8	Tr	0
Sandwich Cookie, w/ filling, 1 ½" dia, round	***	***	*	*	*	*	*	*	*
chocolate w/ creme filling	1	50	2	36	8	Tr	8	Tr	0
chocolate w/ creme filling, chocolate coated	1	80	5	56	11	Tr	11	Tr	0

	Serving Size	Calories	Fat (g)	Calories from Fat (%)	Total Carbs (g)	Fiber (g)	Net Carbs (g)	Protein (g)	Sugar Alcohol (g)
chocolate w/ extra creme filling	1	70	3	39	9	Tr	9	Tr	0
peanut butter sandwich	1	70	3	39	9	Tr	9	1	0
sugar wafer w/ creme filling, sm	1	20	Tr	0	3	0	3	Tr	0
sugar wafer w/ creme filling, lg	1	45	2	40	6	Tr	6	Tr	0
vanilla w/ creme filling	1	50	2	36	7	Tr	7	Tr	0
vanilla w/ creme filling, oval	1	70	3	39	11	Tr	11	Tr	0
Shortbread, plain, 1⅝" square	1	40	2	45	5	Tr	5	Tr	0
Snickerdoodle	1	139	6	39	20	0	20	2	0
Sugar Cookie, regular	1	70	3	39	10	Tr	10	Tr	0
Wafer, chocolate	1	25	Tr	0	4	Tr	4	Tr	0
Wafer, vanilla	1	30	Tr	0	4	Tr	4	Tr	0
Wafer, vanilla, low fat	1	20	Tr	0	3	Tr	3	Tr	0
Cooking Spray, nonstick, ⅓ second spray	1 spray	0	Tr	0	Tr	0	Tr	0	0
Corn	***	***	*	*	*	*	*	*	*
Canned, drained solids	½ cup	70	Tr	0	15	2	13	2	0
Canned, cream style kernels	½ cup	90	Tr	0	23	2	21	2	0
Fresh, sweet white or yellow, 7" cob, cooked	1 ear	110	1	8	26	3	23	3	0
Frozen kernels, cooked	½ cup	70	Tr	0	16	2	14	2	0
Corn Cake, butter flavor (see also Rice Cake)	1	40	Tr	0	8	Tr	8	Tr	0
Corn Chips	***	***	*	*	*	*	*	*	*
Barbecue flavor	1 oz	150	9	54	16	2	14	2	0
Regular	1 oz	150	8	48	18	2	16	2	0

	Serving Size	Calories	Fat (g)	Calories from Fat (%)	Total Carbs (g)	Fiber (g)	Net Carbs (g)	Protein (g)	Sugar Alcohol (g)
Tortilla type	***	***	*	*	*	*	*	*	*
blue corn	1 oz	142	7	44	18	2	16	2	0
low fat or baked	1 oz	120	2	15	23	2	21	3	0
nacho cheese flavor	1 oz	150	7	42	18	1	17	2	0
nacho flavor, reduced fat	1 oz	130	4	28	20	1	19	3	0
ranch flavor	1 oz	140	7	45	18	1	17	2	0
taco flavor	1 oz	140	7	45	18	2	16	2	0
white corn	1 oz	140	7	45	19	2	17	2	0
yellow corn	1 oz	140	6	39	19	1	18	2	0
Corn Grits (hominy) - see Grits	***	***	*	*	*	*	*	*	*
Corn Syrup, light	1 Tbsp	60	Tr	0	17	0	17	0	0
Corn Syrup, dark	1 Tbsp	60	0	0	16	0	16	0	0
Cornbread, 2 x 3"	1 pc	190	6	28	29	1	28	4	0
Corned Beef	3 oz	210	13	56	0	0	0	23	0
Corned Beef Hash, canned, *Hormel*	1 cup	390	24	55	22	3	19	21	0
Cornish Hen, roasted	½ bird	340	24	64	0	0	0	29	0
Cornmeal, yellow or white, dry form	***	***	*	*	*	*	*	*	*
Self rising	1 cup	490	2	4	103	10	93	12	0
Whole grain	1 cup	440	4	8	94	9	85	10	0
Cornstarch	1 Tbsp	30	Tr	0	7	Tr	7	Tr	0
Cottage Cheese - see Cheese	***	***	*	*	*	*	*	*	*
Crab - see Fish/Seafood	***	***	*	*	*	*	*	*	*
Crab cake	1	160	10	56	5	Tr	5	11	0
Cracker Jacks	½ cup	120	2	15	23	1	22	2	0
CRACKERS	***	***	*	*	*	*	*	*	*
Cheese crackers, 1" squares	10	50	3	54	6	Tr	6	1	0
Club crackers, *Keebler*	4	70	3	39	9	Tr	9	Tr	0

	Serving Size	Calories	Fat (g)	Calories from Fat (%)	Total Carbs (g)	Fiber (g)	Net Carbs (g)	Protein (g)	Sugar Alcohol (g)
Graham crackers, 2½" square	3	90	2	20	16	Tr	16	2	0
Matzo, plain, 6" square	1	110	Tr	0	23	Tr	23	3	0
Melba toast, plain	4	45	Tr	0	9	Tr	9	2	0
Oyster crackers	25	110	2	16	19	Tr	19	2	0
Ritz Bitz w/ peanut butter, 1.25 oz bag	1	170	10	53	20	1	19	4	0
Ritz crackers, regular	5	80	4	45	10	Tr	10	1	0
Ritz crackers, reduced fat	5	70	2	26	11	0	11	1	0
Rye crispbread, *Rye Krisp* wafer	1	90	Tr	0	21	4	17	2	0
Rye crispbread, *Wasa Rye*	1	35	Tr	0	8	2	6	Tr	0
Saltine crackers	5	60	1	15	11	Tr	11	1	0
Sandwich crackers, 1½" dia	***	***	*	*	*	*	*	*	*
cheese filled	2	60	3	45	8	Tr	8	1	0
peanut butter filled	2	70	3	39	8	Tr	8	2	0
peanut butter filled, cheese cracker	2	60	3	45	7	Tr	7	2	0
Snack crackers, round, 2" dia	5	80	4	45	10	Tr	10	1	0
Sociables	7	70	4	51	9	0	9	1	0
Triscuits, whole wheat	5	100	3	27	16	2	14	2	0
Town House crackers	5	80	5	56	10	Tr	10	Tr	0
Whole wheat, thin squares	8	80	3	34	10	Tr	10	1	0
Cranberries	***	***	*	*	*	*	*	*	*
Dried, sweetened	¼ cup	90	Tr	0	25	2	23	Tr	0
Fresh, raw	½ cup	25	Tr	0	6	2	4	Tr	0
Cranberry-Orange Relish	2 Tbsp	60	Tr	0	16	0	16	Tr	0
Cranberry Sauce	***	***	*	*	*	*	*	*	*
jellied, canned	1 slice	90	Tr	0	22	Tr	22	Tr	0

	Serving Size	Calories	Fat (g)	Calories from Fat (%)	Total Carbs (g)	Fiber (g)	Net Carbs (g)	Protein (g)	Sugar Alcohol (g)
whole berry, canned	¼ cup	111	0	0	28	1	27	1	0
Cream Cheese - see Cheese, Cream Cheese	***	***	*	*	*	*	*	*	*
Cream of Tartar	1 tsp	10	0	0	2	0	2	0	0
Cream of Wheat cereal, as prep	1 cup	130	Tr	0	28	1	27	4	0
Cream of Wheat cereal, instant, as prep	1 cup	150	Tr	0	32	1	31	4	0
Cream Puff, 2" x 3½"	1	290	18	56	27	Tr	27	7	0
Cream, Whipped Topping	***	***	*	*	*	*	*	*	*
Cool Whip	***	***	*	*	*	*	*	*	*
Extra Creamy	2 Tbsp	25	2	72	2	0	0	2	0
Fat Free	2 Tbsp	15	0	0	3	0	3	0	0
Lite	2 Tbsp	20	1	45	3	0	3	0	0
Original	2 Tbsp	25	1.5	54	3	0	3	0	0
Sugar Free	2 Tbsp	20	1	45	3	0	3	0	0
Heavy, whipped	2 cups	820	88	97	7	0	7	5	0
Heavy, whipped	2 Tbsp	102	11	97	Tr	0	Tr	Tr	0
Light, whipped	2 cups	700	74	95	7	0	7	5	0
Light, whipped	2 Tbsp	45	5	100	Tr	0	Tr	Tr	0
Pressurized, in can	1 Tbsp	10	Tr	0	Tr	0	Tr	Tr	0
Creamer - see Beverages, Creamer	***	***	*	*	*	*	*	*	*
Crème Fraiche	2 Tbsp	110	11	90	1	0	1	1	0
Croissant, butter flavor, 4"	1	230	12	47	26	2	24	5	0
Croissant w/ Egg, Bacon, Cheese - see Breakfast Sandwich	***	***	*	*	*	*	*	*	*
Croutons	***	***	*	*	*	*	*	*	*
plain	½ cup	60	Tr	0	11	Tr	11	2	0
seasoned	½ cup	90	4	40	13	1	12	2	0
Croutons, low carb	***	***	*	*	*	*	*	*	*

	Serving Size	Calories	Fat (g)	Calories from Fat (%)	Total Carbs (g)	Fiber (g)	Net Carbs (g)	Protein (g)	Sugar Alcohol (g)
Linda's Diet Delites Low Carb croutons (all flavors)	½ pkg	90	3.5	35	14	12	2	12	0
Moon Cheese Toppers	***	***	*	*	*	*	*	*	*
Bacon	1 svg	70	5	64	0	0	0	5	0
Italian Herb	1 svg	70	5	64	0	0	0	5	0
Parmesan	1 svg	68	5	66	0	0	0	5	0
Cucumber	***	***	*	*	*	*	*	*	*
Fresh, peeled, diced	½ cup	8	Tr	0	1	Tr	1	0	0
Fresh, peeled, whole, 8 ¼" long	1	35	Tr	0	6	2	4	2	0
Fresh, peeled, sliced	1 cup	15	Tr	0	3	Tr	3	Tr	0
Fresh, unpeeled, whole, 8 ¼" long	1	45	Tr	0	11	2	9	2	0
Fresh, unpeeled, sliced	1 cup	15	Tr	0	4	Tr	4	Tr	0
Cucumber Salad, mayo dressing	¾ cup	120	10	75	9	2	7	2	0
Curry Powder	1 tsp	5	Tr	0	1	Tr	1	Tr	0
Custard, egg	***	***	*	*	*	*	*	*	*
Caramel (flan)	½ cup	220	6	25	35	0	35	7	0
Vanilla	½ cup	150	7	42	15	0	15	7	0
Dandelion Greens, chopped, cooked	1 cup	35	Tr	0	7	3	4	2	0
Danish Pastry, approx 4" dia	***	***	*	*	*	*	*	*	*
Cheese	1	270	16	53	26	Tr	26	6	0
Cinnamon Toast Crunch	1	260	15	52	29	Tr	29	5	0
Fruit filled	1	260	13	45	34	1	33	4	0
Lemon	1	260	13	45	34	1	33	4	0
Nut	1	280	16	51	30	1	29	5	0
Date, Deglet Noor, pitted	***	***	*	*	*	*	*	*	*
chopped	1 cup	420	Tr	0	110	11	99	4	0

	Serving Size	Calories	Fat (g)	Calories from Fat (%)	Total Carbs (g)	Fiber (g)	Net Carbs (g)	Protein (g)	Sugar Alcohol (g)
whole	1	20	Tr	0	5	Tr	5	Tr	0
Date, Medjool, pitted	1	70	Tr	0	18	2	16	Tr	0
Dessert - see Ice Cream, Frozen Dessert, or specific listings	***	***	*	*	*	*	*	*	*
Dessert Topping - see Topping	***	***	*	*	*	*	*	*	*
Dill Seed	1 tsp	5	Tr	0	1	Tr	1	Tr	0
Dill Weed	***	***	*	*	*	*	*	*	*
Dried	1 tsp	0	Tr	0	Tr	Tr	Tr	Tr	0
Raw, sprigs	5	0	Tr	0	Tr	0	Tr	Tr	0
Doughnut	***	***	*	*	*	*	*	*	*
Cake Doughnuts, regular ring type, approx 3" dia	***	***	*	*	*	*	*	*	*
chocolate frosting	1	190	11	52	22	Tr	22	2	0
chocolate, sugared or glazed	1	180	8	40	24	Tr	24	2	0
plain	1	230	13	51	25	Tr	25	3	0
sugared or glazed	1	190	10	47	23	Tr	23	2	0
French Cruller, glazed	1	170	8	42	24	Tr	24	1	0
Yeast Doughnuts, regular ring type, approx 3" dia	***	***	*	*	*	*	*	*	*
creme filled	1	310	21	61	26	Tr	26	5	0
custard filled	1	235	16	61	20	1	19	4	0
glazed	1	240	14	53	27	Tr	27	4	0
jelly filled	1	290	16	50	33	Tr	33	5	0
Dressing - see Salad Dressing	***	***	*	*	*	*	*	*	*
Dried Fruit - see specific listings, and Trail Mix	***	***	*	*	*	*	*	*	*
Duck, roasted	***	***	*	*	*	*	*	*	*
Meat only	½ duck	440	25	51	0	0	0	52	0

	Serving Size	Calories	Fat (g)	Calories from Fat (%)	Total Carbs (g)	Fiber (g)	Net Carbs (g)	Protein (g)	Sugar Alcohol (g)
Meat only, chopped	1 cup	280	16	51	0	0	0	33	0
Éclair, 5" x 2"	1	260	16	55	24	Tr	24	6	0
Edamame - see Soybeans	***	***	*	*	*	*	*	*	*
EGG	***	***	*	*	*	*	*	*	*
Raw	***	***	*	*	*	*	*	*	*
medium, whole	1	60	4	60	Tr	0	Tr	6	0
large, whole	1	70	5	64	Tr	0	Tr	6	0
extra large, whole	1	80	6	68	Tr	0	Tr	7	0
white only, large	1	15	Tr	0	Tr	0	Tr	4	0
yolk only, large	1	50	5	90	Tr	0	Tr	3	0
Prepared (1 lg egg/svg)	***	***	*	*	*	*	*	*	*
fried	1	90	7	70	Tr	0	Tr	6	0
hard boiled, chopped	1 cup	210	14	60	2	0	2	17	0
hard boiled, whole	1	80	5	56	Tr	0	Tr	6	0
omelet, plain	1	100	7	63	Tr	0	Tr	7	0
poached	1	70	5	64	Tr	0	Tr	6	0
scrambled	1	100	8	72	1	0	1	7	0
Egg Substitute or Imitation	***	***	*	*	*	*	*	*	*
frozen	¼ cup	100	7	63	2	0	2	7	0
liquid	1.5 fl oz	40	2	45	Tr	0	Tr	6	0
liquid, egg whites only	3 Tbsp	25	0	0	1	0	1	5	0
powdered	⅓ oz	45	1	20	2	0	2	6	0
Eggplant, cubed, cooked	1 cup	35	Tr	0	9	3	6	Tr	0
Eggplant Parmigiana	½ cup	265	16	54	26	3	23	6	0
Eggroll	***	***	*	*	*	*	*	*	*
Chicken	1	160	4	23	23	2	21	8	0
Pork	1	190	6	28	25	2	23	9	0
Vegetable	1	150	4	24	25	2	23	5	0

	Serving Size	Calories	Fat (g)	Calories from Fat (%)	Total Carbs (g)	Fiber (g)	Net Carbs (g)	Protein (g)	Sugar Alcohol (g)
Enchilada - see Frozen Dinner or individual restaurant listings	***	***	*	*	*	*	*	*	*
Enchirito - see individual restaurant listings	***	***	*	*	*	*	*	*	*
Endive, raw	***	***	*	*	*	*	*	*	*
chopped	1 cup	10	Tr	0	2	2	0	Tr	0
head	1	90	1	10	17	16	1	6	0
Energy Bar, low carb	***	***	*	*	*	*	*	*	*
Atkins Advantage Chocolate Chip Granola Bar	1	200	8	36	18	6	12	17	0
Atkins Advantage S'mores Bar	1	220	9	37	27	12	15	17	0
English Muffin - see Bread	***	***	*	*	*	*	*	*	*
English Muffin w/ Egg, Cheese & Canadian Bacon - see Breakfast Sandwich	***	***	*	*	*	*	*	*	*
Equal sweetener	1 pkt	0	0	0	Tr	0	Tr	Tr	0
Fig	***	***	*	*	*	*	*	*	*
dried	1	20	Tr	0	5	Tr	5	Tr	0
fresh, medium	1	35	Tr	0	10	2	8	Tr	0
FISH/SEAFOOD	***	***	*	*	*	*	*	*	*
Abalone, fried	3 oz	160	6	34	9	0	9	17	0
Anchovy, canned in oil	5	40	2	45	0	0	0	6	0
Bass	***	***	*	*	*	*	*	*	*
freshwater, baked	3 oz	120	4	30	0	0	0	21	0
sea bass, baked	3 oz	110	2	16	0	0	0	20	0
striped, baked	3 oz	110	3	25	0	0	0	19	0
Bluefish, baked	3 oz	140	5	32	0	0	0	22	0
Catfish	***	***	*	*	*	*	*	*	*
breaded, fried	3 oz	200	11	50	7	Tr	7	15	0
farmed, baked	3 oz	130	7	48	0	0	0	16	0

	Serving Size	Calories	Fat (g)	Calories from Fat (%)	Total Carbs (g)	Fiber (g)	Net Carbs (g)	Protein (g)	Sugar Alcohol (g)
wild, baked	3 oz	90	2	20	0	0	0	16	0
Caviar, black or red	1 Tbsp	40	3	68	Tr	0	Tr	4	0
Clams	***	***	*	*	*	*	*	*	*
breaded, fried	¾ cup	450	26	52	39	Tr	39	13	0
canned, drained	3 oz	130	2	14	4	0	4	22	0
canned, drained	1 cup	240	3	11	8	0	8	41	0
raw	3 oz	60	Tr	0	2	0	2	11	0
raw	1 med	10	Tr	0	Tr	0	Tr	2	0
steamed	3 oz	130	2	14	4	0	4	22	0
Cod, baked or broiled	3 oz	90	Tr	0	0	0	0	20	0
Crab, Alaska king	***	***	*	*	*	*	*	*	*
steamed	3 oz	80	1	11	0	0	0	17	0
steamed	1 leg	130	2	14	0	0	0	26	0
Crab, blue	***	***	*	*	*	*	*	*	*
canned	3 oz	80	1	11	0	0	0	17	0
steamed	3 oz	90	2	20	0	0	0	17	0
Crab, Dungeness, steamed	3 oz	90	1	10	Tr	0	Tr	19	0
Crab, imitation	3 oz	80	Tr	0	13	Tr	13	7	0
Crab cake	1	160	10	56	5	Tr	5	11	0
Fish fillet breaded, fried	3 oz	200	11	50	14	Tr	14	13	0
Fish stick, breaded, fried, 4" x 1"	1	70	4	51	6	Tr	6	3	0
Flounder, baked or broiled	3 oz	100	1	9	0	0	0	21	0
Frozen - see Fish, Frozen	***	***	*	*	*	*	*	*	*
Grouper, baked or broiled	3 oz	100	1	9	0	0	0	21	0
Haddock	***	***	*	*	*	*	*	*	*
baked or broiled	3 oz	100	Tr	0	0	0	0	21	0
smoked	3 oz	100	Tr	0	0	0	0	22	0

	Serving Size	Calories	Fat (g)	Calories from Fat (%)	Total Carbs (g)	Fiber (g)	Net Carbs (g)	Protein (g)	Sugar Alcohol (g)
Halibut, baked or broiled	3 oz	120	3	23	0	0	0	23	0
Herring, Atlantic	***	***	*	*	*	*	*	*	*
baked or broiled	3 oz	170	10	53	0	0	0	20	0
kippered, med fillet	1	90	5	50	0	0	0	10	0
pickled	1 oz	70	5	64	3	0	3	4	0
Herring, Pacific, baked or broiled	3 oz	210	15	64	0	0	0	18	0
Lobster, steamed	3 oz	80	Tr	0	1	0	1	17	0
Mackerel	***	***	*	*	*	*	*	*	*
Atlantic, baked or broiled	3 oz	220		0	0	0	20	15	0
jack, canned	1 cup	300	12	36	0	0	0	44	0
king, baked or broiled	3 oz	110	2	16	0	0	0	22	0
Pacific and jack, baked or broiled	3 oz	170	9	48	0	0	0	22	0
salted	1 pc	240	10	38	0	0	0	15	0
Spanish, baked or broiled	3 oz	130	5	35	0	0	0	20	0
Monkfish, baked or broiled	3 oz	80	2	23	0	0	0	16	0
Mussels, steamed	3 oz	150	4	24	6	0	6	20	0
Orange roughy, baked or broiled	3 oz	90	Tr	0	0	0	0	19	0
Oyster, Eastern	***	***	*	*	*	*	*	*	*
breaded, fried	3 oz	170	11	58	10	1	9	8	0
canned	3 oz	60	2	30	3	0	3	6	0
farmed, baked or broiled	6 med	50	1	18	4	0	4	4	0
farmed, raw meat	6 med	50	1	18	5	0	5	4	0
wild, baked or broiled	6 med	40	1	23	3	0	3	5	0
wild, raw meat	6 med	60	2	30	3	0	3	6	0
wild, steamed	6 med	60	2	30	3	0	3	6	0
Oyster, Pacific	***	***	*	*	*	*	*	*	*

	Serving Size	Calories	Fat (g)	Calories from Fat (%)	Total Carbs (g)	Fiber (g)	Net Carbs (g)	Protein (g)	Sugar Alcohol (g)
raw	6 med	240	7	26	15	0	15	28	0
steamed	6 med	250	7	25	15	0	15	28	0
Perch, baked or broiled	3 oz	100	2	18	0	0	0	20	0
Pike, baked or broiled	3 oz	100	Tr	0	0	0	0	21	0
Pollock, baked or broiled	3 oz	100	1	9	0	0	0	21	0
Pompano, baked or broiled	3 oz	180	10	50	0	0	0	20	0
Rockfish, baked or broiled	3 oz	100	2	18	0	0	0	20	0
Salmon, Atlantic	***	***	*	*	*	*	*	*	*
farmed, baked or broiled	3 oz	180	11	55	0	0	0	19	0
wild, baked or broiled	3 oz	160	7	39	0	0	0	22	0
Salmon, chinook, smoked (lox)	3 oz	100	4	36	0	0	0	16	0
Salmon, coho	***	***	*	*	*	*	*	*	*
farmed, baked or broiled	3 oz	150	7	42	0	0	0	21	0
wild, baked or broiled	3 oz	120	4	30	0	0	0	20	0
Salmon, pink, canned	3 oz	120	4	30	0	0	0	20	0
Sardines, canned in oil, drained	2	50	3	54	0	0	0	6	0
Scallop	***	***	*	*	*	*	*	*	*
bay or sea, steamed	3 oz	100	1	9	0	0	0	20	0
breaded, fried	6 large	200	10	45	9	Tr	9	17	0
Shark, battered and fried	3 oz	190	12	57	5	0	5	16	0
Shrimp	***	***	*	*	*	*	*	*	*
breaded, fried	4 large	70	4	51	3	Tr	3	6	0
breaded, fried	3 oz	210	10	43	10	Tr	10	18	0
canned, drained	3 oz	90	1	10	0	0	0	17	0

	Serving Size	Calories	Fat (g)	Calories from Fat (%)	Total Carbs (g)	Fiber (g)	Net Carbs (g)	Protein (g)	Sugar Alcohol (g)
steamed	3 oz	80	Tr	0	0	0	0	18	0
Snapper, baked or broiled	3 oz	110	2	16	0	0	0	22	0
Sole, baked or broiled	3 oz	100	1	9	0	0	0	21	0
Squid, fried	3 oz	150	6	36	7	0	7	15	0
Swordfish, baked or broiled	3 oz	130	4	28	0	0	0	22	0
Trout, baked or broiled	3 oz	160	7	39	0	0	0	23	0
Trout, rainbow	***	***	*	*	*	*	*	*	*
farmed, baked or broiled	3 oz	140		0	0	0	21	6	0
wild, baked or broiled	3 oz	130	5	35	0	0	0	20	0
Tuna	***	***	*	*	*	*	*	*	*
canned in oil, drained	3 oz	160	7	39	0	0	0	23	0
canned in water, chunk light	3 oz	100	Tr	0	0	0	0	22	0
canned in water, solid white	3 oz	110	3	25	0	0	0	20	0
bluefin, baked or broiled	3 oz	160	5	28	0	0	0	25	0
skipjack, baked or broiled	3 oz	110	1	8	0	0	0	24	0
tuna salad, oil packed, w/ mayo	½ cup	190	10	47	10	0	10	16	0
tuna salad, water packed, w/ light mayo type dressing	½ cup	130	5	35	6	0	6	15	0
yellowfin	3 oz	120	1	8	0	0	0	26	0
Whiting, baked or broiled	3 oz	100	1	9	0	0	0	20	0
Fish, Frozen (*Gorton's*)	***	***	*	*	*	*	*	*	*
Grilled Fillets, Cajun	1 fillet	90	3	30	1	0	1	15	0
Grilled Fillets, Garlic Butter	1 fillet	80	3	34	0	0	0	14	0

	Serving Size	Calories	Fat (g)	Calories from Fat (%)	Total Carbs (g)	Fiber (g)	Net Carbs (g)	Protein (g)	Sugar Alcohol (g)
Grilled Fillets, Lemon Butter	1 fillet	90	3	30	0	0	0	14	0
Grilled Fillets, Lemon Pepper	1 fillet	90	3	30	0	0	0	15	0
Grilled Fillets, Italian Herb	1 fillet	90	3	30	2	1	1	13	0
Grilled Cod, Roasted Garlic & Herb	1 fillet	70	2	26	1	0	1	12	0
Grilled Haddock, Signature	1 fillet	80	2.5	28	1	0	1	14	0
Grilled Salmon, Classic	1 fillet	90	2	20	3	0	3	15	0
Grilled Salmon, Lemon Butter	1 fillet	90	2	20	3	0	3	15	0
Grilled Tilapia, Roasted Garlic & Butter	1 fillet	80	2	23	2	1	1	14	0
Grilled Tilapia, Signature	1 fillet	80	2	23	2	0	2	13	0
Skillet Crisp Tilapia, Classic Seasonings	1 fillet	190	9	43	16	1	15	11	0
Skillet Crisp Tilapia, Garlic & Herb	1 fillet	180	8	40	15	0	15	12	0
Simply Bake Haddock, Garlic Herb Butter	1 fillet	130	2.5	17	7	0	7	20	0
Simply Bake Salmon, Roasted Garlic & Butter	1 fillet	140	2.5	16	8	1	7	21	0
Simply Bake Shrimp, Classic Scampi	4 oz (about 9 shrimp)	130	5	35	9	1	8	13	0
Simply Bake Shrimp, Creamy Alfredo	4 oz (about 8 shrimp)	140	6	39	8	1	7	13	0
Simply Bake Tilapia, Signature Seasoning	1 fillet	130	3	21	6	Tr	6	20	0
Fish Sandwich, w/ tartar sauce	1	430	23	48	41	Tr	41	17	0
Fish Sandwich, w/ tartar sauce & cheese	1	520	29	50	48	Tr	48	21	0

	Serving Size	Calories	Fat (g)	Calories from Fat (%)	Total Carbs (g)	Fiber (g)	Net Carbs (g)	Protein (g)	Sugar Alcohol (g)
Flank Steak - see Beef	***	***	*	*	*	*	*	*	*
Flour, unsifted	***	***	*	*	*	*	*	*	*
All purpose, white	1 cup	460	1	2	95	3	92	13	0
Almond, finely ground, *Bob's Red Mill*	1 cup	640	56	79	24	12	12	24	0
Bread	1 cup	500	2	4	99	3	96	16	0
Buckwheat, whole groat	1 cup	400	4	9	85	12	73	15	0
Cake or pastry	1 cup	500	1	2	107	2	105	11	0
Carob	1 cup	230	Tr	0	92	41	51	5	0
Chickpea/garbanzo	1 cup	356	6	15	53	10	43	21	0
Coconut, *Bob's Red Mill*	1 cup	480	16	30	64	40	24	16	0
Gluten-free blend, *King Arthur*	1 cup	563	2	3	127	2	125	8	0
Self-rising, white	1 cup	440	1	2	93	3	90	12	0
Rice	1 cup	580	2	3	127	4	123	9	0
Whole wheat	1 cup	410	2	4	87	15	72	16	0
Frankfurter - see Hot Dog	***	***	*	*	*	*	*	*	*
Freezer Pop - see Frozen Dessert	***	***	*	*	*	*	*	*	*
French Fries, frozen, heated	***	***	*	*	*	*	*	*	*
Regular or crinkle cut	10	120	4	30	19	2	17	2	0
Steak fries	10	200	5	23	36	4	32	3	0
Sweet potato fries	10	98	5	46	19	3	16	1	0
Thin, shoestring strips	10	40	1	23	7	Tr	7	Tr	0
French Toast	2 slices	250	7	25	38	1	37	9	0
Fried Chicken - see Chicken	***	***	*	*	*	*	*	*	*
Fried Rice - see Rice	***	***	*	*	*	*	*	*	*
Frosting	***	***	*	*	*	*	*	*	*
Chocolate	1 oz	120	5	38	19	0	19	0	0

	Serving Size	Calories	Fat (g)	Calories from Fat (%)	Total Carbs (g)	Fiber (g)	Net Carbs (g)	Protein (g)	Sugar Alcohol (g)
Vanilla	1 oz	110	5	41	18	Tr	18	Tr	0
Frozen Dessert	***	***	*	*	*	*	*	*	*
(See also Ice Cream)	***	***	*	*	*	*	*	*	*
Ice Pops 1.75 oz	***	***	*	*	*	*	*	*	*
regular	1	40	Tr	0	10	0	10	0	0
w/ low calorie sweetener	1	15	0	0	3	0	3	0	0
Popsicle pops, sugar free	1	10	0	0	3	0	3	0	0
Fudgesicle bar, fat free	1	70	Tr	0	14	Tr	14	3	0
Fudgesicle bar, no sugar added	1	90	Tr	0	19	1	19	3	0
Frozen Dinner	***	***	*	*	*	*	*	*	*
***Atkins* Frozen Foodie** Meal Kits	***	***	*	*	*	*	*	*	*
Beef Merlot	1 meal	300	21	63	9	3	6	20	0
Beef Teriyaki Stir-Fry	1 meal	260	18	62	10	4	6	18	0
Chicken & Broccoli Alfredo	1 meal	290	18	56	9	5	4	25	0
Chicken Margherita	1 meal	410	30	66	10	3	7	27	0
Chili Con Carne	1 meal	330	23	63	10	5	5	24	0
Crustless Chicken Pot Pie	1 meal	300	19	57	8	3	5	23	0
Orange Chicken	1 meal	410	30	66	10	3	7	27	0
Roasted Turkey w/ Garlic Mashed Cauliflower	1 meal	300	19	57	10	4	6	23	0
***Atkins* Frozen Meals**	***	***	*	*	*	*	*	*	*
Beef Fiesta Taco Bowl	1 meal	310	20	58	14	8	6	21	0
Beef Merlot	1 meal	300	21	63	9	3	6	20	0
Beef Stew	1 meal	260	15	52	13	5	8	18	0
Beef Teriyaki Stir-Fry	1 meal	260	18	62	10	4	6	18	0
Chicken & Broccoli Alfredo	1 meal	290	18	56	9	5	4	25	0

	Serving Size	Calories	Fat (g)	Calories from Fat (%)	Total Carbs (g)	Fiber (g)	Net Carbs (g)	Protein (g)	Sugar Alcohol (g)
Chicken Margherita	1 meal	400	28	63	9	3	6	28	0
Chicken Marsala	1 meal	220	8	33	10	2	8	25	0
Chili Con Carne	1 meal	330	23	63	10	5	5	24	0
Crustless Chicken Pot Pie	1 meal	300	19	57	8	3	5	23	0
Italian-Style Pasta Bake	1 meal	320	18	51	16	8	8	32	0
Meat Lasagna	1 meal	410	24	53	23	12	11	34	0
Meatloaf w/ Portobello Mushroom Gravy	1 meal	330	21	57	11	4	7	23	0
Mexican-Style Chicken & Vegetables	1 meal	320	18	51	10	4	6	31	0
Orange Chicken	1 meal	410	30	66	10	3	7	27	0
Pork Verde	1 meal	300	20	60	10	2	8	23	0
Roasted Turkey w/ Garlic Mashed Cauliflower	1 meal	300	19	57	10	4	6	23	0
Sesame Chicken Stir-Fry	1 meal	330	19	52	19	10	9	29	0
Shrimp Scampi	1 meal	290	19	59	19	11	8	21	0
Swedish Meatballs	1 meal	390	22	51	24	13	11	32	0
Banquet	***	***	*	*	*	*	*	*	*
Boneless Pork Ribs	1 meal	370	17	41	47	4	43	6	0
Chicken Nugget	1 meal	380	19	45	38	4	34	14	0
Crock-Pot Classics, Chicken & Dumplings	⅔ cup	200	8	36	21	6	15	10	0
Crock-Pot Classics, Hearty Beef & Vegetables	⅔ cup	140	6	39	15	4	11	12	0
Crock-Pot Classics, Meatballs in Stroganoff Sauce	⅔ cup	300	14	42	29	5	24	14	0
Fish Sticks	1 meal	360	13	33	46	3	43	13	0
Fried Beef Steak	1 meal	390	19	44	41	3	38	14	0
Meatloaf	1 meal	300	15	45	28	5	23	14	0

	Serving Size	Calories	Fat (g)	Calories from Fat (%)	Total Carbs (g)	Fiber (g)	Net Carbs (g)	Protein (g)	Sugar Alcohol (g)
Original Fried Chicken	1 meal	380	20	47	35	5	30	14	0
Original Fried Chicken Meal	1 meal	430	21	44	39	4	35	21	0
Salisbury Steak	1 meal	300	16	48	25	5	20	14	0
Swedish Meatballs	1 meal	430	23	48	35	5	30	20	0
Turkey Dinner	1 meal	200	8	36	27	5	22	14	0
Gorton's - see Fish, Frozen	***	***	*	*	*	*	*	*	*
Healthy Choice	***	***	*	*	*	*	*	*	*
Bacon & Smokey Cheddar Chicken	1 meal	260	6	21	32	3	29	18	0
Beef Pot Roast	1 meal	260	5	17	40	7	33	14	0
Beef Tips Portobello	1 meal	260	6	21	34	5	29	16	0
Cajun Style Chicken & Shrimp	1 meal	260	4	14	40	3	37	15	0
Chicken Alfredo Florentine	1 meal	230	4	16	31	4	27	17	0
Chicken Fettuccini Alfredo	1 meal	290	6	19	41	7	34	16	0
Chicken Margherita	1 meal	320	7	20	45	5	40	18	0
Chicken Parmigiana	1 meal	340	9	24	49	8	41	16	0
Chicken Pesto Classico	1 meal	320	9	25	39	4	35	19	0
Chicken Red Pepper Alfredo	1 meal	250	5	18	30	4	26	20	0
Classic Meat Loaf	1 meal	300	8	24	40	9	31	15	0
Country Breaded Chicken	1 meal	370	9	22	53	6	47	15	0
Country Herb Chicken	1 meal	240	5	19	34	5	29	15	0
Creamy Garlic Shrimp	1 meal	240	4	15	39	6	33	13	0
Fire Roasted Tomato Chicken	1 meal	320	5	14	48	7	41	19	0
Five-Spice Beef & Vegetables	1 meal	290	5	16	48	4	44	14	0

	Serving Size	Calories	Fat (g)	Calories from Fat (%)	Total Carbs (g)	Fiber (g)	Net Carbs (g)	Protein (g)	Sugar Alcohol (g)
General Tso's Spicy Chicken	1 meal	320	4	11	53	4	49	15	0
Golden Roasted Turkey Breast	1 meal	320	5	14	49	8	41	20	0
Grilled Basil Chicken	1 meal	290	6	19	38	5	33	20	0
Grilled Chicken BBQ	1 meal	270	3	10	43	7	36	15	0
Grilled Chicken Marinara	1 meal	270	5	17	35	5	30	21	0
Grilled Chicken Monterey	1 meal	290	6	19	41	5	36	17	0
Grilled Chicken Teriyaki	1 meal	280	4	13	44	8	36	15	0
Grilled Whiskey Steak	1 meal	250	4	14	34	6	28	18	0
Hearty, Beef Stroganoff	1 meal	300	6	18	43	5	38	18	0
Homestyle Salisbury Steak	1 meal	290	6	19	42	8	34	16	0
Honey Balsamic Chicken	1 meal	360	7	18	59	5	54	15	0
Honey Ginger Chicken	1 meal	310	5	15	53	3	50	14	0
Lemon Pepper Fish	1 meal	310	5	15	53	5	48	13	0
Mandarin Beef Lo Mein	1 meal	360	6	15	60	8	52	16	0
Marinara Manicotti Formaggio	1 meal	350	7	18	61	8	53	13	0
Mediterranean Pasta	1 meal	360	5	13	65	12	53	13	0
Orange Zest Chicken	1 meal	290	4	12	46	6	40	17	0
Oven Roasted Chicken	1 meal	260	5	17	37	6	31	15	0
Portabella Marsala Pasta	1 meal	270	7	23	38	5	33	12	0
Portabella Spinach Parmesan	1 meal	270	7	23	40	5	35	11	0

	Serving Size	Calories	Fat (g)	Calories from Fat (%)	Total Carbs (g)	Fiber (g)	Net Carbs (g)	Protein (g)	Sugar Alcohol (g)
Pumpkin Squash Ravioli	1 meal	300	6	18	52	6	46	9	0
Roasted Beef Merlot	1 meal	230	8	31	21	5	16	17	0
Roasted Chicken Fresca	1 meal	230	5	20	29	6	23	17	0
Roasted Chicken Marsala	1 meal	250	6	22	30	4	26	18	0
Roasted Sesame Chicken	1 meal	340	6	16	53	5	48	18	0
Salisbury Steak	1 meal	190	6	28	18	5	13	14	0
Simply Steamers Chicken & Vegetable Stir Fry	1 meal	190	4	19	15	4	11	23	0
Simply Steamers Grilled Chicken & Broccoli Alfredo	1 meal	190	5	24	8	4	4	28	0
Slow Roasted Turkey Medallions	1 meal	220	5	20	28	5	23	14	0
Sweet & Sour Chicken	1 meal	400	10	23	61	5	56	13	0
Sweet Asian Potstickers	1 meal	380	5	12	75	6	69	8	0
Sweet Bourbon Steak Tips	1 meal	290	7	22	38	6	32	17	0
Sweet Sesame Chicken	1 meal	330	6	16	50	6	44	17	0
Tomato Basil Penne	1 meal	280	6	19	39	7	32	13	0
Turkey Breast & Cranberries	1 meal	320	4	11	53	7	46	16	0
Lean Cuisine	***	***	*	*	*	*	*	*	*
Alfredo Pasta w/ Chicken & Broccoli	1 meal	250	6	22	33	3	30	17	0
Angel Hair Pomodoro	1 meal	250	5	18	42	4	38	8	0
Asian Style Potstickers	1 meal	260	4	14	47	3	44	9	0
Baked Chicken	1 meal	240	5	19	34	3	31	15	0

	Serving Size	Calories	Fat (g)	Calories from Fat (%)	Total Carbs (g)	Fiber (g)	Net Carbs (g)	Protein (g)	Sugar Alcohol (g)
Baked Chicken Florentine	1 meal	200	8	36	14	3	11	18	0
Balsamic Glazed Chicken	1 meal	350	9	23	43	6	37	24	0
Beef & Broccoli	1 meal	260	5	17	39	2	37	14	0
Beef Chow Fun	1 meal	320	5	14	54	3	51	15	0
Beef Portobello	1 meal	220	6	25	25	2	23	16	0
Beef Pot Roast	1 meal	210	6	26	26	3	23	14	0
Butternut Squash Ravioli	1 meal	350	9	23	54	6	48	13	0
Cheddar Bacon Chicken	1 meal	220	8	33	17	2	15	19	0
Cheddar Potatoes w/ Broccoli	1 meal	230	5	20	35	4	31	12	0
Cheese Lasagna w/ Chicken Breast Scaloppini	1 meal	280	8	26	34	4	30	18	0
Cheese Ravioli	1 meal	240	6	23	36	3	33	11	0
Chicken & Vegetables	1 meal	240	5	19	29	3	26	20	0
Chicken Carbonara	1 meal	280	7	23	33	2	31	22	0
Chicken Chow Mein	1 meal	260	4	14	41	3	38	14	0
Chicken Enchilada Suiza	1 meal	270	4	13	47	3	44	12	0
Chicken Fettuccini	1 meal	290	6	19	43	3	40	16	0
Chicken Florentine	1 meal	410	9	20	54	6	48	28	0
Chicken Florentine Lasagna	1 meal	280	6	19	36	3	33	20	0
Chicken Fried Rice Bowl	1 meal	280	6	19	39	3	36	17	0
Chicken in Peanut Sauce	1 meal	280	8	26	30	5	25	22	0
Chicken Marsala	1 meal	250	9	32	29	2	27	14	0
Chicken Mediterranean	1 meal	240	4	15	32	6	26	19	0
Chicken Parmesan	1 meal	310	8	23	39	5	34	21	0
Chicken Pecan	1 meal	260	6	21	32	4	28	19	0

	Serving Size	Calories	Fat (g)	Calories from Fat (%)	Total Carbs (g)	Fiber (g)	Net Carbs (g)	Protein (g)	Sugar Alcohol (g)
Chicken Portobello	1 meal	390	8	18	48	2	46	32	0
Chicken Teriyaki Bowl	1 meal	250	2	7	44	3	41	15	0
Chicken Teriyaki Stir Fry	1 meal	250	2	7	46	3	43	12	0
Chicken Tuscan	1 meal	280	6	19	34	5	29	22	0
Chicken w/ Almonds	1 meal	260	6	21	34	3	31	17	0
Chicken w/ Basil Cream Sauce	1 meal	290	7	22	36	3	33	20	0
Classic Five Cheese Lasagna	1 meal	360	8	20	51	4	47	21	0
Classic Macaroni & Beef	1 meal	310	9	26	38	3	35	20	0
Deluxe Cheddar Potato	1 meal	260	7	24	35	4	31	14	0
Fettuccini Alfredo	1 meal	280	6	19	42	1	41	14	0
Fiesta Grilled Chicken	1 meal	260	6	21	33	4	29	19	0
Five Cheese Rigatoni	1 meal	330	9	25	50	4	46	12	0
Four Cheese Cannelloni	1 meal	240	6	23	30	3	27	17	0
Ginger Garlic Stir Fry w/ Chicken	1 meal	290	4	12	46	4	42	17	0
Glazed Chicken	1 meal	220	4	16	25	1	24	21	0
Glazed Turkey Tenderloins	1 meal	250	5	18	38	3	35	13	0
Grilled Chicken & Penne Pasta	1 meal	330	5	14	52	6	46	20	0
Grilled Chicken Caesar Bowl	1 meal	240	7	26	25	3	22	18	0
Grilled Chicken Primavera	1 meal	220	5	20	24	5	19	18	0
Grilled Chicken w/ Teriyaki Glaze	1 meal	280	3	10	45	2	43	17	0
Herb Roasted Chicken	1 meal	180	4	20	20	3	17	18	0

	Serving Size	Calories	Fat (g)	Calories from Fat (%)	Total Carbs (g)	Fiber (g)	Net Carbs (g)	Protein (g)	Sugar Alcohol (g)
Honey Dijon Grilled Chicken	1 meal	220	7	29	22	2	20	17	0
Hunan Stir Fry w/ Beef	1 meal	270	7	23	37	2	35	15	0
Jumbo Rigatoni w/ Meatballs	1 meal	390	8	18	56	7	49	23	0
Lasagna w/ Meat Sauce	1 meal	320	7	20	23	4	39	20	0
Lemon Chicken	1 meal	300	9	27	41	3	38	13	0
Lemon Garlic Shrimp	1 meal	350	7	18	54	5	49	18	0
Lemon Pepper Fish	1 meal	330	8	22	50	2	48	15	0
Lemongrass Chicken	1 meal	250	6	22	30	4	26	18	0
Linguini Carbonara	1 meal	300	8	24	43	2	41	14	0
Macaroni & Cheese	1 meal	290	7	22	41	1	40	15	0
Meatloaf w/ Gravy & Whipped Potatoes	1 meal	260	8	28	25	3	22	21	0
Orange Chicken	1 meal	300	7	21	46	2	44	14	0
Orange Peel Chicken	1 meal	390	9	21	63	3	60	15	0
Oven Roasted Beef	1 meal	210	8	34	18	2	16	16	0
Oven Roasted Beef Burgundy	1 meal	300	8	24	39	3	36	17	0
Parmesan Crusted Fish	1 meal	290	8	25	40	4	36	15	0
Pasta Romano w/ Bacon	1 meal	280	7	23	43	4	39	12	0
Pesto Chicken w/ Bowtie Pasta	1 meal	340	9	24	42	4	38	23	0
Pomegranate Chicken	1 meal	180	3	15	20	3	17	17	0
Roasted Chicken w/ Lemon Pepper Fettuccini	1 meal	230	6	23	28	2	26	16	0
Roasted Garlic Chicken	1 meal	180	7	35	9	1	8	20	0

	Serving Size	Calories	Fat (g)	Calories from Fat (%)	Total Carbs (g)	Fiber (g)	Net Carbs (g)	Protein (g)	Sugar Alcohol (g)
Roasted Turkey & Vegetables	1 meal	190	6	28	19	4	15	15	0
Roasted Turkey Breast	1 meal	290	7	22	38	5	33	19	0
Roasted Turkey Breast w/ Dressing	1 meal	260	3	10	48	3	45	12	0
Rosemary Chicken	1 meal	210	4	17	27	3	24	17	0
Salisbury Steak	1 meal	270	8	27	27	10	17	22	0
Salisbury Steak w/ Mac & Cheese	1 meal	280	9	29	25	3	22	24	0
Salmon Mediterranean	1 meal	230	4	16	30	3	27	18	0
Salmon w/ Basil	1 meal	220	6	25	23	4	19	19	0
Sante Fe Style Rice & Beans	1 meal	300	5	15	52	5	47	11	0
Sesame Chicken	1 meal	330	9	25	47	2	45	16	0
Sesame Stir Fry w/ Chicken	1 meal	300	6	18	41	5	36	20	0
Shrimp & Angel Hair Pasta	1 meal	220	4	16	32	2	30	14	0
Shrimp Alfredo	1 meal	260	5	17	36	3	33	18	0
Southern Beef Tips	1 meal	250	5	18	36	3	33	15	0
Spaghetti w/ Meat Sauce	1 meal	290	5	16	47	4	43	15	0
Spaghetti w/ Meatballs	1 meal	270	5	17	38	5	33	18	0
Steak Portabella	1 meal	160	5	28	11	3	8	18	0
Steak Tips Dijon	1 meal	280	7	23	33	5	28	21	0
Steak Tips Portobello	1 meal	180	7	35	13	3	10	15	0
Stuffed Cabbage	1 meal	220	4	16	21	5	16	24	0
Sun Dried Tomato Pesto Chicken	1 meal	290	9	28	34	4	30	18	0
Swedish Meatballs	1 meal	300	8	24	34	3	31	22	0
Sweet & Sour Chicken	1 meal	310	3	9	53	2	51	17	0

	Serving Size	Calories	Fat (g)	Calories from Fat (%)	Total Carbs (g)	Fiber (g)	Net Carbs (g)	Protein (g)	Sugar Alcohol (g)
Sweet Sriracha Braised Beef	1 meal	180	5	25	18	3	15	15	0
Szechuan Style Stir Fry w/ Shrimp	1 meal	230	3	12	39	5	34	13	0
Teriyaki Steak Bowl	1 meal	280	6	19	37	3	34	19	0
Thai Style Chicken	1 meal	220	4	16	28	2	26	18	0
Three Cheese Chicken	1 meal	210	10	43	10	3	7	21	0
Three Cheese Stuffed Rigatoni Bowl	1 meal	240	6	23	35	4	31	12	0
Tortilla Crusted Fish	1 meal	330	9	25	45	3	42	16	0
Vegetable Eggroll	1 meal	310	5	15	60	3	57	7	0
Marie Callender's	***	***	*	*	*	*	*	*	*
Beef Tips Dinner	1 meal	360	12	30	35	6	29	26	0
Cheesy Chicken Breast, Rice w/ Broccoli	1 meal	480	18	34	47	5	42	31	0
Fettuccine Chicken & Broccoli	1 meal	630	37	53	43	6	37	30	0
Grilled Chicken Bake	1 meal	610	35	52	43	5	38	30	0
Herb Roasted Chicken	1 meal	460	25	49	26	5	21	30	0
Meat Loaf w/ Gravy	1 meal	480	22	41	39	3	36	31	0
Old Fashioned Beef Pot Roast	1 meal	330	10	27	32	9	23	27	0
Salisbury Steak Dinner	1 meal	400	16	36	38	7	31	27	0
Slow Roasted Beef	1 meal	370	13	32	37	7	30	25	0
Turkey w/ Stuffing	1 meal	400	9	20	45	4	41	32	0
Smart Ones (Weight Watchers)	***	***	*	*	***	*	*	*	*
Angel Hair Marinara	1 meal	230	4	16	40	4	36	9	0
Broccoli & Cheddar Roasted Potatoes	1 meal	240	7	26	35	4	31	10	0

	Serving Size	Calories	Fat (g)	Calories from Fat (%)	Total Carbs (g)	Fiber (g)	Net Carbs (g)	Protein (g)	Sugar Alcohol (g)
Chicken Carbonara	1 meal	250	5	18	32	2	30	20	0
Chicken Enchiladas Monterey	1 meal	310	10	29	41	5	36	12	0
Chicken Enchiladas Suiza	1 meal	290	5	16	49	3	46	11	0
Chicken Fettuccini	1 meal	340	6	16	47	4	43	23	0
Chicken Marsala w/ Broccoli	1 meal	180	7	35	10	2	8	20	0
Chicken Mirabella	1 meal	200	2	9	33	3	30	12	0
Chicken Oriental	1 meal	230	3	12	39	2	37	12	0
Chicken Parmesan	1 meal	290	5	16	35	4	31	26	0
Chicken Santa Fe	1 meal	140	3	19	11	4	7	20	0
Cranberry Turkey Medallions	1 meal	250	2	7	43	4	39	16	0
Creamy Parmesan Chicken	1 meal	250	8	29	24	3	21	21	0
Creamy Rigatoni w/ Chicken & Broccoli	1 meal	290	8	25	33	2	31	20	0
Dragon Shrimp Lo Mein	1 meal	240	4	15	36	3	33	14	0
Fettuccini Alfredo	1 meal	240	4	15	41	4	37	12	0
Home Style Beef Pot Roast	1 meal	180	5	25	20	3	17	17	0
Honey Mango Barbeque Chicken	1 meal	240	4	15	34	0	34	9	0
Lasagna Bake w/ Meat Sauce	1 meal	270	4	13	43	3	40	14	0
Lasagna Florentine	1 meal	290	9	28	35	4	29	15	0
Lemon Herb Chicken Piccata	1 meal	230	2	8	41	2	39	12	0
Macaroni & Cheese	1 meal	270	2	7	52	2	50	11	0
Meatloaf	1 meal	250	8	29	23	3	20	22	0
Orange Sesame Chicken	1 meal	320	8	23	48	2	46	14	0
Pasta Primavera	1 meal	280	6	19	44	6	38	12	0
Picante Chicken & Pasta	1 meal	260	4	14	32	4	28	23	0

	Serving Size	Calories	Fat (g)	Calories from Fat (%)	Total Carbs (g)	Fiber (g)	Net Carbs (g)	Protein (g)	Sugar Alcohol (g)
Pineapple Beef Teriyaki	1 meal	260	5	17	38	0	38	18	0
Ravioli Florentine	1 meal	250	5	18	40	4	36	11	0
Roast Beef w/ Gravy	1 meal	210	9	39	19	2	17	14	0
Roast Turkey Medallions w/ Mushroom Gravy	1 meal	220	2	8	38	3	35	13	0
Roasted Chicken w/ Sour Cream & Chive Mashed Potatoes	1 meal	180	4	20	20	2	18	17	0
Salisbury Steak	1 meal	200	8	36	12	3	9	20	0
Santa Fe Style Rice & Beans	1 meal	310	7	20	51	4	47	10	0
Shrimp Marinara	1 meal	180	2	10	31	4	27	9	0
Sirloin Beef & Asian Style Vegetables	1 meal	220	5	20	27	3	24	17	0
Slow Roasted Turkey Breast	1 meal	210	7	30	18	2	16	18	0
Spaghetti w/ Meat Sauce	1 meal	310	6	17	48	5	43	16	0
Spicy Szechuan Style Vegetable & Chicken	1 meal	240	5	19	36	4	32	11	0
Stuffed Turkey Breast	1 meal	290	6	19	42	4	38	17	0
Swedish Meatballs	1 meal	270	5	17	35	3	32	20	0
Sweet & Sour Chicken	1 meal	210	2	9	31	2	29	16	0
Teriyaki Chicken & Vegetables	1 meal	230	3	12	39	3	36	14	0
Thai Style Chicken & Rice Noodles	1 meal	260	4	14	43	2	41	14	0
Three Cheese Macaroni	1 meal	300	6	18	48	3	45	14	0
Three Cheese Ziti Marinara	1 meal	320	8	23	47	4	43	14	0
Traditional Lasagna w/ Meat Sauce	1 meal	300	6	18	43	5	38	17	0

	Serving Size	Calories	Fat (g)	Calories from Fat (%)	Total Carbs (g)	Fiber (g)	Net Carbs (g)	Protein (g)	Sugar Alcohol (g)
Tuna Noodle Gratin	1 meal	240	5	19	37	3	34	15	0
Turkey Medallions w/ Mushroom Gravy	1 meal	200	10	45	11	3	8	18	0
Stouffer's	***	***	*	*	***	*	*	*	*
Baked Chicken Breast	1 meal	250	10	36	20	1	19	20	0
Beef Pot Roast	1 meal	320	8	23	41	8	33	20	0
Beef Stroganoff	1 meal	380	17	40	34	2	32	22	0
Bourbon Steak Tips	1 meal	570	24	38	65	4	61	23	0
Cheese Manicotti	1 meal	360	14	35	41	2	39	18	0
Cheese Ravioli	1 meal	380	13	31	47	5	42	19	0
Cheesy Spaghetti Bake	1 meal	460	24	47	39	4	35	21	0
Chicken a la King	1 meal	360	12	30	44	0	44	18	0
Chicken Carbonara	1 meal	670	32	43	56	6	50	40	0
Chicken Fettuccini	1 meal	570	27	43	55	5	50	26	0
Chicken Fettuccini Alfredo	1 meal	840	38	41	94	5	89	31	0
Chicken Parmigiana	1 meal	410	14	31	47	4	43	23	0
Classics Meatloaf	1 loaf, no sauce	190	10	47	9	1	8	17	0
Classics Salisbury Steak	1 steak	360	19	48	22	2	20	25	0
Classics Spinach Souffle	½ cup	150	10	60	9	1	8	6	0
Escalloped Chicken & Noodles	1 meal	450	22	44	43	5	38	19	0
Fettuccini Alfredo	1 meal	610	34	50	57	5	52	18	0
Fish Fillet	1 meal	400	16	36	36	4	32	27	0
Five Cheese Lasagna	1 meal	370	14	34	39	4	35	21	0
Fried Chicken Breast	1 meal	360	18	45	30	2	28	20	0
Garlic Chicken Pasta	1 meal	330	9	25	37	5	32	25	0
Green Pepper Steak	1 meal	240	4	15	32	3	29	18	0

	Serving Size	Calories	Fat (g)	Calories from Fat (%)	Total Carbs (g)	Fiber (g)	Net Carbs (g)	Protein (g)	Sugar Alcohol (g)
Grilled Chicken Teriyaki	1 meal	300	4	12	45	3	42	21	0
Grilled Herb Chicken	1 meal	250	6	22	29	3	26	19	0
Grilled Lemon Pepper Chicken	1 meal	240	8	30	24	4	20	19	0
Lasagna Bake w/ Meat Sauce	1 meal	350	10	26	49	5	44	17	0
Lasagna w/ Meat & Sauce	1 meal	350	11	28	38	3	35	24	0
Lasagna w/ Tomato Sauce & Italian Sausage	1 meal	410	19	42	41	4	37	18	0
Macaroni & Beef	1 meal	410	16	35	45	4	41	22	0
Macaroni & Cheese w/ Broccoli	1 meal	480	20	38	52	5	47	22	0
Meatloaf	1 meal	600	31	47	45	5	40	35	0
Monterey Chicken	1 meal	530	21	36	54	5	49	31	0
Pork Cutlet	1 meal	370	21	51	31	3	28	13	0
Rigatoni w/ Roasted White Chicken Meat	1 meal	390	15	35	44	3	41	19	0
Roast Turkey	1 meal	290	12	37	30	2	28	16	0
Roast Turkey Breast	1 meal	460	19	37	51	5	46	22	0
Roasted Chicken	1 meal	460	24	47	34	5	29	26	0
Salisbury Steak	1 meal	710	39	49	48	3	45	41	0
Sesame Chicken	1 meal	590	16	24	87	6	81	25	0
Shrimp Scampi	1 meal	400	12	27	56	5	51	16	0
Spaghetti w/ Meat Sauce	1 meal	350	12	31	44	5	39	17	0
Spaghetti w/ Meatballs	1 meal	360	12	30	45	6	39	19	0
Swedish Meatballs	1 meal	560	27	43	47	3	44	32	0
Tuna Noodle Casserole	1 meal	450	20	40	45	3	42	22	0
Turkey Tetrazzini	1 meal	450	23	46	38	2	36	23	0
Stuffed Pepper	1 meal	210	9	39	23	3	20	10	0

	Serving Size	Calories	Fat (g)	Calories from Fat (%)	Total Carbs (g)	Fiber (g)	Net Carbs (g)	Protein (g)	Sugar Alcohol (g)
Vegetable Lasagna	1 meal	390	18	42	40	4	36	17	0
Veal Parmigiana	1 meal	430	18	38	46	5	41	20	0
Fruit	***	***	*	*	*	*	*	*	*
(See also specific listings)	***	***	*	*	*	*	*	*	*
Mixed, canned, in heavy syrup	1 cup	180	Tr	0	48	3	45	Tr	0
Mixed, frozen, sweetened	1 cup	250	Tr	0	61	5	56	4	0
Fruit Cocktail, canned	***	***	*	*	*	*	*	*	*
In heavy syrup	1 cup	180	Tr	0	47	3	42	Tr	0
In juice	1 cup	110	Tr	0	28	2	26	1	0
In light syrup	1 cup	140	Tr	0	36	2	34	Tr	0
Fruit Salad, canned	***	***	*	*	*	*	*	*	*
In heavy syrup	1 cup	190	Tr	0	49	3	46	Tr	0
In juice	1 cup	130	Tr	0	33	3	30	1	0
In light syrup	1 cup	150	Tr	0	38	3	35	Tr	0
Tropical, in heavy syrup	1 cup	220	Tr	0	58	3	55	1	0
Fudge - see Candy	***	***	*	*	*	*	*	*	*
Funyuns (snacks)	13	140	7	45	18	1	17	2	0
Garlic, raw	1 clove	0	Tr	0	Tr	Tr	Tr	Tr	0
Garlic Powder or Salt	1 tsp	10	Tr	0	2	Tr	2	Tr	0
Gelatin	***	***	*	*	*	*	*	*	*
Reduced calorie, sweetened w/ aspartame, as prep (*Jell-O*)	½ cup	25	0	0	5	0	5	Tr	0
Sweetened w/ sugar, as prep (*Jell-O*)	½ cup	80	0	0	19	0	19	2	0
Unsweetened, 1 envelope	1 Tbsp	25	Tr	0	0	0	0	6	0
Ginger, dried, ground	1 tsp	5	Tr	0	1	Tr	1	Tr	0
Ginger root, fresh	***	***	*	*	*	*	*	*	*
Grated	1 tsp	0	Tr	0	Tr	0	Tr	Tr	0
Slices, 1" dia	5	10	Tr	0	2	Tr	2	Tr	0

	Serving Size	Calories	Fat (g)	Calories from Fat (%)	Total Carbs (g)	Fiber (g)	Net Carbs (g)	Protein (g)	Sugar Alcohol (g)
Gordita - see frozen dinner or individual restaurant listings	***	***	*	*	*	*	*	*	*
Granola - see Cereal	***	***	*	*	*	*	*	*	*
Granola Bar	***	***	*	*	*	*	*	*	*
Hard	***	***	*	*	*	*	*	*	*
Almond	1 oz	140	7	45	18	1	17	2	0
Chocolate chip	1 oz	120	5	38	20	1	19	2	0
Peanut	1 oz	140	6	39	18	1	17	3	0
Peanut butter	1 oz	140	7	45	18	Tr	18	3	0
Plain	1 oz	130	6	42	18	2	16	3	0
Soft	***	***	*	*	*	*	*	*	*
Chocolate chip	1 oz	120	5	38	20	1	19	2	0
Chocolate covered chocolate chip	1 oz	130	7	48	18	1	17	2	0
Chocolate covered coconut	1 oz	150	9	54	16	2	14	2	0
Chocolate covered peanut butter	1 oz	140	9	58	15	Tr	15	3	0
Nonfat, fruit filled	1 oz	100	Tr	0	22	2	20	2	0
Nut & raisin	1 oz	130	6	42	18	2	16	2	0
Oats, fruit & nuts	1 oz	110	2	16	22	2	20	2	0
Peanut butter	1 oz	120	4	30	18	1	17	3	0
Peanut butter & chocolate chip	1 oz	120	6	45	17	1	16	3	0
Plain	1 oz	130	5	35	19	1	18	2	0
Grapefruit, pink, red, or white	***	***	*	*	*	*	*	*	*
Canned, in juice	1 cup	90	Tr	0	23	1	22	2	0
Canned, in light syrup	1 cup	150	Tr	0	39	1	38	1	0
Fresh, 4" dia	1 half	40	Tr	0	10	1	9	Tr	0
Fresh, sections	1 cup	70	Tr	0	19	3	16	2	0
Grapes, seeded	***	***	*	*	*	*	*	*	*
Fresh, medium size, all types	10 ea	35	Tr	0	9	Tr	9	Tr	0

	Serving Size	Calories	Fat (g)	Calories from Fat (%)	Total Carbs (g)	Fiber (g)	Net Carbs (g)	Protein (g)	Sugar Alcohol (g)
Fresh, medium size, all types	1 cup	100	Tr	0	27	1	26	1	0
Gravy, canned	***	***	*	*	*	*	*	*	*
Au jus	¼ cup	10	Tr	0	2	0	2	Tr	0
Beef	¼ cup	30	1	30	3	Tr	3	2	0
Chicken	¼ cup	45	3	60	3	Tr	3	1	0
Low sodium, meat or poultry	¼ cup	30	1	30	4	Tr	4	2	0
Mushroom	¼ cup	30	2	60	3	Tr	3	Tr	0
Turkey	¼ cup	30	1	30	4	Tr	4	2	0
Grits, corn, as prep	1 cup	140	Tr	0	31	Tr	31	3	0
Ground Beef - see Beef	***	***	*	*	*	*	*	*	*
Guava	***	***	*	*	*	*	*	*	*
Fresh, chopped	1 cup	110	2	16	24	9	15	4	0
Fresh, whole	1	35	Tr	0	8	3	5	1	0
Strawberry guava, whole	1	0	Tr	0	1	Tr	1	Tr	0
Gum - see Chewing Gum	***	***	*	*	*	*	*	*	*
HAM	***	***	*	*	*	*	*	*	*
(See also Pork)	***	***	*	*	*	*	*	*	*
Canned, roasted	3 oz	190	13	62	Tr	0	Tr	18	0
Canned, roasted, extra lean	3 oz	120	4	30	Tr	0	Tr	18	0
Cured, roasted, lean & fat	3 oz	210	14	60	0	0	0	18	0
Cured, roasted, lean only	3 oz	130	5	35	0	0	0	21	0
Diced	2 oz	70	3	39	1	0	1	9	0
Leg, roasted, lean & fat	3 oz	230	15	59	0	0	0	23	0
Leg, roasted, lean only	3 oz	180	8	40	0	0	0	25	0
Lunch meat, ⅛" slices	***	***	*	*	*	*	*	*	*
extra lean	2 oz	60	2	30	Tr	0	Tr	11	0

	Serving Size	Calories	Fat (g)	Calories from Fat (%)	Total Carbs (g)	Fiber (g)	Net Carbs (g)	Protein (g)	Sugar Alcohol (g)
regular	2 oz	90	5	50	2	Tr	2	9	0
Steak, cured, extra lean, 1 slice	2 oz	70	2	26	0	0	0	11	0
Boarshead	***	***	*	*	*	*	*	*	*
Black Forest brand smoked	2 oz	60	1	15	2	0	2	10	0
Branded Deluxe ham	2 oz	60	1	15	2	0	2	9	0
Canadian style bacon, extra lean	2 oz	70	2	26	1	0	1	12	0
Cappy brand ham	2 oz	60	2	30	3	0	3	10	0
Seasoned fresh ham	2 oz	80	3	34	0	0	0	14	0
Smoked Virginia ham	2 oz	60	1	15	2	0	2	9	0
Oscar Mayer	***	***	*	*	*	*	*	*	*
Baked	2.25 oz	70	2	26	Tr	0	Tr	11	0
Baked, 96 fat free, 3 slices	2.25 oz	70	2	26	1	0	1	10	0
Chopped, 1 slice	1 oz	50	3	54	1	0	1	5	0
Honey	2.25 oz	70	2	26	2	0	2	11	0
Smoked	2.25 oz	60	2	30	Tr	0	Tr	11	0
Hamburger & Cheeseburger	***	***	*	*	*	*	*	*	*
(See Beef, Ground & Dining Out)	***	***	*	*	*	*	*	*	*
Hash Browns - see Potatoes	***	***	*	*	*	*	*	*	*
Hearts of Palm, canned	1 cup	40	Tr	0	7	4	3	4	0
Honey, Real, 1 pkt	1 Tbsp	60	0	0	17	0	17	T	0
Honey, Sugar Free	***	***	*	*	*	*	*	*	*
HoneyTree's Sugar Free Imitation Honey	1 Tbsp	50	0	0	17	0	17	0	17
Honeydew Melon, fresh, avg size 6½" melon	***	***	*	*	*	*	*	*	*
Cubed or balls	1 cup	60	Tr	0	16	1	15	Tr	0

	Serving Size	Calories	Fat (g)	Calories from Fat (%)	Total Carbs (g)	Fiber (g)	Net Carbs (g)	Protein (g)	Sugar Alcohol (g)
Wedge, ⅛ of melon	1	60	Tr	0	15	1	14	Tr	0
Horseradish, as prep	1 tsp	0	Tr	0	Tr	Tr	Tr	Tr	0
Hot Dog (Frankfurter)	***	***	*	*	*	*	*	*	*
Beef	1	150	13	78	2	0	2	5	0
Beef, low fat	1	130	11	76	Tr	0	Tr	7	0
Beef & pork	1	140	13	84	Tr	0	Tr	5	0
Beef & pork, low fat	1	90	6	60	3	0	3	6	0
Boarshead	***	***	*	*	*	*	*	*	*
Lite Beef Frankfurters	1	90	6	60	0	0	0	7	0
Pork & Beef Frankfurters	1	150	14	84	0	0	0	7	0
Chicken	1	100	7	63	1	Tr	1	7	0
Pork	1	200	18	81	Tr	Tr	Tr	10	0
Turkey	1	100	8	72	2	0	2	6	0
Hummus, commercial	1 Tbsp	25	1	36	2	Tr	2	1	0
Hush Puppies	1	70	3	39	10	Tr	10	2	0
Ice Cream	***	***	*	*	*	*	*	*	*
Chocolate	***	***	*	*	*	*	*	*	*
light	½ cup	140	5	32	18	Tr	18	3	0
light, no sugar added	½ cup	110	4	33	18	Tr	18	3	0
regular	½ cup	140	7	45	19	Tr	19	3	0
rich	½ cup	190	13	62	15	Tr	15	4	0
Low Carb	***	***	*	*	*	*	*	*	*
chocolate	½ cup	130	8	55	11	3	8	3	0
vanilla	½ cup	130	8	55	11	3	8	2	0
Sherbet, Orange	½ cup	110	2	16	23	1	22	Tr	0
Strawberry	½ cup	130	6	42	18	Tr	18	2	0
Vanilla	***	***	*	*	*	*	*	*	*
light	½ cup	130	4	28	20	Tr	20	4	0
light, no sugar added	½ cup	110	5	41	15	Tr	15	3	0
regular	½ cup	140	7	45	16	Tr	16	2	0

	Serving Size	Calories	Fat (g)	Calories from Fat (%)	Total Carbs (g)	Fiber (g)	Net Carbs (g)	Protein (g)	Sugar Alcohol (g)
rich	½ cup	270	17	57	24	0	24	4	0
soft serve	½ cup	190	11	52	19	Tr	19	4	0
soft serve, light	½ cup	110	2	16	19	0	19	4	0
Ice Cream Cone, cake or wafer	1	15	Tr	0	3	Tr	3	Tr	0
Sugar cone	1	40	Tr	0	80	Tr	8	Tr	0
Waffle cone, large	1	120	2	15	23	Tr	23	2	0
Ice Cream Sandwich, vanilla	1	220	9	37	31	1	30	4	0
Ice Pop - see Frozen Dessert	***	***	*	*	*	*	*	*	*
Italian Ices	½ cup	60	Tr	0	16	0	16	Tr	0
Jalapeno - see Peppers	***	***	*	*	*	*	*	*	*
Jam, all flavors	***	***	*	*	*	*	*	*	*
Regular	1 Tbsp	60	Tr	0	14	Tr	14	Tr	0
Restaurant size packet	½ oz	40	Tr	0	10	Tr	10	Tr	0
Sugar free	1 Tbsp	35	0	0	13	0	1	0	12
Sweetened w/ sodium saccharin	1 Tbsp	20	Tr	0	8	Tr	8	Tr	0
Jell-O - see Gelatin	***	***	*	*	*	*	*	*	*
Jelly, all flavors	***	***	*	*	*	*	*	*	*
Reduced sugar	1 Tbsp	35	Tr	0	9	Tr	9	Tr	0
Regular	1 Tbsp	60	0	0	15	Tr	15	Tr	0
Restaurant size packet	½ oz	35	0	0	10	Tr	10	Tr	0
Kale	***	***	*	*	*	*	*	*	*
Fresh, chopped	1 cup	35	Tr	0	7	1	6	2	0
Fresh, chopped, cooked	1 cup	35	Tr	0	7	3	4	3	0
Frozen, chopped, cooked	1 cup	40	Tr	0	7	3	4	3	0
Ketchup	***	***	*	*	*	*	*	*	*
Low sodium	1 Tbsp	15	Tr	0	4	0	4	Tr	0
Regular	1 Tbsp	15	Tr	0	4	0	4	Tr	0

	Serving Size	Calories	Fat (g)	Calories from Fat (%)	Total Carbs (g)	Fiber (g)	Net Carbs (g)	Protein (g)	Sugar Alcohol (g)
Restaurant size packet	1	5	Tr	0	2	0	2	Tr	0
Sugar free	1 Tbsp	0	0	0	6	0	2	0	4
Kiwi Fruit, fresh, medium size	1	45	Tr	0	11	2	9	Tr	0
Knockwurst	1 link	220	20	82	2	0	2	8	0
Kohlrabi, cooked, slices	1 cup	50	Tr	0	11	2	9	3	0
Lamb	***	***	*	*	*	*	*	*	*
Cubed, braised	3 oz	190	8	38	0	0	0	29	0
Cubed, broiled	3 oz	160	6	34	0	0	0	24	0
Ground, broiled	3 oz	240	17	64	0	0	0	21	0
Leg of lamb, roasted	***	***	*	*	*	*	*	*	*
lean & fat	3 oz	240	14	53	0	0	0	26	0
lean only	3 oz	160	7	39	0	0	0	24	0
Loin chop, broiled	***	***	*	*	*	*	*	*	*
lean & fat	3 oz	250	18	65	0	0	0	22	0
lean only	3 oz	180	8	40	0	0	0	26	0
Rib roast, lean & fat	3 oz	290	23	71	0	0	0	19	0
lean only	3 oz	200	11	50	0	0	0	22	0
Shoulder, braised	***	***	*	*	*	*	*	*	*
lean & fat	3 oz	290	20	62	0	0	0	25	0
lean only	3 oz	240	14	53	0	0	0	28	0
Lard	1 cup	1850	205	100	0	0	0	0	0
Lard	1 Tbsp	120	13	98	0	0	0	0	0
Lasagna	***	***	*	*	*	*	*	*	*
w/ meat sauce	1 pc	380	14	33	38	4	34	25	0
vegetable	1 pc	320	14	39	32	4	28	16	0
Leek, chopped, cooked	¼ cup	10	Tr	0	2	Tr	2	Tr	0
Whole, cooked	1	40	Tr	0	10	1	9	1	0
Lemon, fresh, 2 ¼" dia	1	20	Tr	0	12	5	7	1	0
Lentils, cooked (see also Peas)	½ cup	120	Tr	0	20	8	12	9	0
Lettuce, fresh, raw	***	***	*	*	*	*	*	*	*

	Serving Size	Calories	Fat (g)	Calories from Fat (%)	Total Carbs (g)	Fiber (g)	Net Carbs (g)	Protein (g)	Sugar Alcohol (g)
Bibb, Boston, Butterhead	***	***	*	*	*	*	*	*	*
single leaf	1	0	Tr	0	Tr	Tr	Tr	Tr	0
whole head, 5" dia	1	20	Tr	0	4	2	2	2	0
Green leaf	***	***	*	*	*	*	*	*	*
inner leaf	1	0	Tr	0	Tr	Tr	Tr	Tr	0
pieces, shredded	1 cup	5	Tr	0	1	Tr	1	Tr	0
whole head	1	50	Tr	0	10	5	5	5	0
Iceberg, Crisphead	***	***	*	*	*	*	*	*	*
pieces, shredded	1 cup	10	Tr	0	2	Tr	2	Tr	0
single leaf	1	0	Tr	0	Tr	Tr	Tr	Tr	0
wedge slice, ⅛ of 6" head	1	15	Tr	0	3	1	2	Tr	0
whole head, 6" dia	1	80	Tr	0	16	7	9	5	0
Red leaf	***	***	*	*	*	*	*	*	*
inner leaf	1	0	Tr	0	Tr	0	Tr	Tr	0
pieces, shredded	1 cup	0	Tr	0	Tr	Tr	Tr	Tr	0
whole head	1	50	Tr	0	7	3	4	4	0
Romaine or cos	***	***	*	*	*	*	*	*	*
inner leaf	1	0	Tr	0	Tr	Tr	Tr	Tr	0
pieces, shredded	1 cup	10	Tr	0	2	1	1	Tr	0
whole head	1	110	2	16	21	13	8	8	0
Lime, fresh, 2" dia	1	20	Tr	0	7	2	5	Tr	0
Liver	***	***	*	*	*	*	*	*	*
Beef, fried	3 oz	150	4	24	4	0	4	23	0
Chicken, simmered	3 oz	140	6	39	Tr	0	Tr	21	0
Veal, braised	3 oz	160	5	28	3	0	3	24	0
Liverwurst, pork	2 oz	190	16	76	1	0	1	8	0
Lobster - see Fish/ Seafood	***	***	*	*	*	*	*	*	*
Lunch Meat (thin ⅛" slices)	***	***	*	*	*	*	*	*	*
(see also specific listings)	***	***	*	*	*	*	*	*	*

	Serving Size	Calories	Fat (g)	Calories from Fat (%)	Total Carbs (g)	Fiber (g)	Net Carbs (g)	Protein (g)	Sugar Alcohol (g)
Beef or pork, regular	2 slices	200	18	81	1	0	1	7	0
Chicken, roasted	2 slices	35	Tr	0	Tr	0	Tr	7	0
Chicken, smoked	2 slices	35	Tr	0	Tr	0	Tr	7	0
Ham, extra lean	2 slices	60	1	15	Tr	0	Tr	10	0
Ham, regular	2 slices	90	5	50	2	Tr	2	9	0
Turkey, regular	2 slices	45	Tr	0	2	0	2	7	0
Macaroni, elbows	***	***	*	*	*	*	*	*	*
Plain, cooked	1 cup	220	1	4	43	3	40	8	0
Whole wheat, cooked	1 cup	170	Tr	0	37	4	33	8	0
Macaroni & Cheese	1 cup	300	10	30	40	3	37	10	0
Mackerel - see Fish/Seafood	***	***	*	*	*	*	*	*	*
Malt-O-Meal - see Cereal	***	***	*	*	*	*	*	*	*
Mandarin Orange	***	***	*	*	*	*	*	*	*
Canned, in juice	1 cup	70	Tr	0	18	2	16	1	0
Canned, in light syrup	1 cup	150	Tr	0	41	2	39	1	0
Fresh, whole, 2½"	1	45	Tr	0	12	2	10	Tr	0
Fresh, sections	1 cup	100	Tr	0	26	4	22	2	0
Mango	***	***	*	*	*	*	*	*	*
Fresh, peeled, sliced	1 cup	110	Tr	0	28	3	25	Tr	0
Fresh, whole	1	140	Tr	0	35	4	31	1	0
Margarine - see also Butter	***	***	*	*	*	*	*	*	*
Fat free	1 cup	100	7	63	10	0	10	Tr	0
Fat free	1 Tbsp	5	Tr	0	Tr	0	Tr	Tr	0
Regular, 4 sticks/lb	1 stick	810	91	100	Tr	0	Tr	Tr	0
Regular, hard or soft	1 cup	1630	183	100	2	0	2	Tr	0
Regular, hard or soft	1 Tbsp	100	11	99	Tr	0		Tr	0
Regular, hard or soft	1 pat	35	4	100	Tr	0		Tr	0
Vegetable oil spread, 60 fat	1 cup	1220	137	100	2	0	2	Tr	0
Vegetable oil spread, 60 fat	1 Tbsp	80	8	90	Tr	0	Tr	Tr	0

	Serving Size	Calories	Fat (g)	Calories from Fat (%)	Total Carbs (g)	Fiber (g)	Net Carbs (g)	Protein (g)	Sugar Alcohol (g)
Vegetable oil spread, 20 fat	1 cup	420	47	100	Tr	0		Tr	0
Vegetable oil spread, 20 fat	1 Tbsp	25	3	100	Tr	0		Tr	0
Marjoram, dried spice	1 tsp	0	Tr	0	Tr	Tr	Tr	Tr	0
Marmalade	1 Tbsp	50	0	0	13	Tr	13	Tr	0
Restaurant size packet	½ oz	35	0	0	9	Tr	9	Tr	0
Marshmallow	***	***	*	*	*	*	*	*	*
Miniature size	1 cup	160	Tr	0	41	Tr	41	Tr	0
Regular size	1	25	Tr	0	6	0	6	Tr	0
Peeps marshmallow bunny	1	25	0	0	7	0	7	Tr	0
Marshmallow Topping	1 oz	90	Tr	0	22	0	22	Tr	0
Mayonnaise	***	***	*	*	*	*	*	*	*
Dressing, no cholesterol	1 Tbsp	100	12	100	Tr	0	Tr	0	0
Fat free	1 Tbsp	15	Tr	0	3	Tr	3	Tr	0
Light/reduced calorie	1 Tbsp	50	5	90	1	0	1	Tr	0
w/ olive oil, reduced fat	1 Tbsp	54	6	100	0	0	0	0	0
w/ olive oil, regular	1 Tbsp	100	11	99	0	0	0	0	0
Regular	1 Tbsp	100	11	99	Tr	0	Tr	Tr	0
Regular	1 cup	1580	175	100	7	0	7	2	0
Meat - see specific listings	***	***	*	*	*	*	*	*	*
Meatless Burger - see Soy Burger or Vegetable Burger	***	***	*	*	*	*	*	*	*
Meatloaf - see Frozen Dinner	***	***	*	*	*	*	*	*	*
Meatloaf, vegetarian	1 slice	110	5	41	5	3	2	12	0
Minestrone - see Soup	***	***	*	*	*	*	*	*	*
MIXES, Low Carb	***	***	*	*	*	*	*	*	*
Baking	***	***	*	*	*	*	*	*	*

	Serving Size	Calories	Fat (g)	Calories from Fat (%)	Total Carbs (g)	Fiber (g)	Net Carbs (g)	Protein (g)	Sugar Alcohol (g)
Caulipower Cauliflower-Based Baking Mix	¼ cup	80	0	0	17	3	14	2	0
Caulipower Paleo Cauliflower-Based Baking Mix	¼ cup	90	3	30	15	4	11	3	0
Bread	***	***	*	*	*	*	*	*	*
Julian Bakery PaleoThin Sandwich Bread Mix	⅟₁₆ loaf	80	6	68	7	4	3	3	0
Brownie	***	***	*	*	*	*	*	*	*
Diabetic Kitchen Gourmet Chocolate Brownie Mix	1 svg mix	60	2.5	38	17	15	2	1	0
Keto and Co Fudge Brownie Mix	1 svg mix	45	1	20	16	8	2	2	6
Cake	***	***	*	*	*	*	*	*	*
Diabetic Kitchen Gourmet Chocolate Cake & Cupcake Mix	1 slice or cupcake	120	7	53	20	15	5	4	0
Cocoa	***	***	*	*	*	*	*	*	*
Diabetic Kitchen Gourmet Drinking Chocolate	2 Tbsp	35	2	51	10	8	2	2	0
Kiss My Keto Keto Cocoa	1 scoop	70	7	90	3	3	0	1	0
Donut	***	***	*	*	*	*	*	*	*
Diabetic Kitchen Cinnamon Donut Mix	1 svg mix	50	3	54	10	8	2	1	0
Muffin	***	***	*	*	*	*	*	*	*
Diabetic Kitchen Banana Muffin Mix	1 svg mix	100	6	54	21	15	6	3	0
Diabetic Kitchen Cheesy Bread Muffin Mix	1 svg mix	60	3.5	53	10	7	3	2	0

	Serving Size	Calories	Fat (g)	Calories from Fat (%)	Total Carbs (g)	Fiber (g)	Net Carbs (g)	Protein (g)	Sugar Alcohol (g)
Diabetic Kitchen Cinnamon Muffin Mix	1 svg mix	110	6	49	22	17	5	3	0
Pancake	***	***	*	*	*	*	*	*	*
Diabetic Kitchen Pancake & Waffle Mix	1 svg mix	90	5	50	16	10	6	3	0
Julian Bakery PaleoThin Pancake & Waffle Mix	1 pancake	170	13	69	7	1	6	9	0
Pizza Crust	***	***	*	*	*	*	*	*	*
Julian Bakery Paleo Thin Pizza Crust Mix	1 slice	130	7	48	15	2	13	4	0
Molasses	1 Tbsp	60	Tr	0	15	0	15	0	0
Molasses	1 cup	980	Tr	0	252	0	252	0	0
Mortadella	1 slice	50	4	72	Tr	0	Tr	3	0
Muffin, sm size, 2 ¾" dia	***	***	*	*	*	*	*	*	*
Blueberry	1	260	13	45	33	1	32	4	0
Blueberry, low fat	1	180	3	15	36	3	33	3	0
Corn	1	200	6	27	34	2	32	4	0
Oat bran	1	180	5	25	32	3	29	5	0
Plain	1	170	7	37	24	2	22	4	0
Muffin, Low Carb	***	***	*	*	*	*	*	*	*
ThinSlim Foods	***	***	*	*	*	*	*	*	*
Banana	1	40	1	23	20	8	2	6	10
Blueberry	1	40	1	23	20	8	2	6	10
Chocolate	1	45	1	20	20	8	2	6	10
Chocolate Bliss	1	50	1	18	21	8	3	6	10
Cinnamon	1	40	1	23	20	8	2	6	10
Peanut Butter Chocolate Chip	1	45	1	20	20	8	2	6	10
Pumpkin Spice	1	40	1	23	20	8	2	6	10
Vanilla	1	40	1	23	20	8	2	6	10

	Serving Size	Calories	Fat (g)	Calories from Fat (%)	Total Carbs (g)	Fiber (g)	Net Carbs (g)	Protein (g)	Sugar Alcohol (g)
Mulberries	1 cup	60	Tr	0	14	2	12	2	0
Mushroom	***	***	*	*	*	*	*	*	*
Chanterelle, fresh	1 cup	21	Tr	0	4	2	2	1	0
Cremini (baby bella), fresh, sliced	1 cup	20	Tr	0	3	Tr	3	2	0
Enoki, fresh, whole	1 cup	30	Tr	0	5	2	3	2	0
Maitake, fresh, diced	1 cup	25	Tr	0	5	2	3	1	0
Morel, fresh	1 cup	21	Tr	0	3	2	1	2	0
Oyster, fresh, sliced	1 cup	35	Tr	0	6	2	4	3	0
Porcini, dried	1 oz	100	1	9	14	5	9	9	0
Portobello, fresh, cap	3 oz	18	Tr	0	3	1	2	2	0
Portobello, fresh, chopped	1 cup	19	Tr	0	3	1	2	2	0
Shiitake, fresh	4 ea	26	Tr	0	5	2	3	2	0
Straw, canned, drained	1 cup	60	1	15	8	5	3	7	0
White Button	***	***	*	*	*	*	*	*	*
Canned, drained solids	1 cup	40	Tr	0	8	4	4	3	0
Diced	1 cup	20	Tr	0	4	1	3	2	0
Dried, whole	4	45	Tr	0	11	2	9	1	0
Fresh, cooked, pieces	1 cup	80	Tr	0	21	3	18	2	0
Fresh, raw, slices	1 cup	15	Tr	0	2	Tr	2	2	0
Fresh, sliced, cooked	1 cup	45	Tr	0	8	3	5	3	0
Grilled, sliced	1 cup	40	Tr	0	6	3	3	5	0
Whole	1	20	Tr	0	4	1	3	2	0
Mussels - see Fish/Seafood	***	***	*	*	*	*	*	*	*
Mustard	***	***	*	*	*	*	*	*	*
Brown, spicy	1 tsp	5	0	0	0	0	0	0	0
Dijon	1 tsp	5	0	0	0	0	0	0	0
Honey	1 tsp	7	Tr	0	1	Tr	1	Tr	0

	Serving Size	Calories	Fat (g)	Calories from Fat (%)	Total Carbs (g)	Fiber (g)	Net Carbs (g)	Protein (g)	Sugar Alcohol (g)
Whole grain, honey	1 tsp	12	Tr	0	2	Tr	2	Tr	0
Yellow	1 tsp	0	Tr	0	Tr	Tr	Tr	Tr	0
Mustard Seed, ground, yellow	1 tsp	15	Tr	0	1	Tr	1	Tr	0
Mustard Greens	***	***	*	*	*	*	*	*	*
Fresh, chopped, cooked	1 cup	20	Tr	0	3	3	0	3	0
Frozen, chopped, cooked	1 cup	30	Tr	0	5	4	1	3	0
Nectarine, fresh, med, 2½" dia	1	60	Tr	0	15	2	13	2	0
Fresh, sliced	1 cup	60	Tr	0	15	2	13	2	0
Noodles	***	***	*	*	*	*	*	*	*
Chow mein noodles	1 cup	240	14	53	26	2	24	4	0
Egg noodles, dry, uncooked	1 cup	150	2	12	27	1	26	5	0
Egg noodles, plain, cooked	1 cup	220	3	12	40	2	38	7	0
Rice noodles, cooked	1 cup	190	Tr	0	44	2	42	2	0
Shirataki noodles	4 oz	10	0	0	3	3	0	0	0
Spinach noodles, dry	1 cup	150	2	12	27	3	24	6	0
Spinach noodles, cooked	1 cup	210	3	13	39	4	35	8	0
NUTS	***	***	*	*	*	*	*	*	*
Almonds	***	***	*	*	*	*	*	*	*
blanched, whole	1 oz	170	14	74	6	3	3	6	0
dry roasted, whole	1 oz	170	15	79	6	3	3	6	0
honey roasted, whole	1 oz	170	14	74	8	4	4	5	0
sliced	¼ cup	130	11	76	5	3	2	5	0
slivered	¼ cup	156	13	75	6	3	3	6	0
whole, about 23	1 oz	160	14	79	6	4	2	6	0
Brazil nuts, whole, about 6	1 oz	190	19	90	4	2	2	4	0

	Serving Size	Calories	Fat (g)	Calories from Fat (%)	Total Carbs (g)	Fiber (g)	Net Carbs (g)	Protein (g)	Sugar Alcohol (g)
Cashews, whole, dry roasted, about 18	1 oz	160	13	73	9	Tr	9	4	0
Chestnuts, roasted, shelled, about 3	1 oz	70	Tr	0	15	1	14	Tr	0
Coconut - see Coconut	***	***	*	*	*	*	*	*	*
Hazelnuts, about 21	1 oz	180	17	85	5	3	2	4	0
Macadamia nuts, about 11	1 oz	200	22	99	4	2	2	2	0
Mixed nuts w/ peanuts, dry roasted	1 oz	170	15	79	7	3	4	5	0
Mixed nuts w/ peanuts, oil roasted	1 oz	180	16	80	6	3	3	5	0
Mixed nuts w/o peanuts, oil roasted	1 oz	170	16	85	6	2	4	4	0
Peanuts	***	***	*	*	*	*	*	*	*
boiled	1 oz	90	6	60	6	3	3	4	0
dry roasted	1 cup	850	73	77	31	12	19	35	0
dry roasted	1 oz	170	14	74	6	2	4	7	0
oil roasted	1 oz	170	14	74	5	2	3	8	0
Pecans	***	***	*	*	*	*	*	*	*
chopped	½ cup	380	39	92	8	5	3	5	0
halves, about 19 or 20	1 oz	200	20	90	4	3	1	3	0
Pine nuts	1 oz	190	19	90	4	1	3	4	0
Pistachio nuts, shelled, about 49	1 oz	160	13	73	8	3	5	6	0
Walnuts, English	***	***	*	*	*	*	*	*	*
chopped	¼ cup	190	19	90	4	2	2	5	0
halves, about 14	1 oz	190	19	90	4	2	2	4	0
Nut Butter	***	***	*	*	*	*	*	*	*
Adapt Your Life Chocolate Praline	1 pkt	144	10	63	2	2	0	12	0
Adapt Your Life Salted Caramel	1 pkt	148	10	61	2	1	1	13	0
Almond	1 Tbsp	100	10	90	3	Tr	3	2	0

	Serving Size	Calories	Fat (g)	Calories from Fat (%)	Total Carbs (g)	Fiber (g)	Net Carbs (g)	Protein (g)	Sugar Alcohol (g)
Justin's Classic Almond Butter	2 Tbsp	190	18	85	6	3	3	7	0
Cashew	1 Tbsp	90	8	80	4	Tr	4	3	0
Hazelnut	1 Tbsp	90	8	80	3	2	1	3	0
Peanut - see Peanut Butter	***	***	*	*	*	*	*	*	*
Perfect Keto Nut Butter	2 Tbsp	210	20	86	7	5	2	4	0
Sunflower Seed - see Sunflower Seed Butter	***	***	*	*	*	*	*	*	*
Oat Bran	***	***	*	*	*	*	*	*	*
Cooked	1 cup	90	2	20	25	6	19	7	0
Uncooked	1 cup	230	7	27	62	15	47	16	0
Oatmeal, plain, as prep w/ water	¾ cup	120	3	23	21	3	18	5	0
Oats, steel cut, dry	1 cup	610	11	16	103	17	86	26	0
Oats, traditional, old fashioned, rolled, dry	1 cup	371	6	15	66	9	57	13	0
OIL (for cooking & salads)	***	***	*	*	*	*	*	*	*
Avocado	1 cup	1980	224	100	0	0	0	0	0
Avocado	1 Tbsp	124	14	100	0	0	0	0	0
Canola	1 cup	1930	218	100	0	0	0	0	0
Canola	1 Tbsp	120	14	100	0	0	0	0	0
Cooking spray - see *PAM*	***	***	*	*	*	*	*	*	*
Corn	1 cup	1930	218	100	0	0	0	0	0
Corn	1 Tbsp	120	14	100	0	0	0	0	0
Cottonseed/soybean blend	1 cup	1930	218	100	0	0	0	0	0
Cottonseed/soybean blend	1 Tbsp	120	14	100	0	0	0	0	0
Grapeseed	1 cup	1930	218	100	0	0	0	0	0
Grapeseed	1 Tbsp	120	14	100	0	0	0	0	0
MCT oil, *Piping Rock*	1 Tbsp	100	14	100	0	0	0	0	0

	Serving Size	Calories	Fat (g)	Calories from Fat (%)	Total Carbs (g)	Fiber (g)	Net Carbs (g)	Protein (g)	Sugar Alcohol (g)
Olive, regular or extra virgin	1 cup	1910	216	100	0	0	0	0	0
Olive, regular or extra virgin	1 Tbsp	120	14	100	0	0	0	0	0
Peanut	1 cup	1910	216	100	0	0	0	0	0
Peanut	1 Tbsp	120	14	100	0	0	0	0	0
Safflower	1 cup	1930	218	100	0	0	0	0	0
Safflower	1 Tbsp	120	14	100	0	0	0	0	0
Sesame, light or dark	1 cup	1930	218	100	0	0	0	0	0
Sesame, light or dark	1 Tbsp	120	14	100	0	0	0	0	0
Soybean	1 cup	1930	218	100	0	0	0	0	0
Soybean	1 Tbsp	120	14	100	0	0	0	0	0
Sunflower	1 cup	1930	218	100	0	0	0	0	0
Sunflower	1 Tbsp	120	14	100	0	0	0	0	0
Vegetable	1 cup	1928	218	100	0	0	0	0	0
Vegetable	1 Tbsp	121	14	100	0	0	0	0	0
Okra	***	***	*	*	*	*	*	*	*
Fresh, sliced, cooked	½ cup	20	Tr	0	4	2	2	2	0
Frozen, slices, cooked	½ cup	25	Tr	0	5	3	2	2	0
Whole, 3" pods, cooked	8 ea	20	Tr	0	4	2	2	2	0
Olive	***	***	*	*	*	*	*	*	*
Black, canned, lg size	5	25	2	72	1	Tr	1	Tr	0
Pickled, green, med size	5	20	2	90	Tr	Tr	Tr	Tr	0
Olive Loaf, 2 slices	2 oz	130	9	62	5	0	5	7	0
Onion	***	***	*	*	*	*	*	*	*
Pearl, frozen, cooked	1 cup	52	0	0	12	2	10	1	0
Round red, white, or yellow	***	***	*	*	*	*	*	*	*
Cooked, boiled, sliced or chopped	1 cup	90	Tr	0	21	3	18	3	0

	Serving Size	Calories	Fat (g)	Calories from Fat (%)	Total Carbs (g)	Fiber (g)	Net Carbs (g)	Protein (g)	Sugar Alcohol (g)
Cooked, boiled, whole, 2½" dia	1	40	Tr	0	10	1	9	1	0
Cooked, sautéed, chopped	1 cup	120	9	68	7	2	5	Tr	0
Fresh, chopped	1 cup	60	Tr	0	15	3	12	2	0
Fresh, raw, whole, 2½" dia	1	45	Tr	0	10	2	8	1	0
Fresh, sliced, ⅛" thick	1 slice	5	Tr	0	1	Tr	1	Tr	0
Frozen, cooked, boiled, whole	1 cup	60	Tr	0	14	3	11	2	0
Spring onion w/ green tops & bulb	***	***	*	*	*	*	*	*	*
Fresh, chopped	1 whole	10	Tr	0	2	Tr	2	Tr	0
Fresh, chopped	1 cup	30	Tr	0	7	3	4	2	0
Fresh, tops only, chopped	1 Tbsp	0	Tr	0	Tr	Tr	Tr	Tr	0
Sweet onion, raw	1 whole	110	Tr	0	25	3	22	3	0
Onion Flakes, dried	1 Tbsp	15	Tr	0	4	Tr	4	Tr	0
Onion Powder or Salt	1 tsp	10	Tr	0	2	Tr	2	Tr	0
Onion Rings, breaded, fried, med size	5 ea	120	8	60	12	Tr	12	2	0
Orange	***	***	*	*	*	*	*	*	*
Fresh, large size, 3" dia	1	90	Tr	0	22	4	18	2	0
Fresh, sections	1 cup	90	Tr	0	21	4	17	2	0
Oregano, dried, leaves	1 tsp	0	Tr	0	Tr	Tr	Tr	Tr	0
Dried, ground	1 tsp	5	Tr	0	1	Tr	1	Tr	0
PAM, nonstick cooking spray, ⅓ second spray	1 spray	0	0	0	0	0	0	0	0
PAM, Baking, ⅓ second spray	1 spray	0	0	0	0	0	0	0	0
Pancake, 4" dia	***	***	*	*	*	*	*	*	*
Frozen	1	90	2	20	16	1	15	2	0
Kellogg's Eggo Buttermilk Pancake	1	90	3	30	15	Tr	15	2	0

	Serving Size	Calories	Fat (g)	Calories from Fat (%)	Total Carbs (g)	Fiber (g)	Net Carbs (g)	Protein (g)	Sugar Alcohol (g)
Paleo, grain free, mix, *Bob's Red Mill*	⅓ cup	192	9	42	20	3	17	7	0
Regular, from mix	1	80	3	34	11	Tr	11	3	0
Whole wheat, from mix	1	90	3	30	13	1	12	4	0
Pancake Syrup - see Syrup	***	***	*	*	*	*	*	*	*
Papaya	***	***	*	*	*	*	*	*	*
Fresh, peeled, 5" long x 3" dia	1	120	Tr	0	30	6	24	2	0
Fresh, peeled, cubed	1 cup	60	Tr	0	14	3	11	Tr	0
Paprika, dried powder	1 tsp	5	Tr	0	1	Tr	1	Tr	0
Parsley	***	***	*	*	*	*	*	*	*
Dried, leaves	1 Tbsp	0	Tr	0	Tr	Tr	Tr	Tr	0
Freeze dried, leaves	1 Tbsp	0	Tr	0	Tr	Tr	Tr	Tr	0
Fresh, chopped	¼ cup	5	Tr	0	Tr	Tr	Tr	Tr	0
Fresh, whole sprigs	10	0	Tr	0	Tr	Tr	Tr	Tr	0
Parsnip	***	***	*	*	*	*	*	*	*
Sliced, cooked	½ cup	60	Tr	0	13	3	10	1	
Whole, 9" long, cooked	1	110	Tr	0	27	6	21	2	
Passion Fruit, raw, avg size	1	15	Tr	0	4	2	2	Tr	
PASTA, Alternative	***	***	*	*	*	*	*	*	*
Cali'flour Foods Cauliflower & Yellow Lentil Penne Pasta	2 oz	190	0	0	34	3	31	14	0
Explore Cuisine Edamame Spaghetti, dry	2 oz	180	3.5	18	20	13	7	24	0
Explore Cuisine Black Bean Spaghetti, dry	2 oz	180	3	15	19	11	8	25	0
Julian Bakery PaleoThin Fettuccine	3.5 oz	10	0	0	3	2	1	0	0

	Serving Size	Calories	Fat (g)	Calories from Fat (%)	Total Carbs (g)	Fiber (g)	Net Carbs (g)	Protein (g)	Sugar Alcohol (g)
Julian Bakery PaleoThin Noodles (Angel Hair)	3.5 oz	10	0	0	3	2	1	0	0
ThinSlim Foods Impastable Low Carb Pasta, all shapes	2 oz	55	0.5	8	44	36	8	4	0
PASTA, Regular (see also Noodles & specific listings)	***	***	*	*	*	*	*	*	*
Rice pasta, cooked	1 cup	250	6	22	43	5	38	5	0
Small shells, cooked	1 cup	180	1	5	36	2	34	7	0
Spaghetti	***	***	*	*	*	*	*	*	*
Plain, cooked	1 cup	220	1	4	43	3	40	8	0
Plain, dry	2 oz	210	Tr	0	43	2	41	7	0
Spinach, dry	2 oz	210	Tr	0	43	6	37	8	0
Whole wheat, cooked	1 cup	170	Tr	0	37	6	31	8	0
Spiral shaped, cooked	1 cup	210	1	4	41	2	39	8	0
Tortellini, cheese filled	¾ cup	250	6	22	38	2	36	11	0
Pastrami	***	***	*	*	*	*	*	*	*
Regular, beef	2 oz	80	3	34	0	0	0	12	0
Regular, beef, 98 fat free	2 oz	50	Tr	0	Tr	0	Tr	11	0
Turkey	2 oz	80	4	45	1	Tr	1	9	0
Pastry - see Danish Pastry & specific listings	***	***	*	*	*	*	*	*	*
Peach	***	***	*	*	*	*	*	*	*
Canned, in heavy syrup	1 cup	190	Tr	0	52	3	49	1	0
Canned, in heavy syrup	1 half	70	Tr	0	20	1	19	Tr	0
Canned, in juice	1 cup	110	Tr	0	29	3	26	2	0
Canned, in juice	1 half	45	Tr	0	11	1	10	Tr	0
Canned, in light syrup	1 cup	140	Tr	0	37	3	34	1	0

	Serving Size	Calories	Fat (g)	Calories from Fat (%)	Total Carbs (g)	Fiber (g)	Net Carbs (g)	Protein (g)	Sugar Alcohol (g)
Canned, in light syrup	1 half	50	Tr	0	14	1	13	Tr	0
Dried, halves	3	90	Tr	0	24	3	21	1	0
Fresh, sliced	1 cup	60	1	15	15	2	13	1	0
Fresh, whole, med, 2⅔" dia	1	60	Tr	0	14	2	12	1	0
Frozen, sweetened slices, thawed	1 cup	240	Tr	0	60	5	55	2	0
Peanut - see Nuts	***	***	*	*	*	*	*	*	*
Peanut Butter	***	***	*	*	*	*	*	*	*
Powdered, *PB2*	2 Tbsp	50	1.5	27	5	2	3	5	0
Reduced fat, smooth	2 Tbsp	170	11	58	11	2	9	8	0
Regular, chunky	2 Tbsp	190	16	76	7	3	4	8	0
Regular, smooth	2 Tbsp	190	16	76	6	2	4	8	0
Pear	***	***	*	*	*	*	*	*	*
Canned, in heavy syrup	1 cup	200	Tr	0	51	4	47	Tr	0
Canned, in heavy syrup	1 half	60	Tr	0	15	1	14	Tr	0
Canned, in juice	1 cup	120	Tr	0	32	4	28	Tr	0
Canned, in juice	1 half	40	Tr	0	10	1	9	Tr	0
Canned, in light syrup	1 cup	140	Tr	0	38	4	34	Tr	0
Canned, in light syrup	1 half	45	Tr	0	12	1	11	Tr	0
Fresh, Asian, 3" dia	1	120	Tr	0	29	10	19	1	0
Fresh, other varieties, sliced	1 cup	80	Tr	0	22	4	18	Tr	0
Fresh, other varieties, whole, med	1	100	Tr	0	28	6	22	Tr	0
Peas (cooked w/o fats)	***	***	*	*	*	*	*	*	*
Green peas, baby, canned	½ cup	60	Tr	0	10	4	6	4	0
Green peas, canned	½ cup	60	Tr	0	11	4	7	4	0
Green peas, fresh, shelled	½ cup	70	Tr	0	13	4	9	4	0

	Serving Size	Calories	Fat (g)	Calories from Fat (%)	Total Carbs (g)	Fiber (g)	Net Carbs (g)	Protein (g)	Sugar Alcohol (g)
Green peas, frozen	½ cup	60	Tr	0	11	4	7	4	0
Lentils	½ cup	120	Tr	0	20	8	12	9	0
Pigeon peas (red gram)	½ cup	100	Tr	0	20	6	14	6	0
Split peas	½ cup	120	Tr	0	21	8	13	8	0
Pea Pods	***	***	*	*	*	*	*	*	*
Fresh, cooked	½ cup	35	Tr	0	6	2	4	3	0
Fresh, raw, chopped	½ cup	20	Tr	0	4	1	3	1	0
Fresh, raw, whole	1 cup	25	Tr	0	5	2	3	2	0
Frozen, cooked	½ cup	40	Tr	0	7	3	4	3	0
Peas and Carrots	***	***	*	*	*	*	*	*	*
Canned	½ cup	50	Tr	0	11	3	8	3	0
Frozen, cooked	½ cup	40	Tr	0	8	3	5	3	0
Peas and Onions	***	***	*	*	*	*	*	*	*
Canned	½ cup	30	Tr	0	5	1	4	2	0
Frozen, cooked	½ cup	40	Tr	0	8	2	6	2	0
Pecan - see Nuts	***	***	*	*	*	*	*	*	*
Pecan Pie	1 slice	540	22	37	79	3	76	6	0
Pepper, dried powder or granules	***	***	*	*	*	*	*	*	*
Black	1 tsp	5	Tr	0	1	Tr	1	Tr	0
Cayenne or red	1 tsp	5	Tr	0	1	Tr	1	Tr	0
White	1 tsp	5	Tr	0	2	Tr	2	Tr	0
Pepperoni, 14 slices	1 oz	140	12	77	0	0	0	6	0
Peppers	***	***	*	*	*	*	*	*	*
Banana, sliced	¼ cup	10	0	0	2	0	2	0	0
Chili, hot, red or green	***	***	*	*	*	*	*	*	*
canned, chopped	½ cup	15	Tr	0	4	4	4	Tr	0
fresh, chopped	½ cup	30	Tr	0	7	1	6	2	0
fresh, whole	1	20	Tr	0	4	Tr	4	Tr	0
Green, sweet	***	***	*	*	*	*	*	*	*
canned, chopped	1 cup	25	Tr	0	6	2	4	1	0

	Serving Size	Calories	Fat (g)	Calories from Fat (%)	Total Carbs (g)	Fiber (g)	Net Carbs (g)	Protein (g)	Sugar Alcohol (g)
raw, chopped	1 cup	30	Tr	0	7	3	4	1	0
raw, sliced	1 cup	20	Tr	0	4	2	2	Tr	0
raw, whole, lg, 3" dia	1	35	Tr	0	8	3	5	1	0
Jalapeno	***	***	*	*	*	*	*	*	*
canned, sliced	1 cup	30	Tr	0	5	3	2	Tr	0
fresh, sliced	1 cup	25	1	36	5	3	2	1	0
fresh, whole	1	0	Tr	0	Tr	Tr	Tr	Tr	0
Pasilla, dried, whole	1	25	Tr	0	4	2	2	Tr	0
Red, sweet	***	***	*	*	*	*	*	*	*
canned, diced or pieces	½ cup	60	0	0	13	2	11	1	0
canned, halves	1 cup	25	Tr	0	6	2	4	1	0
raw, chopped	1 cup	45	Tr	0	9	3	6	2	0
raw, sliced	1 cup	30	Tr	0	6	2	4	Tr	0
raw, whole, lg, 3" dia	1	50	Tr	0	10	3	7	2	0
Red or green, sweet, chopped, cooked	1 cup	40	Tr	0	9	2	7	1	0
Yellow, sweet, raw	***	***	*	*	*	*	*	*	*
strips	10	15	Tr	0	3	Tr	3	Tr	0
whole, lg, 3" dia	1	50	Tr	0	12	2	10	2	0
Persimmon	***	***	*	*	*	*	*	*	*
Japanese, fresh, whole	1	120	Tr	0	31	6	25	Tr	0
Native, fresh, whole	1	30	Tr	0	8	2	6	Tr	0
Pickle	***	***	*	*	*	*	*	*	*
Bread & Butter slices	6	40	Tr	0	10	Tr	10	Tr	0
Dill, spear	1	0	Tr	0	Tr	Tr	Tr	Tr	0
Dill, whole, 4" long	1	15	Tr	0	4	2	2	Tr	0
Sour, spear	1	0	Tr	0	Tr	Tr	Tr	Tr	0
Sour, whole, 4" long	1	15	Tr	0	3	2	1	Tr	0
Sweet Gherkin, whole, lg, 3" long	1	30	Tr	0	7	Tr	7	Tr	0

	Serving Size	Calories	Fat (g)	Calories from Fat (%)	Total Carbs (g)	Fiber (g)	Net Carbs (g)	Protein (g)	Sugar Alcohol (g)
Sweet Gherkin, whole, sm, 2⅛" long	1	5	Tr	0	1	Tr	1	Tr	0
Pickle Relish	1 Tbsp	20	Tr	0	5	Tr	5	Tr	0
Restaurant size packet	1	15	Tr	0	4	Tr	4	Tr	0
Pie (⅛ of 9" pie, unless noted)	***	***	*	*	*	*	*	*	*
Apple	1 slice	300	14	42	43	2	41	2	0
Banana Cream, ⅙ of 8" pie	1 slice	397	20	45	49	1	48	6	0
Blueberry	1 slice	290	13	40	44	1	43	2	
Boston Cream - see Cake	***	***	*	*	*	*	*	*	*
Cherry	1 slice	330	14	38	50	1	49	3	0
Cherry, fried pie, 5" x 3¾"	1	400	21	47	55	3	52	4	0
Chocolate Cream, ⅙ of 8" pie	1 slice	340	22	58	38	2	36	3	0
Coconut Creme, ⅙ of 7" pie	1 slice	190	11	52	24	Tr	24	1	0
Coconut Custard, ⅙ of 8" pie	1 slice	270	14	47	31	2	29	6	0
Dutch Apple	1 slice	400	16	36	61	2	59	3	0
Lemon Meringue, ⅙ of 8" pie	1 slice	300	10	30	53	1	52	2	0
Lemon, fried pie, 5" x 3¾"	1	400	21	47	55	3	52	4	0
Peach, ⅙ of 8" pie	1 slice	260	12	42	39	Tr	39	2	0
Pecan	1 slice	540	22	37	79	3	76	6	0
Pumpkin	1 slice	320	13	37	46	2	44	5	0
Pie Crust, 9" dia	***	***	*	*	*	*	*	*	*
Chocolate wafer, from recipe	1 crust	1130	69	55	121	3	118	11	0
Chocolate wafer, ready crust	1 crust	880	41	42	117	5	112	11	0
Graham cracker, from recipe	1 crust	1180	60	46	156	4	152	10	0

	Serving Size	Calories	Fat (g)	Calories from Fat (%)	Total Carbs (g)	Fiber (g)	Net Carbs (g)	Protein (g)	Sugar Alcohol (g)
Graham cracker, ready crust	1 crust	920	45	44	118	4	114	9	0
Regular, from dry mix	1 crust	800	49	55	81	3	78	11	0
Regular, from frozen	1 crust	78087		0	5	82	10	44	0
Regular, from recipe	1 crust	950	62	59	86	3	83	12	0
Vanilla wafer, from recipe	1 crust	940	64	61	88	Tr	88	7	0
Pilaf - see Rice Pilaf	***	***	*	*	*	*	*	*	*
Pineapple	***	***	*	*	*	*	*	*	*
Canned, in heavy syrup	***	***	*	*	*	*	*	*	*
chunks or crushed	1 cup	200	Tr	0	51	2	49	Tr	0
sliced, 3" dia	1	40	Tr	0	10	Tr	10	Tr	0
Canned, in juice	***	***	*	*	*	*	*	*	*
chunks or crushed	1 cup	150	Tr	0	39	2	37	1	0
sliced, 3" dia	1	30	Tr	0	7	Tr	7	Tr	0
Canned, in light syrup	***	***	*	*	*	*	*	*	*
chunks or crushed	1 cup	130	Tr	0	34	2	32	Tr	0
sliced, 3" dia	1	25	Tr	0	7	Tr	7	Tr	0
Fresh, chunks	1 cup	80	Tr	0	22	2	22	Tr	0
Fresh, slice, ½" dia	1	30	Tr	0	7	Tr	7	Tr	0
Frozen, chunks, sweetened	1 cup	210	Tr	0	54	3	51	Tr	0
PIZZA (Listings for an avg size slice, ⅛ of 14" pizza)	***	***	*	*	*	*	*	*	*
Thin Crust, Cheese	1 slice	190	10	47	17	1	16	9	0
Regular Crust	***	***	*	*	*	*	*	*	*
Cheese	1 slice	270	10	33	34	2	32	12	0
Meat & Vegetables	1 slice	330	15	41	35	3	32	15	0
Pepperoni & Cheese	1 slice	300	12	36	34	2	32	13	0
Thick Crust, Cheese	1 slice	290	12	37	33	2	31	13	0
Frozen/Refrigerated	***	***	*	*	*	*	*	*	*

	Serving Size	Calories	Fat (g)	Calories from Fat (%)	Total Carbs (g)	Fiber (g)	Net Carbs (g)	Protein (g)	Sugar Alcohol (g)
Caulipower, Three Cheese	½ pie	380	18	43	37	3	34	16	0
Caulipower, Margherita	½ pie	330	15	41	37	3	34	12	0
Caulipower, Veggie	½ pie	310	14	41	37	3	34	10	0
Caulipower, Uncured Pepperoni	⅓ pie	270	14	47	26	2	24	9	0
Caulipower, Uncured Turkey Pepperoni	⅓ pie	250	11	40	27	2	25	10	0
Healthy Choice, cheese	1 pizza	350	5	13	55	5	50	20	0
Healthy Choice, pepperoni	1 pizza	350	5	13	54	5	49	22	0
Healthy Choice, supreme	1 pizza	340	4	11	53	4	49	20	0
Lean Cuisine, deluxe	1 pizza	350	8	21	50	3	47	19	0
Lean Cuisine, margherita	1 pizza	340	9	24	50	3	47	14	0
Lean Cuisine, pepperoni	1 pizza	370	9	22	53	4	49	20	0
Quest Thin Crust, 4 Cheese	½ pie	330	21	57	24	18	6	27	0
Quest Thin Crust, Supreme Thin	⅓ pie	260	17	59	17	12	5	20	0
Quest Thin Crust, Uncured Pepperoni	½ pie	340	21	56	24	18	6	28	0
Smart Ones, four cheese	1 pizza	370	7	17	57	4	53	18	0
Smart Ones, pepperoni	1 pizza	390	8	18	58	4	54	20	0
Pizza Crust	***	***	*	*	*	*	*	*	*
Cali'Flour Foods Cali'Lite Pizza Crust, all flavors	⅓ crust	60	3	45	2	1	1	5	0
Cali'flour Foods Cauliflower Pizza Crust, all flavors	⅓ crust	150	10	60	8	4	4	8	0

	Serving Size	Calories	Fat (g)	Calories from Fat (%)	Total Carbs (g)	Fiber (g)	Net Carbs (g)	Protein (g)	Sugar Alcohol (g)
Cali'Flour Foods Traditional Pizza Crust, all flavors	⅓ crust	90	6	60	2	1	1	8	0
Caulipower Paleo Cauliflower Pizza Crust	⅓ crust	170	10	53	17	3	14	4	0
Caulipower Cauliflower Pizza Crust	⅓ crust	170	6	32	26	2	24	2	0
Outer Aisle Gourmet Cauliflower Pizza Crust	1 crust	120	6	45	4	1	3	10	0
ThinSlim Foods Love-the-Taste Low Carb Pizza Crust	¼ crust	90	4	40	14	14	0	14	0
Trader Joe's Cauliflower Pizza Crust	⅙ crust	80	0	0	17	1	16	1	0
Plantain, peeled	***	***	*	*	*	*	*	*	*
Cooked, mashed	1 cup	230	Tr	0	62	5	57	2	0
Cooked, slices	1 cup	180	Tr	0	48	4	44	1	0
Fresh, whole, medium size	1	220	Tr	0	57	4	53	2	0
Plum	***	***	*	*	*	*	*	*	*
Canned, in heavy syrup	1 cup	230	Tr	0	60	2	58	Tr	0
Canned, in juice	1 cup	150	Tr	0	38	2	36	1	0
Canned, in light syrup	1 cup	160	Tr	0	41	2	39	Tr	0
Dried - see Prunes	***	***	*	*	*	*	*	*	*
Fresh, sliced	1 cup	80	Tr	0	19	2	17	1	0
Fresh, whole, med, 2⅛" dia	1	30	Tr	0	8	Tr	8	Tr	0
Pomegranate	***	***	*	*	*	*	*	*	*
Fresh, seeds	½ cup	70	1	13	16	4	12	2	0
Fresh, whole, 4" dia	1	230	3	12	53	11	42	5	0
Pop Tart - see Toaster Pastry	***	***	*	*	*	*	*	*	*
Popcorn	***	***	*	*	*	*	*	*	*
Air popped	1 cup	30	Tr	0	6	1	5	1	0

	Serving Size	Calories	Fat (g)	Calories from Fat (%)	Total Carbs (g)	Fiber (g)	Net Carbs (g)	Protein (g)	Sugar Alcohol (g)
Caramel coated w/ peanuts	⅔ cup	110	2	16	23	1	22	2	0
Cheese flavored	1 cup	60	4	60	6	1	5	1	0
Microwave, butter flavor	1 cup	40	2	45	5	Tr	5	Tr	0
Microwave, butter, reduced fat	1 cup	30	Tr	0	6	1	5	1	0
Microwave, 94 fat free	1 cup	30	Tr	0	6	1	5	Tr	0
Popped in oil	1 cup	60	3	45	6	1	5	Tr	0
Popcorn Cake, plain	1	60	3	45	6	1	5	Tr	0
Popsicle - see Frozen Dessert	***	***	*	*	*	*	*	*	*
PORK	***	***	*	*	*	*	*	*	*
(Weights for meat w/o bones)	***	***	*	*	*	*	*	*	*
Bacon	***	***	*	*	*	*	*	*	*
Canadian	2 slices	90	4	40	Tr	0	Tr	11	0
regular	1 slice	45	3	60	Tr	0	Tr	3	0
thick cut	2 slices	110	9	74	0	0	0	8	0
Boston Butt, braised	***	***	*	*	*	*	*	*	*
lean & fat	3 oz	230	15	59	0	0	0	21	0
lean only	3 oz	200	11	50	0	0	0	23	0
Chopped, cooked	2 oz	70	3	39	1	0	1	9	0
Picnic Pork, roasted	***	***	*	*	*	*	*	*	*
lean & fat	3 oz	270	20	67	0	0	0	20	0
lean only	3 oz	190	11	52	0	0	0	23	0
Pork Chop, loin cut	***	***	*	*	*	*	*	*	*
broiled, lean & fat	3 oz	220	13	53	0	0	0	24	0
broiled, lean only	3 oz	180	9	45	0	0	0	25	0
pan fried, lean & fat	3 oz	230	15	59	0	0	0	22	0
pan fried, lean only	3 oz	190	10	47	0	0	0	24	0
Rib Roast, lean & fat	3 oz	210	10	43	0	0	0	24	0

	Serving Size	Calories	Fat (g)	Calories from Fat (%)	Total Carbs (g)	Fiber (g)	Net Carbs (g)	Protein (g)	Sugar Alcohol (g)
lean only	3 oz	180	9	45	0	0	0	25	0
Ribs, country style, roasted	***	***	*	*	*	*	*	*	*
lean & fat	3 oz	280	22	71	0	0	0	20	0
lean only	3 oz	210	13	56	0	0	0	23	0
Sausage	***	***	*	*	*	*	*	*	*
breakfast, link	1	65	5	69	Tr	0	Tr	4	0
liver (braunschweiger), ¼" slice	1	60	5	75	Tr	0	Tr	3	0
liverwurst, ¼" slice	1	60	5	75	Tr	0	Tr	3	0
Oscar Mayer, pork sausage links	2	170	15	79	Tr	0	Tr	8	0
Polish kielbasa	2 oz	190	16	76	Tr	0	Tr	8	0
regular sausage	2 oz	190	16	76	0	0	0	11	0
smoked, 4" link	1	210	19	81	Tr	0	Tr	8	0
Vienna sausage, 2" links	2	70	6	77	Tr	0	Tr	3	0
Scrapple, cooked	2 oz	129	8	56	8	0	8	5	0
Shoulder, roasted	***	***	*	*	*	*	*	*	*
lean & fat	3 oz	250	18	65	0	0	0	20	0
lean only	3 oz	200	12	54	0	0	0	22	0
Spareribs, braised	3 oz	340	26	69	0	0	0	25	0
(Other Pork Products, see:	***	***	*	*	*	*	*	*	*
Bologna, Ham, Hot Dog, Salami & specific entrées)	***	***	*	*	*	*	*	*	*
Pork Rinds	1 oz	150	9	54	0	0	0	17	0
Pot Pie, frozen, heated	***	***	*	*	*	*	*	*	*
Beef	1 pie	590	31	47	59	2	57	19	0
Chicken	1 pie	500	25	45	54	3	51	14	0
Turkey	1 pie	700	35	45	70	4	66	26	0
Banquet	***	***	*	*	*	*	*	*	*
Beef	1 pie	450	27	54	36	2	34	14	0

	Serving Size	Calories	Fat (g)	Calories from Fat (%)	Total Carbs (g)	Fiber (g)	Net Carbs (g)	Protein (g)	Sugar Alcohol (g)
Chicken	1 pie	370	21	51	34	2	32	10	0
Chicken w/ Broccoli	1 pie	350	20	51	32	2	30	10	0
Turkey	1 pie	390	21	48	36	2	34	10	0
Marie Callender's	***	***	*	*	*	*	*	*	*
Beef	1 pie	540	32	53	46	3	43	16	0
Cheesy Chicken	1 pie	600	37	56	46	3	43	17	0
Chicken	1 pie	530	31	53	48	3	45	14	0
Creamy Mushroom & Chicken	1 cup	560	35	56	45	3	42	15	0
Creamy Parmesan Chicken	1 cup	530	32	54	43	2	41	17	0
Honey Roasted Chicken	1 cup	530	30	51	47	3	44	16	0
Turkey	1 cup	530	32	54	45	4	41	15	0
Stouffer's	***	***	*	*	*	*	*	*	*
White Meat Chicken	1 pie	660	37	50	62	2	60	19	0
White Meat Turkey	1 pie	710	41	52	61	2	59	23	0
Pot Roast - see Frozen Dinner	***	***	*	*	*	*	*	*	*
POTATO (see also Sweet Potatoes)	***	***	*	*	*	*	*	*	*
Au Gratin	1 cup	320	19	53	28	4	24	12	0
Baked, med	***	***	*	*	*	*	*	*	*
whole potato, w/ skin	1	160	Tr	0	37	4	33	4	0
whole potato, w/o skin	1	150	Tr	0	34	2	32	3	0
skin only	1	120	Tr	0	27	5	22	3	0
peeled, whole potato	1	120	Tr	0	27	2	25	3	0
peeled, diced	½ cup	70	Tr	0	16	1	15	2	0
French Fries, frozen, heated	***	***	*	*	*	*	*	*	*
regular or crinkle cut	10 ea	120	4	30	19	2	17	2	0

	Serving Size	Calories	Fat (g)	Calories from Fat (%)	Total Carbs (g)	Fiber (g)	Net Carbs (g)	Protein (g)	Sugar Alcohol (g)
steak fries	10 ea	200	5	23	36	4	32	3	0
thin shoestring	10 ea	40	1	23	7	Tr	7	Tr	0
Hash Browns, frozen, heated, 3" x 1½" patty	1	60	3	45	8	Tr	8	Tr	0
Hash Browned potatoes	1 cup	410	20	44	55	5	50	5	0
Mashed, dehydrated, as prep w/ milk & butter	1 cup	230	10	39	30	5	25	4	0
Mashed, w/ milk & butter	1 cup	240	9	34	35	3	32	4	0
Scalloped	1 cup	220	9	37	26	5	21	7	0
Tater Tots/potato puffs, frozen, heated	10	150	7	42	22	2	20	2	0
Potato Chips (about 14 chips, unless noted)	***	***	*	*	*	*	*	*	*
Baked	½ oz	79	3	34	12	1	11	1	0
Barbecue flavor	1 oz	140	9	58	15	1	14	2	0
Cheese flavored	1 oz	140	8	51	16	2	14	2	0
Fat free	1 oz	80	Tr	0	18	2	16	2	0
Plain, regular	1 oz	150	10	60	15	1	14	2	0
Pringles, regular (about 16)	1 oz	150	9	54	15	1	14	1	0
Reduced fat	1 oz	130	6	42	19	2	17	2	0
Ruffles, original	1 oz	160	10	56	14	1	13	2	0
Ruffles, reduced fat	1 oz	140	7	45	18	1	17	2	0
Sour cream & onion flavor	1 oz	150	10	60	15	2	13	2	0
Potato Pancakes, 2¾" dia	1	60	3	45	6	Tr	6	1	0
Potato Salad	1 cup	260	21	73	28	3	25	7	0
Potato Sticks, fried, crunchy	½ cup	90	6	60	10	Tr	10	1	0
Preserves	***	***	*	*	*	*	*	*	*
All flavors, regular	1 Tbsp	60	Tr	0	14	Tr	14	Tr	0

	Serving Size	Calories	Fat (g)	Calories from Fat (%)	Total Carbs (g)	Fiber (g)	Net Carbs (g)	Protein (g)	Sugar Alcohol (g)
Restaurant size packet	½ oz	40	Tr	0	10	Tr	10	Tr	0
Pretzels	***	***	*	*	*	*	*	*	*
Twists	10	230	2	8	48	2	46	6	0
Soft, twisted, med	1	390	4	9	80	2	78	9	0
Soft, *Auntie Anne's*, original	1	310	1	3	65	2	63	8	0
Prickly Pear	***	***	*	*	*	*	*	*	*
Fresh, sliced	1 cup	60	Tr	0	14	5	9	1	0
Fresh, whole	1	40	Tr	0	10	4	6	Tr	0
Prosciutto, Boarshead	1 oz	60	3	45	0	0	0	8	0
Prunes, dried, pitted	***	***	*	*	*	*	*	*	*
Stewed, unsweetened	1 cup	270	Tr	0	70	8	62	2	0
Uncooked, unsweetened	5 ea	110	Tr	0	30	3	27	1	0
Pudding	***	***	*	*	*	*	*	*	*
Banana, regular	4 oz	130	3	21	21	0	21	3	0
instant	4 oz	130	3	21	22	0	22	3	0
Chocolate, regular	½ cup	170	5	26	28	1	27	5	0
fat free	½ cup	110	Tr	0	24	Tr	24	2	0
instant	½ cup	160	5	28	28	2	26	5	0
Coconut Cream, regular	½ cup	160	5	28	25	Tr	25	4	0
instant	½ cup	170	5	26	28	Tr	28	4	0
Lemon, instant	½ cup	170	4	21	30	0	30	4	0
Rice pudding, regular	4 oz	130	3	21	22	1	21	4	0
Tapioca, regular	4 oz	140	4	26	24	0	24	2	0
fat free	4 oz	110	Tr	0	24	0	24	2	0
Vanilla, regular	½ cup	160	4	23	26	Tr	26	4	0
fat free	4 oz	100	0	0	23	0	23	2	0
instant	½ cup	160	4	23	28	0	28	4	0
Puff Pastry, frozen, baked	1 sheet	1370	94	62	112	4	108	18	0
individual shell	1	220	15	61	18	Tr	18	3	0

	Serving Size	Calories	Fat (g)	Calories from Fat (%)	Total Carbs (g)	Fiber (g)	Net Carbs (g)	Protein (g)	Sugar Alcohol (g)
Pumpkin	***	***	*	*	*	*	*	*	*
Canned	1 cup	80	Tr	0	20	7	13	3	0
Fresh, cooked, mashed	1 cup	50	Tr	0	12	3	9	2	0
Pumpkin Pie Mix, canned	1 cup	280	Tr	0	71	22	49	3	0
Pumpkin Pie Spice	1 tsp	5	Tr	0	1	Tr	1	Tr	0
Quesadilla - see individual restaurant listings	***	***	*	*	*	*	*	*	*
Radish, fresh, raw, med	5	0	Tr	0	Tr	Tr	Tr	Tr	0
Sliced	1 cup	20	Tr	0	4	2	2	Tr	0
Raisin	***	***	*	*	*	*	*	*	*
Golden, not packed	1 cup	440	Tr	0	115	6	109	5	0
Regular, not packed	1 cup	430	Tr	0	115	5	110	5	0
small box	1½ oz	130	Tr	0	34	2	32	1	0
miniature box	½ oz	40	Tr	0	11	Tr	11	Tr	0
Raisin Bran - see Cereal	***	***	*	*	*	*	*	*	*
Raspberry	***	***	*	*	*	*	*	*	*
Fresh	1 cup	60	Tr	0	15	8	7	2	0
Frozen, sweetened, unthawed	1 cup	260	Tr	0	65	11	54	2	0
Ravioli, Chef Boyardee	***	***	*	*	*	*	*	*	*
Beef	1 cup	220	7	29	33	1	32	8	0
Beef, mini	1 cup	230	8	31	31	3	28	8	0
Relish - see Pickle Relish or specific listings	***	***	*	*	*	*	*	*	*
Rhubarb	***	***	*	*	*	*	*	*	*
Fresh, diced	1 cup	25	Tr	0	6	2	4	1	0
Frozen, cooked, sweetened	1 cup	280	Tr	0	75	5	70	Tr	0
RICE	***	***	*	*	*	*	*	*	*
Low Carb	***	***	*	*	*	*	*	*	*
Full Green Cauliflower Rice	7 oz	40	0.5	11	8	5	3	3	0

	Serving Size	Calories	Fat (g)	Calories from Fat (%)	Total Carbs (g)	Fiber (g)	Net Carbs (g)	Protein (g)	Sugar Alcohol (g)
Green Giant Cauliflower Crumbles	¾ cup	20	0	0	4	2	2	2	0
Julian Bakery PaleoThin Rice	3.5 oz	10	0	0	3	2	1	0	0
Plain Rice Dishes	***	***	*	*	*	*	*	*	*
Brown rice, med grain, cooked	1 cup	220	2	8	46	4	42	5	0
Brown rice, long grain, cooked	1 cup	220	2	8	45	4	41	5	0
White rice, med grain, cooked	1 cup	240	Tr	0	53	Tr	53	4	0
White rice, long grain, cooked	1 cup	210	Tr	0	45	Tr	45	4	0
White rice, parboiled, cooked	1 cup	190	Tr	0	42	1	41	5	0
White rice, instant, as prep	1 cup	190	Tr	0	41	1	40	4	0
White rice, glutinous, cooked	1 cup	170	Tr	0	37	2	35	4	0
Wild rice, cooked	1 cup	170	Tr	0	35	3	32	7	0
Rice Cake, brown rice	1	35	Tr	0	7	Tr	7	Tr	0
Rice Krispies Treat	1	150	3	18	30	Tr	30	1	0
Rice Pilaf	1 cup	280	6	19	50	1	49	7	0
Roast Beef - see Beef	***	***	*	*	*	*	*	*	*
Rolls - see Bread/Bread Products	***	***	*	*	*	*	*	*	*
Rosemary	***	***	*	*	*	*	*	*	*
Dried spice	1 tsp	0	Tr	0	Tr	Tr	Tr	Tr	0
Fresh, chopped	1 tsp	0	Tr	0	Tr	Tr	Tr	Tr	0
Rutabaga	***	***	*	*	*	*	*	*	*
Cubed, cooked	1 cup	70	Tr	0	15	3	12	2	0
Mashed, cooked	1 cup	90	Tr	0	21	4	17	3	0
Saccharin Sweetener	1 pkt	0	0	0	Tr	0	Tr	Tr	0
Sage, dried ground	1 tsp	0	Tr	0	Tr	Tr	Tr	Tr	0
Salad Dressing	***	***	*	*	*	*	*	*	*
Blue cheese, fat free	1 Tbsp	20	Tr	0	4	Tr	4	Tr	0

	Serving Size	Calories	Fat (g)	Calories from Fat (%)	Total Carbs (g)	Fiber (g)	Net Carbs (g)	Protein (g)	Sugar Alcohol (g)
Blue cheese, low calorie	1 Tbsp	15	1	60	Tr	0	Tr	Tr	0
Blue cheese, regular	1 Tbsp	70	8	100	Tr	Tr	Tr	Tr	0
Buttermilk, lite	1 Tbsp	30	2	60	3	Tr	3	Tr	0
Caesar, low calorie	1 Tbsp	15	Tr	0	3	0	3	Tr	0
Caesar, regular	1 Tbsp	80	9	100	Tr	Tr	Tr	Tr	0
French, fat free	1 Tbsp	20	Tr	0	5	Tr	5	Tr	0
French, low calorie	1 Tbsp	30	2	60	4	0	4	Tr	0
French, low fat	1 Tbsp	35	2	51	5	Tr	5	Tr	0
French, regular	1 Tbsp	70	7	90	3	0	3	Tr	0
Honey mustard, low calorie	1 Tbsp	60	3	45	9	Tr	9	Tr	0
Italian, fat free	1 Tbsp	5	Tr	0	1	Tr	1	Tr	0
Italian, low calorie	1 Tbsp	30	3	90	Tr	0	Tr	Tr	0
Italian, low fat	1 Tbsp	10	Tr	0	Tr	0	Tr	Tr	0
Italian, regular	1 Tbsp	40	4	90	2	0	2	Tr	0
Mayonnaise, fat free	1 Tbsp	15	Tr	0	3	Tr	3	Tr	0
Mayonnaise, light	1 Tbsp	50	5	90	1	0	1	Tr	0
Mayonnaise, regular	1 Tbsp	100	11	99	Tr	0	Tr	Tr	0
Ranch, fat free	1 Tbsp	15	Tr	0	4	0	4	Tr	0
Ranch, low fat	1 Tbsp	30	2	60	3	Tr	3	Tr	0
Ranch, regular	1 Tbsp	70	8	100	1	Tr	1	Tr	0
Russian, low calorie	1 Tbsp	25	Tr	0	4	0	4	Tr	0
Russian, regular	1 Tbsp	50	4	72	5	Tr	5	Tr	0
Thousand Island, fat free	1 Tbsp	20	Tr	0	5	Tr	5	Tr	0
Thousand Island, low fat	1 Tbsp	30	2	60	4	Tr	4	Tr	0
Thousand Island, regular	1 Tbsp	60	6	90	2	Tr	2	Tr	0
Salami	***	***	*	*	*	*	*	*	*
Beef, cooked	1 oz	70	6	77	70	0	Tr	4	0
Pork, hard or dry	1 oz	110	9	74	110	0	Tr	6	0
sliced, 3" x 1/16" slices	2	80	7	79	80	0	Tr	5	0

	Serving Size	Calories	Fat (g)	Calories from Fat (%)	Total Carbs (g)	Fiber (g)	Net Carbs (g)	Protein (g)	Sugar Alcohol (g)
Pork, Italian	1 oz	120	10	75	120	0	Tr	6	0
Turkey, cooked	1 oz	45	3	60	45	0	Tr	5	0
Salsa	1 Tbsp	0	Tr	0	0	Tr	1	Tr	0
Salt, kosher	½ tsp	0	0	0	0	0	0	0	0
Salt, table	½ tsp	0	0	0	0	0	0	0	0
Sandwich Meat - see Lunch Meat	***	***	*	*	*	*	*	*	*
Sandwich Spread	***	***	*	*	*	*	*	*	*
Pork or beef	1 Tbsp	35	3	77	2	0	2	1	0
Poultry	1 Tbsp	25	2	72	Tr	0	Tr	2	0
SAUCE	***	***	*	*	*	*	*	*	*
A1 Steak Sauce	1 Tbsp	30	0	0	8	Tr	8	Tr	0
Barbecue sauce	1 Tbsp	25	Tr	0	6	Tr	6	0	0
Catsup	1 Tbsp	15	Tr	0	4	0	4	Tr	0
Cheese sauce	¼ cup	110	8	65	4	Tr	4	4	0
Chili sauce	¼ cup	70	Tr	0	14	4	10	2	0
Hoisin sauce	1 Tbsp	35	Tr	0	7	Tr	7	Tr	0
Horseradish, prepared	1 tsp	0	Tr	0	Tr	Tr	Tr	Tr	0
Hot sauce	1 tsp	0	Tr	0	Tr	0	Tr	Tr	0
Marinara sauce	½ cup	110	3	25	18	3	15	2	0
Mayonnaise, fat free	1 Tbsp	15	Tr	0	3	Tr	3	Tr	0
Mayonnaise, light	1 Tbsp	50	5	90	1	0	1	Tr	0
Mayonnaise, regular	1 Tbsp	100	11	99	Tr	0	Tr	Tr	0
Mustard, regular (see also Mustard)	1 tsp	0	Tr	0	Tr	Tr	Tr	Tr	0
Oyster sauce	1 Tbsp	10	Tr	0	2	Tr	2	Tr	0
Pasta sauce	½ cup	110	3	25	18	3	15	2	0
Pepper sauce, hot	1 tsp	0	Tr	0	Tr	0	Tr	Tr	0
Pickle relish	1 Tbsp	20	Tr	0	5	Tr	5	Tr	0
Pizza sauce	¼ cup	35	Tr	0	6	1	5	1	0
Plum sauce	1 Tbsp	35	Tr	0	8	Tr	8	Tr	0
Salsa	1 Tbsp	0	Tr	0	1	Tr	1	Tr	0

	Serving Size	Calories	Fat (g)	Calories from Fat (%)	Total Carbs (g)	Fiber (g)	Net Carbs (g)	Protein (g)	Sugar Alcohol (g)
Sofrito	½ cup	240	19	71	6	2	4	13	0
Soy sauce	1 Tbsp	10	Tr	0	1	Tr	1	1	0
Spaghetti sauce	½ cup	110	3	25	18	3	15	2	0
Sweet & sour sauce	1 Tbsp	15	Tr	0	3	Tr	3	Tr	0
Tabasco sauce	1 tsp	0	Tr	0	Tr	0	Tr	Tr	0
Tamari sauce	1 Tbsp	10	Tr	0	1	Tr	1	2	0
Teriyaki sauce	1 Tbsp	15	0	0	3	0	3	1	0
Tomato sauce	½ cup	30	Tr	0	7	2	5	2	0
White sauce	½ cup	180	13	65	12	Tr	12	5	0
Worcestershire sauce	1 Tbsp	15	0	0	3	0	3	0	0
Sauerkraut	1 cup	45	Tr	0	10	7	3	2	0
Sausage	***	***	*	*	*	*	*	*	*
(See also Pork)	***	***	*	*	*	*	*	*	*
Beef	2 oz	190	16	76	Tr	0	Tr	10	0
Beef, cured, smoked	1 oz	90	8	80	Tr	0	Tr	4	0
Beef & pork	2 oz	220	20	82	2	0	2	8	0
Beef & pork, smoked	2 oz	180	16	80	1	0	1	7	0
Blood	2 oz	210	19	81	Tr	0	Tr	8	0
Chicken & beef, smoked	2 oz	170	13	69	0	0	0	10	0
Low fat, beef, pork & turkey	2 oz	60	1	15	6	Tr	6	5	0
Polish, kielbasa	2 oz	130	10	69	2	0	2	7	0
Sweet Italian, 3 oz link	1	130	7	48	2	0	2	14	0
Turkey	2 oz	110	6	49	0	0	0	13	0
Turkey & pork	2 oz	170	13	69	Tr	0	Tr	13	0
Vienna, 2" links	2	70	6	77	Tr	0	Tr	3	0
Scallop - see Fish/ Seafood	***	***	*	*	*	*	*	*	*
Seafood - see Fish/ Seafood	***	***	*	*	*	*	*	*	*
Seasoning - see specific listings	***	***	*	*	*	*	*	*	*
Poultry	1 tsp	5	Tr	0	Tr	Tr	Tr	Tr	0

	Serving Size	Calories	Fat (g)	Calories from Fat (%)	Total Carbs (g)	Fiber (g)	Net Carbs (g)	Protein (g)	Sugar Alcohol (g)
Seaweed	***	***	*	*	*	*	*	*	*
Agar, dried	¼ oz	20	Tr	0	6	Tr	6	Tr	0
Agar, raw	2 Tbsp	0	0	0	Tr	Tr	Tr	Tr	0
Kelp, raw	2 Tbsp	0	Tr	0	Tr	Tr	Tr	Tr	0
Spirulina, dried	1 Tbsp	20	Tr	0	2	Tr	2	4	0
Wakame, raw	2 Tbsp	5	Tr	0	Tr	Tr	Tr	Tr	0
Seeds	***	***	*	*	*	*	*	*	*
(See also specific listings)	***	***	*	*	*	*	*	*	*
Chia	1 Tbsp	51	3	53	4	3	1	2	0
Flaxseed, whole	1 Tbsp	60	4	60	3	3	0	2	0
Flaxseed, ground	1 Tbsp	35	3	77	2	2	0	1	0
Hemp, hulled	1 Tbsp	53	5	85	1	Tr	Tr	3	0
Pumpkin seeds, kernels, roasted	1 oz	150	12	72	4	1	3	9	0
Sesame seeds, plain	1 Tbsp	50	5	90	2	1	1	2	0
Sesame seeds, toasted	1 oz	160	14	79	7	4	3	5	0
Sunflower seeds, dry roasted	1 oz	170	14	74	7	3	4	6	0
Shakes	***	***	*	*	*	*	*	*	*
Atkins Shakes	***	***	*	*	*	*	*	*	*
Café Caramel	1 carton	160	10	56	3	1	2	15	0
Chocolate Banana Energy	1 carton	170	9	48	9	5	4	15	0
Creamy Chocolate	1 carton	240	14	53	7	4	3	23	0
Dark Chocolate Royale	1 carton	160	10	56	6	4	2	15	0
French Vanilla	1 carton	160	9	51	2	1	1	15	0
Milk Chocolate Delight	1 carton	160	9	51	5	3	2	15	0
Mocha Latte	1 carton	160	10	56	5	2	3	15	0
Strawberry	1 carton	160	9	51	2	1	1	15	0
Vanilla Cream	1 carton	230	14	55	4	1	3	23	0

	Serving Size	Calories	Fat (g)	Calories from Fat (%)	Total Carbs (g)	Fiber (g)	Net Carbs (g)	Protein (g)	Sugar Alcohol (g)
Atkins Plus Protein & Fiber Shakes	***	***	*	*	*	*	*	*	*
Creamy Milk Chocolate	1 carton	190	5	24	9	7	2	30	0
Creamy Vanilla	1 carton	180	5	25	8	7	1	30	0
Atkins Protein Powder, chocolate or vanilla	1 scoop	100	3	27	7	5	2	15	0
KetoChow Meal Replacement Shakes	***	***	*	*	*	*	*	*	*
Banana	1 scoop	124	1	7	7	6	1	26	0
Chocolate	1 scoop	133	1	7	9	7	2	27	0
Chocolate Mint	1 scoop	130	1	7	8	7	1	26	0
Chocolate Peanut Butter	1 scoop	184	4	20	11	9	2	31	0
Chocolate Toffee	1 scoop	126	1	7	8	7	1	26	0
Cookies & Cream	1 scoop	124	1	7	7	6	1	26	0
Eggnog	1 scoop	127	1	7	8	7	1	26	0
Mocha	1 scoop	134	1	7	9	7	2	27	0
Orange Cream	1 scoop	126	1	7	8	7	1	26	0
Pumpkin Spice Caramel	1 scoop	127	1	7	8	7	1	26	0
Raspberry Cheesecake	1 scoop	126	1	7	8	7	1	26	0
Root Beer Float	1 scoop	131	1	7	8	7	1	26	0
Salted Caramel	1 scoop	124	1	7	7	6	1	26	0
Savory Chicken Soup	1 scoop	126	1	7	7	1	6	26	0
Snickerdoodle	1 scoop	127	1	7	8	7	1	26	0
Strawberry	1 scoop	124	1	7	6	1	5	26	0
Strawberry, Natural	1 scoop	124	1	7	7	6	1	26	0
Vanilla	1 scoop	124	1	7	7	6	1	26	0
SlimFast Keto Meal Shakes	***	***	*	*	*	*	*	*	*
Fudge Brownie Batter	2 scoops	190	15	71	9	2	4	8	3

	Serving Size	Calories	Fat (g)	Calories from Fat (%)	Total Carbs (g)	Fiber (g)	Net Carbs (g)	Protein (g)	Sugar Alcohol (g)
Vanilla Cake Batter	2 scoops	190	15	71	8	0	5	8	3
Shallot, raw, chopped	1 Tbsp	5	Tr	0	2	Tr	2	Tr	0
Freeze dried	1 Tbsp	0	0	0	Tr	Tr	Tr	Tr	0
Shark - see Fish/Seafood	***	***	*	*	*	*	*	*	*
Sherbet, orange	½ cup	110	2	16	23	1	22	Tr	0
Shortening, regular	1 cup	1810	205	100	0	0	0	0	0
Cottonseed & soybean blend	1 Tbsp	110	13	100	0	0	0	0	0
Shrimp - see Fish/ Seafood & specific entrées	***	***	*	*	*	*	*	*	*
Sirloin Steak - see Beef	***	***	*	*	*	*	*	*	*
Snack Mix, Chex Mix	¾ cup	120	5	38	18	2	16	3	0
Oriental mix, rice based	1 oz	140	7	45	15	4	11	5	0
SNACKS	***	***	*	*	*	*	*	*	*
Cali'flour Foods Cauliflower Thins, all flavors	6 crackers	90	7	70	2	2	0	5	0
Chomps Meat Bars	***	***	*	*	*	*	*	*	*
Beef, Crankin' Cranberry	1 stick	110	6	49	4	0	4	9	0
Beef, Hoppin' Jalapeno	1 stick	100	6	54	1	0	1	9	0
Beef, Original	1 stick	100	6	54	0	0	0	9	0
Original Beef Chomplings	1 stick	43	3	63	0	0	0	4	0
Original Turkey Chomplings	1 stick	29	1	31	0	0	0	5	0
Turkey, Jalapeno	1 stick	70	2	26	1	0	1	10	0
Turkey, Original	1 stick	70	2	26	0	0	0	10	0
Venison, Salt & Pepper	1 stick	100	6	54	0	0	0	9	0
Jimmy Dean Protein Packs	***	***	*	*	*	*	*	*	*
Roasted Almond	1 pkg	290	23	71	5	3	2	15	0
Smoked Ham	1 pkg	180	12	60	4	0	4	14	0

	Serving Size	Calories	Fat (g)	Calories from Fat (%)	Total Carbs (g)	Fiber (g)	Net Carbs (g)	Protein (g)	Sugar Alcohol (g)
Turkey Sausage	1 pkg	170	11	58	2	0	2	14	0
Julian Bakery	6 crackers	70	4.5	58	5	2	3	3	0
PaleoThin Crackers, Salt & Pepper	6 crackers	70	4.5	58	7	2	5	2	0
PrimalThin Crackers, Organic Parmesan	6 crackers	70	4.5	58	7	2	5	2	0
Just the Cheese Bars, all flavors	2 bars	150	12	72	Tr	0	Tr	8	0
Just the Cheese Minis, all flavors	1 pkg	95	8	76	1	0	1	5	0
Linda's Diet Delites Low Carb Bagel Chips, Plain	5 chips	100	4	36	16	14	2	14	0
Moon Cheese	***	***	*	*	*	*	*	*	*
Cheddar	6-7 pc	70	5	64	1	0	1	5	0
Gouda	6-7 pc	70	5	64	0	0	0	5	0
Mozzarella	6-7 pc	67	5	67	1	0	1	5	0
Pepper Jack	6-7 pc	70	5	64	0	0	0	4	0
Sriracha	6-7 pc	67	5	67	1	0	1	5	0
P3 Portable Protein Packs	***	***	*	*	*	*	*	*	*
Chicken, Cashews, Monterey Jack	1 pkg	180	12	60	5	0	5	12	0
Chicken, Peanuts, Cheddar	1 pkg	200	14	63	3	1	2	13	0
Ham, Almonds, Cheddar	1 pkg	190	14	66	4	1	3	12	0
Ham, Cashews, Colby Jack	1 pkg	180	12	60	5	0	5	12	0
Turkey, Almonds, Colby Jack	1 pkg	180	13	65	4	1	3	13	0
Turkey, Peanuts, Cheddar	1 pkg	190	14	66	3	1	2	13	0
P3 Portable Protein Pack: Deli Snackers	***	***	*	*	*	*	*	*	*

	Serving Size	Calories	Fat (g)	Calories from Fat (%)	Total Carbs (g)	Fiber (g)	Net Carbs (g)	Protein (g)	Sugar Alcohol (g)
Turkey, Bacon, Colby Jack	1 pkg	180	13	65	Tr	0	Tr	15	0
Turkey, Ham, Cheddar	1 pkg	150	10	60	2	0	2	14	0
Paleovalley Beef Sticks, all flavors	1 stick	70	5	64	0	0	0	6	0
Quest Protein Chips	***	***	*	*	*	*	*	*	*
BBQ Original Style	1 bag	130	3.5	24	4	1	3	21	0
Cheddar & Sour Cream Original Style	1 bag	140	4.5	29	5	1	4	21	0
Chili Lime Tortilla Style	1 bag	140	4.5	29	4	1	3	20	0
Nacho Cheese Tortilla Style	1 bag	140	6	39	5	1	4	18	0
Ranch Tortilla Style	1 bag	140	4.5	29	5	1	4	19	0
Sour Cream & Onion Original Style	1 bag	140	4	26	5	1	4	21	0
Shrewd Food Protein Crisps	***	***	*	*	*	*	*	*	*
Baked Cheddar	1 pkg	90	3	30	2	0	2	14	0
Brickoven Pizza	1 pkg	90	3	30	2	0	2	14	0
Cookies & Cream	1 pkg	90	3.5	35	3	0	3	13	0
Smokehouse Maple	1 pkg	90	3	30	3	0	3	14	0
Sriracha Cheddar	1 pkg	90	3	30	2	0	2	14	0
Whisps Cheese Crisps	***	***	*	*	*	*	*	*	*
Asiago & Pepper Jack	½ bag	150	11	66	1	0	1	12	0
Bacon BBQ	½ bag	170	14	74	2	0	2	10	0
Cheddar	½ bag	170	14	74	1	0	1	10	0
Parmesan	½ bag	150	11	60	1	0	1	13	0
Tomato Basil	½ bag	150	11	66	2	1	1	12	0
SOUP (as prep)	***	***	*	*	*	*	*	*	*
Bouillon cube, beef	1	10	Tr	0	Tr	0	Tr	Tr	0
Bouillon cube, chicken	1	10	Tr	0	Tr	0	Tr	Tr	0

	Serving Size	Calories	Fat (g)	Calories from Fat (%)	Total Carbs (g)	Fiber (g)	Net Carbs (g)	Protein (g)	Sugar Alcohol (g)
Bouillon cube, low sodium	1	15	Tr	0	2	0	2	Tr	0
Broth, beef	1 cup	15	Tr	0	Tr	0	Tr	3	0
Broth, beef consommé, as prep	1 cup	30	0	0	2	0	2	5	0
Broth, chicken	1 cup	10	Tr	0	Tr	0	Tr	Tr	0
Broth, chicken, low sodium	1 cup	40	1	23	3	0	3	5	0
Bean w/ ham	1 cup	230	9	35	27	11	16	13	0
Bean w/ pork	1 cup	170	6	32	22	8	14	8	0
Beef noodle	1 cup	80	3	34	9	Tr	9	5	0
Beef noodle tomato	1 cup	140	4	26	21	2	19	4	0
Black bean	1 cup	110	2	16	19	8	11	6	0
Cheese, prep w/ water	1 cup	160	11	62	11	1	10	5	0
Cheese, prep w/ milk	1 cup	230	15	59	16	1	15	10	0
Chicken noodle, canned	1 cup	60	2	30	7	Tr	7	3	0
Chicken noodle, chunky	1 cup	90	2	20	10	1	9	8	0
Chicken noodle, dry mix, as prep	1 cup	60	1	15	9	Tr	9	2	0
Chicken & rice	1 cup	60	2	30	7	Tr	7	4	0
Chicken & rice, chunky	1 cup	130	3	21	13	1	12	12	0
Chicken & vegetable	1 cup	80	3	34	9	1	8	4	0
Chicken & vegetable, chunky	1 cup	170	5	26	19	1	18	12	0
Clam chowder, Manhattan	1 cup	80	2	23	12	2	10	2	0
Clam chowder, Manhattan, chunky	1 cup	130	3	21	19	3	16	7	0
Clam chowder, New England	***	***	*	*	*	*	*	*	*
prep w/ water	1 cup	90	3	30	13	Tr	13	4	0
prep w/ milk	1 cup	150	5	30	19	Tr	19	8	0
Cream of Asparagus	***	***	*	*	*	*	*	*	*
prep w/ water	1 cup	90	4	40	11	Tr	11	2	0

	Serving Size	Calories	Fat (g)	Calories from Fat (%)	Total Carbs (g)	Fiber (g)	Net Carbs (g)	Protein (g)	Sugar Alcohol (g)
prep w/ milk	1 cup	160	8	45	16	Tr	16	6	0
Cream of Celery	***	***	*	*	*	*	*	*	*
prep w/ water	1 cup	90	6	60	9	Tr	9	2	0
prep w/ milk	1 cup	160	10	56	15	Tr	15	6	0
Cream of Chicken	***	***	*	*	*	*	*	*	*
prep w/ water	1 cup	120	7	53	9	Tr	9	3	0
prep w/ milk	1 cup	190	12	57	15	Tr	15	8	0
Cream of Mushroom	***	***	*	*	*	*	*	*	*
prep w/ water	1 cup	100	7	63	8	0	8	2	0
prep w/ milk	1 cup	170	10	53	14	0	14	6	0
Cream of Onion	***	***	*	*	*	*	*	*	*
prep w/ water	1 cup	110	5	41	13	1	12	3	0
prep w/ milk	1 cup	190	9	43	18	Tr	18	7	0
Cream of Potato	***	***	*	*	*	*	*	*	*
prep w/ water	1 cup	70	2	26	12	Tr	12	2	0
prep w/ milk	1 cup	150	7	42	17	Tr	17	6	0
Minestrone	1 cup	80	3	34	11	1	10	4	0
Minestrone, chunky	1 cup	130	3	21	21	6	15	5	0
Miso, as prep	1 cup	20	Tr	0	3	Tr	3	1	0
Onion, canned	1 cup	60	2	30	8	Tr	8	4	0
Onion, dry mix, as prep	1 cup	30	Tr	0	6	Tr	6	Tr	0
Pea, green	1 cup	160	3	17	26	5	21	8	0
Ramen beef noodle	½ pkg	190	7	33	27	Tr	27	4	0
Ramen chicken noodle	½ pkg	190	7	33	27	1	26	5	0
Split pea w/ ham	1 cup	190	4	19	28	2	26	10	0
Split pea w/ ham, chunky	1 cup	190	4	19	27	4	23	11	0
Tomato	***	***	*	*	*	*	*	*	*
prep w/ water	1 cup	70	Tr	0	16	2	14	2	0
prep w/ milk	1 cup	140	3	19	22	2	20	6	0
Tomato bisque	***	***	*	*	*	*	*	*	*
prep w/ water	1 cup	120	3	23	27	Tr	24	2	0

	Serving Size	Calories	Fat (g)	Calories from Fat (%)	Total Carbs (g)	Fiber (g)	Net Carbs (g)	Protein (g)	Sugar Alcohol (g)
prep w/ milk	1 cup	200	7	32	29	Tr	29	6	0
Tomato rice	1 cup	120	3	23	21	2	19	2	0
Tomato vegetable	1 cup	50	Tr	0	10	Tr	10	2	0
Turkey vegetable	1 cup	70	3	39	9	Tr	9	3	0
Vegetable	1 cup	70	2	26	12	Tr	12	2	0
Vegetable beef	1 cup	80	2	23	10	2	8	5	0
Sour Cream	***	***	*	*	*	*	*	*	*
Regular	1 cup	440	45	92	7	0	7	5	0
Regular	1 Tbsp	25	2	72	Tr	0	Tr	Tr	0
Reduced fat	1 Tbsp	20	2	90	Tr	0	Tr	Tr	0
Fat free	1 Tbsp	12	0	0	3	0	3	Tr	0
Soy Burger (see also Vegetable Burger)	1	120	4	30	10	3	7	11	0
Soybeans (Edamame)	***	***	*	*	*	*	*	*	*
Green, cooked	½ cup	130	6	42	10	4	6	11	0
Mature seeds, cooked	½ cup	150	8	48	9	5	4	14	0
Spaghetti - see Pasta	***	***	*	*	*	*	*	*	*
Spare Ribs - see Pork	***	***	*	*	*	*	*	*	*
Spice - see specific listings	***	***	*	*	*	*	*	*	*
Spinach	***	***	*	*	*	*	*	*	*
Canned, cooked	1 cup	50	1	18	7	5	2	6	0
Fresh, baby	1 cup	13	0	0	2	1	1	1	0
Fresh, chopped, cooked	1 cup	40	Tr	0	7	4	3	5	0
Fresh, raw	1 cup	5	Tr	0	1	Tr	1	Tr	0
Frozen, chopped, cooked	1 cup	70	2	26	9	7	2	8	0
Spinach Soufflé	1 cup	230	18	70	8	1	7	11	0
Splenda (sucralose)	1 pkt	4	0	0	1	0	1	0	0
Spread	***	***	*	*	*	*	*	*	*
(See also spreads in Margarine)	***	***	*	*	*	*	*	*	*
Cheese, pasteurized	1 Tbsp	80	6	68	3	0	3	5	0

	Serving Size	Calories	Fat (g)	Calories from Fat (%)	Total Carbs (g)	Fiber (g)	Net Carbs (g)	Protein (g)	Sugar Alcohol (g)
Cheese, cream cheese base	1 Tbsp	45	4	80	Tr	0	Tr	1	0
Ham & cheese	1 Tbsp	40	3	68	Tr	0	Tr	2	0
Ham salad	1 Tbsp	30	2	60	2	0	2	1	0
Liverwurst	1 Tbsp	40	4	90	Tr	Tr	Tr	2	0
Sandwich, pork or beef	1 Tbsp	35	3	77	2	Tr	2	1	0
Sandwich, poultry salad	1 Tbsp	26	2	69	Tr	0	Tr	2	0
Squash	***	***	*	*	*	*	*	*	*
Acorn, baked, cubes	1 cup	120	Tr	0	30	9	21	2	0
Butternut, baked, cubes	1 cup	82	Tr	0	22	7	15	2	0
Butternut, raw, cubed	1 cup	60	Tr	0	16	3	13	1	0
Hubbard, cooked, mashed	1 cup	70	Tr	0	15	7	8	4	0
Spaghetti, cooked	1 cup	40	Tr	0	10	2	8	1	0
Summer, cooked, slices	1 cup	35	Tr	0	8	3	5	2	0
Summer, raw, sliced	1 cup	20	Tr	0	4	1	3	1	0
Winter, baked, cubes	1 cup	80	Tr	0	18	6	12	2	0
Starfruit - see Carambola	***	***	*	*	*	*	*	*	*
Steak - see Beef	***	***	*	*	*	*	*	*	*
Steak Sauce, A1	1 Tbsp	30	0	0	8	Tr	8	Tr	0
Strawberries	***	***	*	*	*	*	*	*	*
Fresh, med size, 1¼" dia	10	40	Tr	0	9	2	7	Tr	0
Fresh, sliced	1 cup	50	Tr	0	13	3	10	1	0
Frozen, unsweetened, thawed	1 cup	80	Tr	0	20	5	15	Tr	0
Frozen, sweetened, thawed	1 cup	250	Tr	0	66	5	61	1	0
Strawberry Topping - see Topping	***	***	*	*	*	*	*	*	*
Strudel, Apple	1 pc	200	8	36	29	2	27	2	0
Stuffing	***	***	*	*	*	*	*	*	*

	Serving Size	Calories	Fat (g)	Calories from Fat (%)	Total Carbs (g)	Fiber (g)	Net Carbs (g)	Protein (g)	Sugar Alcohol (g)
Bread, dry mix, as prep	½ cup	180	9	45	22	3	19	3	0
Cornbread, dry mix, as prep	½ cup	180	9	45	22	3	19	3	0
Succotash	***	***	*	*	*	*	*	*	*
Canned	½ cup	80	Tr	0	18	3	15	3	0
Fresh, cooked	½ cup	110	Tr	0	23	4	19	5	0
Frozen, cooked	½ cup	80	Tr	0	17	4	13	4	0
SUGAR	***	***	*	*	*	*	*	*	*
White, granulated	***	***	*	*	*	*	*	*	*
One cup	1 cup	770		0	200	0	200	0	0
One tablespoon	1 Tbsp	50	0	0	13	0	13	0	0
One teaspoon	1 tsp	15	0	0	4	0	4	0	0
Cube	1	10	0	0	2	0	2	0	0
Restaurant size packet	1	10	0	0	3	0	3	0	0
Confectioners' (Powdered)	***	***	*	*	*	*	*	*	*
Unsifted cup	1 cup	470	Tr	0	120	0	120	0	0
Sifted cup	1 cup	390	Tr	0	100	0	100	0	0
Unsifted tablespoon	1 Tbsp	30	Tr	0	8	0	8	0	0
Brown sugar	***	***	*	*	*	*	*	*	*
Packed cup	1 cup	840	0	0	216	0	216	Tr	0
Packed tablespoon	1 Tbsp	50	0	0	14	0	14	Tr	0
Brownulated	1 Tbsp	35	0	0	9	0	9	Tr	0
Sugar Substitute	***	***	*	*	*	*	*	*	*
Aspartame sweetener	1 pkt	0	0	0	Tr	0	Tr	Tr	0
Saccharin sweetener	1 pkt	0	0	0	Tr	0	Tr	Tr	0
Sugar Twin	1 pkt	0	0	0	Tr	0	Tr	Tr	0
Sundae (sm svg)	***	***	*	*	*	*	*	*	*
Caramel	1	300	9	27	49	0	49	7	0
Hot fudge	1	280	9	29	48	0	48	6	0
Strawberry	1	270	8	27	45	0	45	6	0
Sunflower Seed Butter	2 Tbsp	197	18	82	7	2	5	6	0

	Serving Size	Calories	Fat (g)	Calories from Fat (%)	Total Carbs (g)	Fiber (g)	Net Carbs (g)	Protein (g)	Sugar Alcohol (g)
Swedish Meatballs - see Frozen Dinner	***	***	*	*	*	*	*	*	*
Sweet 'N Low	1 pkt	0	0	0	Tr	0	Tr	Tr	0
Sweet Potato	***	***	*	*	*	*	*	*	*
Baked w/ skin, whole, med, 5" x 2"	1	110	Tr	0	24	4	20	2	0
Candied, 2½" x 2"	1 pc	15	3	180	29	3	26	Tr	0
Canned, in syrup, drained	1 cup	210	Tr	0	50	6	44	3	0
Canned, mashed, vacuum pack	1 cup	230	Tr	0	54	5	49	4	0
Cooked, mashed	½ cup	90	Tr	0	21	3	18	2	0
Frozen, baked, cubes	1 cup	180	Tr	0	41	3	38	3	0
Sweet Potato Chips	1 oz	140	7	45	18	1	17	Tr	0
Sweet Roll - see specific listings	***	***	*	*	*	*	*	*	*
SWEETS, LOW CARB	***	***	*	*	*	*	*	*	*
Bars & Cakes	***	***	*	*	*	*	*	*	*
Atkins Endulge	***	***	*	*	*	*	*	*	*
Caramel Nut Chew Bar	1	130	8	55	17	6	11	5	9
Chocolate Caramel Mousse Bar	1 pkt	120	4.5	34	23	9	14	3	12
Chocolate Coconut Bar	1	170	12	64	19	9	10	4	8
Peanut Caramel Cluster Bar	1 pkt	140	10	64	13	6	7	7	4
ThinSlim Foods Cloud Cakes	***	***	*	*	*	*	*	*	*
Blueberry Bliss	1 cake	20	1	45	10	3	0	2	7
Cinnamon	1 cake	20	1	45	10	3	0	2	7
Cinnamon Crumb	1 cake	40	3	68	11	3	0	2	8
Chocolate	1 cake	20	1	45	10	3	0	2	7
Pumpkin Spice (insufficient info available)	1 cake	20	*	*	*	3	*	*	*

	Serving Size	Calories	Fat (g)	Calories from Fat (%)	Total Carbs (g)	Fiber (g)	Net Carbs (g)	Protein (g)	Sugar Alcohol (g)
ThinSlim Foods Squares	***	***	*	*	*	*	*	*	*
Almond	1	40	1	23	20	8	2	6	10
Brownie	1	45	1	20	20	8	2	6	10
Lemon	1	40	1	23	20	8	2	6	10
Peanut Butter Chocolate Chip	1	45	1	20	20	8	2	6	10
Pumpkin Spice	1	40	1	23	20	8	2	6	10
Brownies	***	***	*	*	*	*	*	*	*
Atkins Endulge Nutty Fudge Brownie	1	170	12	64	18	6	2	7	10
ThinSlim Foods Keto Brownie	1	120	10	75	20	9	1	5	10
Candy	***	***	*	*	*	*	*	*	*
Atkins Endulge	***	***	*	*	*	*	*	*	*
Chocolate Candies	1 pkt	110	7	57	19	4	15	1	14
Chocolate Covered Almonds	1 pkt	140	12	77	12	1	11	3	9
Chocolate Peanut Candies	1 pkt	150	11	66	18	2	16	4	15
Pecan Caramel Clusters	2 pkt	120	10	75	15	8	7	1	5
Peanut Butter Cups	2 pc	160	13	73	18	4	14	2	12
ChocZero Chocolate Keto Bark	***	***	*	*	*	*	*	*	*
Dark Chocolate Varieties	1 bar	120	10	75	15	13	2	0	0
Milk Chocolate Varieties	1 bar	150	14	84	11	8	3	3	0
SlimFast Keto Peanut Butter Cup Fat Bomb	1	90	9	90	6	3	3	1	0
Chocolate & Chocolate Bars	***	***	*	*	*	*	*	*	*
Atkins Endulge Milk Chocolate Caramel Squares	3 pc	140	9	58	22	5	17	1	15

	Serving Size	Calories	Fat (g)	Calories from Fat (%)	Total Carbs (g)	Fiber (g)	Net Carbs (g)	Protein (g)	Sugar Alcohol (g)
ChocZero Chocolate Squares	***	***	*	*	*	*	*	*	*
70 Dark Chocolate	1 square	45	4.5	90	5	4	1	0	0
50 Dark Chocolate	1 square	40	4.5	100	6	5	1	0	0
Milk Chocolate	1 square	50	4.5	81	4	3	1	0	0
Julian Bakery PaleoThin Dark Chocolate, plain or Sea Salt & Almond	½ bar	99	9	82	9	6	3	2	0
Ketomanna Ketogenic Chocolate Fudge	1.2 oz	224	22	88	8	5	3	3	0
Kiss My Keto Ketogenic Chocolate Bars	***	***	*	*	*	*	*	*	*
Original Dark Chocolate	⅓ bar	130	13	90	14	7	2	1	5
Pumpkin Seeds & Sea Salt Dark Chocolate	⅓ bar	130	13	90	12	7	1	2	4
Roasted Almonds Dark Chocolate	⅓ bar	130	13	90	13	7	2	2	4
Toasted Hazelnut Dark Chocolate	⅓ bar	130	13	90	13	7	2	2	4
Cookies	***	***	*	*	*	*	*	*	*
Fat Snax Cookies	***	***	*	*	*	*	*	*	*
Chocolate Chip	1	90	8	80	7	2	5	2	3
Double Chocolate Chip	1	100	9	81	7	2	5	2	3
Lemony Lemon	1	90	8	80	6	2	4	2	3
Peanut Butter	1	110	9	74	6	2	4	3	3
Julian Bakery ProCookie Peanut Butter Chocolate Chip	1	190	12	57	26	22	4	12	0
Nui Cookies	***	***	*	*	*	*	*	*	*
Chocolate Chip	2	240	23	86	20	3	4	6	13
Double Chocolate	2	240	23	86	20	4	4	6	12

	Serving Size	Calories	Fat (g)	Calories from Fat (%)	Total Carbs (g)	Fiber (g)	Net Carbs (g)	Protein (g)	Sugar Alcohol (g)
Ginger Something	2	240	23	86	19	3	2	6	14
Peanut Butter	2	270	24	80	18	3	4	8	11
Snickerdoodle	2	240	24	90	18	2	2	6	14
Quest Protein Cookies	***	***	*	*	*	*	*	*	*
Chocolate Chip	1	250	17	61	19	9	4	15	6
Double Chocolate Chip	1	240	16	60	20	10	5	15	5
Oatmeal Raisin	1	250	14	50	25	12	9	15	4
Peanut Butter	1	250	17	61	18	9	5	15	4
Peanut Butter Chocolate Chip	1	220	13	53	21	11	5	16	5
Snickerdoodle	1	250	17	61	19	11	4	15	4
ThinSlim Foods Cookies	***	***	*	*	*	*	*	*	*
Caramel	1	40	1	23	20	8	2	6	10
Chocolate Bliss	1	50	1	18	21	8	3	6	10
Chocolate Chip	1	45	1	20	20	8	2	6	10
Chocolate Glazed	1	65	1	14	36	20	3	6	13
Coconut	1	40	1	23	20	8	2	6	10
Peanut Butter Chocolate Chip	1	45	1	20	20	8	2	6	10
Vanilla	1	40	1	23	20	8	2	6	10
Vanilla Glazed	1	60	1	15	36	20	3	6	13
SYRUP	***	***	*	*	*	*	*	*	*
Chocolate fudge, thick	1 Tbsp	130	3	21	24	0	23	2	0
Corn, dark	1 Tbsp	60	0	0	16	0	16	0	0
Corn, light	1 Tbsp	60	Tr	0	17	0	17	0	0
Grenadine	1 Tbsp	50	0	0	13	0	13	0	0
Malt	1 Tbsp	80	0	0	17	0	17	0	0
Maple	1 Tbsp	50	Tr	0	13	0	13	0	0
Molasses	1 Tbsp	60	Tr	0	15	0	15	0	0
Molasses	1 cup	980	Tr	0	252	0	252	0	0
Pancake Syrup/ Table Syrup	***	***	*	*	*	*	*	*	*

	Serving Size	Calories	Fat (g)	Calories from Fat (%)	Total Carbs (g)	Fiber (g)	Net Carbs (g)	Protein (g)	Sugar Alcohol (g)
Hungry Jack Sugar Free Butter Flavor Syrup	2 Tbsp	10	0	0	4	0	4	0	4
Light, reduced calorie	1 Tbsp	25	0	0	7	0	7	0	0
Log Cabin Sugar Free Syrup	¼ cup	20	0	0	8	0	8	0	7
Mrs. Butterworth's Sugar Free Syrup	¼ cup	20	0	0	8	0	8	0	8
Regular	1 Tbsp	45	0	0	12	0	12	0	0
Walden Farms Calorie Free Pancake Syrup	¼ cup	0	0	0	0	0	0	0	0
Sugar Free Syrup	***	***	*	*	*	*	*	*	*
ChocZero Sugar Free, Low Carb syrups	***	***	*	*	*	*	*	*	*
Banana	1 Tbsp	30	0	0	13	11	2	0	0
Caramel	1 Tbsp	32	0	0	15	14	1	0	0
Chocolate	1 Tbsp	37	0	0	15	14	1	0	0
Maple	1 Tbsp	32	0	0	15	14	1	0	0
Maple Pecan	1 Tbsp	32	0	0	15	14	1	0	0
Maple Vanilla	1 Tbsp	32	0	0	15	14	1	0	0
Peach	1 Tbsp	30	0	0	13	11	2	0	0
Vanilla	1 Tbsp	32	0	0	15	14	1	0	0
DaVinci Gourmet Sugar Free Syrups, all flavors	2 Tbsp	0	0	0	0	0	0	0	0
Monin Sugar Free Syrups, most flavors	2 Tbsp	0	0	0	3	0	3	0	0
Torani Sugar Free Syrups, most flavors	2 Tbsp	0	0	0	0	0	0	0	0
Walden Farms Calorie Free Syrup, all flavors	2 Tbsp	0	0	0	0	0	0	0	0
Taco - see individual restaurant listings	***	***	*	*	*	*	*	*	*
Taco Shell, med, 5" dia	1	60	3	45	8	Tr	8	Tr	0

	Serving Size	Calories	Fat (g)	Calories from Fat (%)	Total Carbs (g)	Fiber (g)	Net Carbs (g)	Protein (g)	Sugar Alcohol (g)
Tahini, from toasted kernels	1 Tbsp	90	8	80	3	1	2	3	0
Tangerine, fresh, med, 2½" dia	1	45	Tr	0	12	2	10	Tr	0
Tapioca, pearl dry	1 cup	540	Tr	0	135	1	134	Tr	0
Tapioca, prep from dry w/ 2 milk	½ cup	134	2	13	25	0	25	4	0
Tapioca, prep from dry w/ whole milk	½ cup	147	4	24	25	0	25	4	0
Taro, cooked, sliced	1 cup	190	Tr	0	46	7	31	Tr	0
Taro Chips	1 oz	140	7	45	19	2	17	Tr	0
Taro Leaf, steamed	½ cup	15	Tr	0	3	2	1	2	0
Tarragon	***	***	*	*	*	*	*	*	*
Dried, leaves	1 tsp	0	Tr	0	Tr	0	Tr	Tr	0
Dried, ground	1 tsp	5	Tr	0	Tr	Tr	Tr	Tr	0
T-bone Steak - see Beef	***	***	*	*	*	*	*	*	*
Thyme	***	***	*	*	*	*	*	*	*
Dried, leaves	1 tsp	0	Tr	0	Tr	Tr	Tr	Tr	0
Dried, ground	1 tsp	0	Tr	0	Tr	Tr	Tr	Tr	0
Fresh	1 tsp	0	Tr	0	Tr	Tr	Tr	Tr	0
Toaster Pastry (Pop Tart)	***	***	*	*	*	*	*	*	*
Apple, frosted	1	220	6	25	39	Tr	39	2	0
Apple, unfrosted	1	210	6	26	37	Tr	37	2	0
Blueberry, frosted	1	220	6	25	39	Tr	39	2	0
Blueberry, unfrosted	1	210	6	26	37	Tr	37	2	0
Brown sugar cinnamon	1	210	7	30	34	Tr	34	3	0
Cherry, frosted	1	220	6	25	39	Tr	39	2	0
Cherry, unfrosted	1	210	6	26	37	Tr	37	2	0
Strawberry, frosted	1	220	6	25	39	Tr	39	2	0
Strawberry, unfrosted	1	210	6	26	37	Tr	37	2	0
Tofu, raw	½ cup	90	6	60	2	Tr	2	10	0
Tofu, silken, raw	2 oz	24	1	38	Tr	0	Tr	3	0
Tomatillos, raw	***	***	*	*	*	*	*	*	*

	Serving Size	Calories	Fat (g)	Calories from Fat (%)	Total Carbs (g)	Fiber (g)	Net Carbs (g)	Protein (g)	Sugar Alcohol (g)
Whole, medium size	2	20	Tr	0	4	1	3	Tr	0
Chopped or diced	½ cup	20	Tr	0	4	1	3	Tr	0
Tomato	***	***	*	*	*	*	*	*	*
Fresh, raw, avg size, 2½" dia	1 whole	20	Tr	0	5	2	3	1	0
Fresh, raw, cherry or grape tomato	1 cup	25	Tr	0	6	2	4	1	0
Fresh, slices ¼" thick	1 slice	0	Tr	0	Tr	Tr	Tr	Tr	
Fresh, chopped or sliced	1 cup	30	Tr	0	7	2	5	2	0
Fresh, cooked	1 cup	45	Tr	0	10	2	8	2	0
Fresh, stewed	1 cup	80	3	34	13	2	11	2	0
Canned, diced, *Hunt's*	1 cup	60	0	0	12	4	8	2	0
Canned, diced, w/ chiles, *Ro-Tel*	1 cup	20	0	0	4	1	3	1	0
Canned, packed in juice	1 cup	40	Tr	0	10	2	8	2	0
Canned, stewed	1 cup	70	Tr	0	16	3	13	2	0
Sundried	***	***	*	*	*	*	*	*	*
plain	1 pc	5	Tr	0	1	Tr	1	Tr	0
packed in oil, drained	1 pc	5	Tr	0	Tr	Tr	Tr	Tr	0
Tomato Paste	1 Tbsp	15	Tr	0	3	Tr	3	Tr	0
Tomato Puree	1 cup	100	Tr	0	23	5	18	4	0
Tomato Sauce, canned	1 cup	60	Tr	0	13	4	9	3	0
Topping, for dessert	***	***	*	*	*	*	*	*	*
Butterscotch	2 Tbsp	100	Tr	0	27	Tr	27	Tr	0
Caramel	2 Tbsp	100	Tr	0	27	Tr	27	Tr	0
Chocolate	2 Tbsp	109	Tr	0	25	1	24	1	0
Cream, Whipped Topping (see also Cream, Whipped Topping)	***	***	*	*	*	*	*	*	*
heavy cream	1 cup	410	44	97	3	0	3	3	0
heavy cream	2 Tbsp	50	6	100	Tr	0	Tr	Tr	0

	Serving Size	Calories	Fat (g)	Calories from Fat (%)	Total Carbs (g)	Fiber (g)	Net Carbs (g)	Protein (g)	Sugar Alcohol (g)
light cream	1 cup	350	37	95	4	0	4	4	0
light cream	2 Tbsp	45	5	100	Tr	0	Tr	Tr	0
pressurized, in can	1 Tbsp	10	Tr	0	Tr	0	Tr	Tr	0
Magic Shell	2 Tbsp	207	15	65	17	1	16	1	0
Marshmallow cream	1 oz	90	Tr	0	22	0	22	Tr	0
Maraschino cherries	3 ea	21	0	0	5	0	5	0	0
Pineapple	2 Tbsp	110	Tr	0	28	Tr	28	Tr	0
Strawberry	2 Tbsp	110	Tr	0	28	Tr	28	Tr	0
Sprinkles (jimmies)	1 Tbsp	60	3	45	9	0	9	0	0
Tortellini, cheese filled	¾ cup	250	6	22	38	2	36	11	0
Tortilla, 6" dia, ready to cook	***	***	*	*	*	*	*	*	*
Corn	1	50	Tr	0	11	2	9	1	0
Flour	1	90	2	20	15	Tr	15	3	0
Tortillas & Wraps, Low Carb	***	***	*	*	*	*	*	*	*
Caulipower Tortillas, original cauliflower	2	120	1	8	25	3	22	3	0
Caulipower Tortillas, grain-free cauliflower	2	140	4	26	19	3	16	7	0
La Banderita Carb Counter 8" tortillas	1	81	2	22	11	6	5	5	0
La Tortilla Factory low-carb tortillas	***	***	*	*	*	*	*	*	*
Flour burrito	1	110	3.5	29	23	13	10	7	0
Flour fajita	1	45	1.5	30	10	6	4	3	0
Flour soft taco	1	70	2.5	32	15	9	6	5	0
Whole wheat fajita	1	40	1.5	34	9	6	3	4	0
Whole wheat original size	1	50	2	36	11	8	3	5	0
Whole wheat large	1	90	3	30	19	13	6	8	0
Mama Lupe's low-carb tortillas	1	60	3	45	7	4	3	5	0
Mission Carb Balance tortillas	***	***	*	*	*	*	*	*	*
Fajitas	1	45	1.5	30	13	9	4	3	0

	Serving Size	Calories	Fat (g)	Calories from Fat (%)	Total Carbs (g)	Fiber (g)	Net Carbs (g)	Protein (g)	Sugar Alcohol (g)
Multi-grain fajita	1	110	3	25	17	3	14	3	0
Multi-grain soft taco	1	150	4	24	23	5	18	4	0
Soft taco	1	70	2.5	32	19	13	6	5	0
Whole wheat fajita	1	45	1.5	30	13	9	4	3	0
Whole wheat soft taco	1	60	2.5	38	19	14	5	5	0
NUCO Organic Coconut Wraps (all flavors)	1	70	5	64	6	2	4	1	0
Tortilla Chips	***	***	*	*	*	*	*	*	*
(see also Corn Chips)	***	***	*	*	*	*	*	*	*
Low fat, baked	1 oz	120	2	15	23	2	21	3	0
Nacho flavor, regular	1 oz	150	7	42	18	1	17	2	0
Nacho flavor, reduced fat, baked	1 oz	125	4	29	20	1	19	2	0
Regular, blue corn	1 oz	142	7	44	18	2	16	2	0
Regular, white corn	1 oz	140	7	45	19	2	17	2	0
Regular, yellow corn	1 oz	140	6	39	19	1	18	2	0
Tostada - see individual restaurant listings	***	***	*	*	*	*	*	*	*
Tuna - see Fish/Seafood	***	***	*	*	*	*	*	*	*
Tuna Dishes - see Frozen Dinner	***	***	*	*	*	*	*	*	*
Tuna Salad .	½ cup	190	10	47	10	0	10	16	0
TURKEY	***	***	*	*	*	*	*	*	*
Giblets, simmered, chopped	1 cup	290	17	53	1	0	1	30	0
Ground Turkey, 4 oz patty, cooked	1	190	11	52	0	0	0	22	0
Neck, simmered	3 oz	150	6	36	0	0	0	23	0
Roast Turkey	***	***	*	*	*	*	*	*	*
dark meat only	3 oz	160	6	34	0	0	0	24	0
light & dark meat	3 oz	150	4	24	0	0	0	25	0
light meat only	3 oz	130	3	21	0	0	0	25	0

	Serving Size	Calories	Fat (g)	Calories from Fat (%)	Total Carbs (g)	Fiber (g)	Net Carbs (g)	Protein (g)	Sugar Alcohol (g)
(Other Turkey Products, see:	***	***	*	*	*	*	*	*	*
Bologna, Hot Dog, Salami, Sausage & specific entrées)	***	***	*	*	*	*	*	*	*
Turmeric, ground	1 tsp	10	Tr	0	1	Tr	1	Tr	0
Turnip, cooked	***	***	*	*	*	*	*	*	*
Cubes	½ cup	15	Tr	0	4	2	2	Tr	0
Mashed	½ cup	25	Tr	0	6	2	4	Tr	0
Turnip Greens, cooked, chopped	1 cup	30	Tr	0	6	5	1	1	0
Vanilla Extract	***	***	*	*	*	*	*	*	*
Alcohol free	1 tsp	0	0	0	Tr	0	Tr	0	0
Real or imitation	1 tsp	10	0	0	Tr	0	Tr	0	0
VEAL	***	***	*	*	*	*	*	*	*
Chop, loin, braised	***	***	*	*	*	*	*	*	*
lean & fat	3 oz	240	18	68	0	0	0	26	0
lean only	3 oz	190	8	38	0	0	0	29	0
Leg (top round), braised, lean & fat	3 oz	180	5	25	0	0	0	31	0
Liver, braised	3 oz	160	5	28	0	0	0	24	0
Rib, roasted	***	***	*	*	*	*	*	*	*
lean & fat	3 oz	190	12	57	0	0	0	20	0
lean only	3 oz	150	6	36	0	0	0	22	0
Shank, braised	***	***	*	*	*	*	*	*	*
lean & fat	3 oz	160	5	28	0	0	0	27	0
lean only	3 oz	150	4	24	0	0	0	27	0
Shoulder, braised	***	***	*	*	*	*	*	*	*
lean & fat	3 oz	190	9	43	0	0	0	27	0
lean only	3 oz	170	5	26	0	0	0	29	0
Vegetable Burger (see also Soy Burger)	1	120	4	30	10	3	7	11	0
Beyond Meat	1	300	20	60	7	4	3	23	0
Boca	1	124	4	29	10	3	7	11	0
Gardein	1	120	1	8	7	2	5	21	0

	Serving Size	Calories	Fat (g)	Calories from Fat (%)	Total Carbs (g)	Fiber (g)	Net Carbs (g)	Protein (g)	Sugar Alcohol (g)
Morningstar Farms Grillers	1	136	6	40	5	2	3	15	0
Vegetables, mixed	***	***	*	*	*	*	*	*	*
(See specific listings for individual vegetables)	***	***	*	*	*	*	*	*	*
Frozen, cooked	1 cup	120	Tr	0	24	8	16	5	0
Mixed, canned, drained, heated	1 cup	80	Tr	0	15	5	10	4	0
Vinegar	***	***	*	*	*	*	*	*	*
Balsamic	1 Tbsp	15	0	0	3	Tr	3	Tr	0
Cider (apple cider)	1 Tbsp	0	0	0	Tr	0	Tr	0	0
Distilled (white)	1 Tbsp	0	0	0	Tr	0	Tr	0	0
Red wine	1 Tbsp	0	0	0	Tr	0	Tr	Tr	0
Rice	1 Tbsp	0	0	0	0	0	0	0	0
White wine/ champagne	1 Tbsp	0	0	0	0	0	0	0	0
Waffle	***	***	*	*	*	*	*	*	*
Frozen, plain, 4" dia	1	100	3	27	16	Tr	16	2	0
Frozen, buttermilk, 4" dia	1	100	3	27	16	Tr	16	3	0
Whole wheat, 7" dia	1	176	6	31	25	2	23	7	0
Walnut - see Nuts	***	***	*	*	*	*	*	*	*
Water Chestnut, canned, slices	½ cup	35	Tr	0	9	2	7	Tr	0
Watercress, raw, chopped	½ cup	0	Tr	0	Tr	Tr	Tr	Tr	0
Raw, sprigs	10	0	Tr	0	Tr	Tr	Tr	Tr	0
Watermelon	***	***	*	*	*	*	*	*	*
Fresh, diced or balls	1 cup	45	Tr	0	12	Tr	12	Tr	0
Fresh, wedge, 1" thick, ⅟₁₆ of melon, 15" long x 7½" dia	1 wedge	90	Tr	0	22	1	21	2	0
Wheat Bran	¼ cup	30	Tr	0	9	6	3	2	0
Wheat Germ, toasted, plain	1 Tbsp	25	Tr	0	4	1	3	2	0

	Serving Size	Calories	Fat (g)	Calories from Fat (%)	Total Carbs (g)	Fiber (g)	Net Carbs (g)	Protein (g)	Sugar Alcohol (g)
Whipped Cream - see Cream, Whipped Topping	***	***	*	*	*	*	*	*	*
Wiener - see Hot Dog	***	***	*	*	*	*	*	*	*
Yam - see Sweet Potato	***	***	*	*	*	*	*	*	*
Yeast	***	***	*	*	*	*	*	*	*
Compressed	1 cake	20	Tr	0	3	1	2	1	0
Dry, active, regular size pkg	1	20	Tr	0	3	2	1	3	0
Dry, active	1 tsp	10	Tr	0	2	Tr	2	2	0
Yeast Extract Spread	1 tsp	10	0	0	Tr	Tr	Tr	Tr	0
Yogurt	***	***	*	*	*	*	*	*	*
Fruit, low fat	½ cup	120	1	8	23	0	23	5	0
Fruit, nonfat	½ cup	120	Tr	0	23	0	23	5	0
Fruit, w/ low calorie sweetener	½ cup	130	2	14	23	0	23	6	0
Plain	***	***	*	*	*	*	*	*	*
made w/ whole milk	½ cup	80	4	45	6	0	6	4	0
made w/ low fat milk	½ cup	80	2	23	9	0	9	6	0
made w/ skim milk	½ cup	70	Tr	0	9	0	9	7	0
Vanilla, low fat	½ cup	100	2	18	17	0	17	6	0
Yogurt, Frozen	***	***	*	*	*	*	*	*	*
Chocolate, soft serve	½ cup	120	4	30	18	2	16	3	0
Regular	½ cup	110	3	25	19	0	19	3	0
Regular, chocolate	½ cup	110	3	25	19	1	18	3	0
Vanilla, soft serve	½ cup	120	4	30	17	0	17	3	0
Zucchini	***	***	*	*	*	*	*	*	*
Cooked	1 cup	48	1	19	10	3	7	2	0
Fresh, med size	1	30	Tr	0	7	2	5	2	0
Spirals	¾ cup	15	0	0	2	1	1	1	0

Dining Out

	Serving Size	Calories	Fat (g)	Calories from Fat (%)	Total Carbs (g)	Fiber (g)	Net Carbs (g)	Protein (g)
A&W	***	***	*	*	*	*	*	*
A&W diet root beer float	16 oz	170	5	26	30	0	30	2
A&W diet root beer, lg	22 fl oz	0	0	0	0	0	0	0
A&W diet root beer, med	14 fl oz	0	0	0	0	0	0	0
A&W diet root beer, sm	11 fl oz	0	0	0	0	0	0	0
A&W regular root beer, lg	22 fl oz	460	0	0	121	0	121	0
A&W regular root beer, med	14 fl oz	290	0	0	76	0	76	0
A&W regular root beer, sm	11 fl oz	220	0	0	57	0	57	0
A&W root beer float	16 oz	330	5	14	70	0	70	2
A&W root beer freeze	16 oz	430	9	19	79	0	79	9
BBQ dipping sauce	1 oz	40	0	0	10	0	10	0
Breaded onion rings, lg	1	480	27	51	62	3	59	7
Breaded onion rings, reg	1	350	16	41	45	2	43	5
Burger patty, extra	1	170	12	64	2	0	2	15
Caramel sundae	1	340	9	24	57	0	57	8
Cheese curds	1	570	40	63	27	2	25	27
Cheese fries	1	390	18	42	50	4	46	4
Cheeseburger	1	420	21	45	37	4	33	23
Chicken strips	3 pc	500	29	52	32	2	30	28
Chili cheese fries	1	410	17	37	52	5	47	8
Chocolate milkshake	16 oz	700	29	37	100	2	98	11
Chocolate sundae	1	320	8	23	53	0	53	8
Coney (chili) cheese dog	1	380	23	54	28	2	26	14
Coney (chili) dog	1	340	20	53	26	2	24	14
Corn dog nuggets, reg	8 pc	280	13	42	32	2	30	9
Corn dog nuggets, sm	5 pc	180	8	40	20	1	19	5
Crispy chicken sandwich	1	550	25	41	52	5	47	30
French fries, lg	1	430	17	36	61	6	55	5
French fries, reg	1	310	12	35	45	4	41	3
French fries, sm	1	200	8	36	28	3	25	2
Grilled chicken sandwich	1	400	15	34	31	4	27	35
Hamburger	1	380	19	45	33	3	30	21

	Serving Size	Calories	Fat (g)	Calories from Fat (%)	Total Carbs (g)	Fiber (g)	Net Carbs (g)	Protein (g)
Honey mustard dipping sauce	1 oz	100	6	54	12	0	12	0
Hot dog plain	1	310	19	55	23	1	22	11
Hot fudge sundae	1	350	11	28	54	1	53	8
M&M's Polar Swirl	12 oz	710	25	32	107	2	105	15
Oreo Polar Swirl	12 oz	690	24	31	107	3	104	14
Original bacon cheeseburger	1	530	30	51	39	4	35	26
Original bacon double cheeseburger	1	760	45	53	45	4	41	44
Original double cheeseburger	1	680	38	50	44	4	40	40
Papa burger	1	690	39	51	44	4	40	40
Papa single burger	1	470	25	48	38	4	34	23
Ranch dipping sauce	1 oz	160	17	96	2	0	2	0
Reese's Polar Swirl	12 oz	740	31	38	97	3	94	18
Strawberry milkshake	16 oz	670	29	39	90	0	90	11
Strawberry sundae	1	300	8	24	47	0	47	12
Vanilla cone	16 oz	260	7	24	41	0	41	7
Vanilla milkshake	16 oz	720	31	39	97	0	97	12
Applebee's	***	***	*	*	*	*	*	*
Insufficient information	***	***	*	*	*	*	*	*
Arby's	***	***	*	*	*	*	*	*
All American Roastburger	1	420	18	39	46	2	44	19
Apple turnover, no icing	1	250	14	50	35	2	33	4
Arby's Melt	1	300	12	36	36	2	34	16
Bacon & Bleu Roastburger	1	470	23	44	44	2	42	22
Bacon, add-on	1	80	6	68	1	0	1	5
Balsamic vinaigrette dressing	1 svg	130	12	83	5	0	5	0
BBQ sauce	1 svg	45	0	0	11	0	11	0
Beef 'n cheddar sandwich, lg	1	660	36	49	46	3	43	43
Beef 'n cheddar sandwich, med	1	540	27	45	44	2	42	33
Beef 'n cheddar sandwich, reg	1	440	20	41	43	2	41	22
Brewed Iced Tea	12 fl oz	5	0	0	1	0	1	0
Buffalo sauce	1 svg	10	1	90	2	0	2	0
Buttermilk ranch dressing	1 svg	230	24	94	2	0	2	0
Cheddar cheese sauce for curly fries	1 svg	50	4	72	4	0	4	1

	Serving Size	Calories	Fat (g)	Calories from Fat (%)	Total Carbs (g)	Fiber (g)	Net Carbs (g)	Protein (g)
Arby's (cont.)	***	***	*	*	*	*	*	*
Cherry turnover, no icing	1	250	14	50	35	2	33	4
Chicken cordon bleu, crispy	1	570	25	39	47	2	45	36
Chicken cordon bleu, roast	1	460	18	35	37	2	35	33
Chicken fillet sandwich, crispy	1	480	23	43	47	2	45	25
Chicken fillet sandwich, roast	1	380	16	38	37	2	35	23
Chicken, bacon & swiss sandwich, crispy	1	540	23	38	50	2	48	31
Chicken, bacon & swiss sandwich, roast	1	440	16	33	40	2	38	30
Chocolate swirl shake	1	650	17	24	110	Tr	110	16
Chopped farmhouse chicken salad, crispy	1	390	19	44	26	22	4	25
Chopped farmhouse chicken salad, grilled	1	250	12	43	10	7	3	22
Chopped farmhouse salad, roast turkey	1	230	13	51	8	2	6	22
Chopped Italian salad	1	430	31	65	11	3	8	23
Chopped side salad	1	70	5	64	4	1	3	5
Chopped turkey club salad	1	250	12	43	10	3	7	23
Classic Italian toasted sub	1	600	27	41	61	3	58	25
Corned beef Reuben sandwich	1	610	33	49	55	3	52	31
Curly fries, lg	1	600	36	54	70	7	63	8
Curly fries, med	1	500	29	52	58	6	52	7
Curly fries, sm	1	360	21	53	42	4	38	5
Dijon honey mustard dressing	1 svg	150	17	100	8	0	8	1
French dip & swiss toasted sub w/ au jus	1	510	16	28	63	3	60	29
Ham & Swiss Melt	1	280	6	19	35	1	34	18
Icing for turnovers	1 svg	130	2	14	29	0	29	0
Jalapeno bites, lg	8 pc	490	34	62	47	3	44	9
Jalapeno bites, reg	5 pc	310	21	61	29	2	27	5
Jamocha swirl shake	1	640	17	24	107	Tr	107	16
Light Italian dressing	1 svg	20	1	45	2	0	2	0
Loaded potato bites, lg	8 pc	570	35	55	43	4	39	18
Loaded potato bites, reg	5 pc	350	22	57	27	2	25	11

	Serving Size	Calories	Fat (g)	Calories from Fat (%)	Total Carbs (g)	Fiber (g)	Net Carbs (g)	Protein (g)
Mozzarella sticks, lg	6 pc	640	42	59	57	3	54	27
Mozzarella sticks, reg	4 pc	430	28	59	38	2	36	18
Pecan chicken salad sandwich	1	870	47	49	92	6	86	25
Philly beef toasted sub	1	590	26	40	59	3	56	29
Popcorn chicken, lg	1	410	18	40	34	3	31	27
Popcorn chicken, reg	1	330	15	41	27	2	25	22
Potato cakes, lg	4	490	37	68	52	5	47	3
Potato cakes, med	3	370	28	68	39	3	36	3
Potato cakes, sm	2	250	18	65	26	2	24	2
Roast beef & swiss sandwich	1	760	40	47	73	6	67	36
Roast beef sandwich, lg	1	550	28	46	41	3	38	42
Roast beef sandwich, med	1	415	21	46	34	2	32	31
Roast beef sandwich, reg	1	320	14	39	34	2	32	21
Roast chicken club	1	500	17	31	46	2	44	30
Roast ham & swiss sandwich	1	690	31	40	75	5	70	33
Roast turkey & swiss sandwich	1	710	30	38	74	5	69	41
Roast turkey, ranch & bacon sandwich	1	820	38	42	74	5	69	46
Super Roast Beef	1	400	19	43	41	5	36	21
Turkey bacon club toasted sub	1	582	21	32	60	3	57	35
Ultimate BLT sandwich	1	780	45	52	75	6	69	23
Vanilla shake	1	550	17	28	83	0	83	16
Au Bon Pain	***	***	*	*	*	*	*	*
Almond croissant	1	600	38	57	55	4	51	13
Apple croissant	1	280	11	35	44	3	41	5
Apple croissants tart	1 oz	80	4	45	12	1	11	1
Apple strudel	1	440	24	49	50	1	49	5
Arizona chicken sandwich	1	690	28	37	60	4	56	47
Asiago cheese bagel	1	340	6	16	56	2	54	15
Bacon & bagel sandwich	1	340	6	16	58	2	56	16
Bacon & egg melt sandwich, on ciabatta	1	510	26	46	41	2	39	26
Baja turkey sandwich	1	700	27	35	71	5	66	46
Baked potato	1 oz	25	0	0	5	1	4	1
Baked stuffed potato soup	12 oz	350	20	51	29	2	27	9

	Serving Size	Calories	Fat (g)	Calories from Fat (%)	Total Carbs (g)	Fiber (g)	Net Carbs (g)	Protein (g)
Au Bon Pain (cont.)	***	***	*	*	*	*	*	*
Balsamic vinaigrette dressing	2 oz	120	9	68	8	0	8	0
Banana nut pound cake	1	480	26	49	56	1	55	7
BBQ beef salad	1 oz	35	1	26	4	0	4	2
BBQ brisket harvest rice bowl	1	790	19	22	118	10	108	37
BBQ brisket harvest rice bowl w/ brown rice	1	740	21	26	103	12	91	37
BBQ brisket sandwich	1	660	21	29	81	5	76	36
BBQ brisket wrap	1	690	28	37	82	8	74	32
BBQ chicken & beef stew	12 oz	300	10	30	35	3	32	19
BBQ chicken harvest rice bowl	1	690	11	14	120	12	108	31
BBQ chicken harvest rice bowl w/ brown rice	1	350	12	31	105	13	92	31
BBQ chicken sandwich	1	560	13	21	83	6	77	29
BBQ chicken wrap	1	640	24	34	83	9	74	29
Beef & vegetable stew	12 oz	310	16	46	25	3	22	18
Beef stroganoff penne	1 oz	40	2	45	4	0	4	2
Black bean soup	12 oz	260	1	3	46	26	20	15
Blondie	1	460	33	65	59	2	57	5
Blue cheese dressing	2 oz	310	33	96	2	0	2	2
Blueberry muffin	1	490	17	31	74	2	72	9
Broccoli cheddar soup	12 oz	300	21	63	20	2	18	11
Brown rice	1 oz	30	0	0	6	0	6	1
Brown rice Waldorf salad	1 oz	45	3	60	5	0	5	0
Caesar dressing	2 oz	270	28	93	4	0	4	1
Caprese sandwich	1	680	32	42	65	4	61	30
Carrot ginger soup	12 oz	140	5	32	22	3	19	1
Carrot walnut muffin	1	560	27	43	72	4	68	9
Chef's salad	1	250	15	54	7	3	4	24
Cherry Danish	1	420	20	43	54	1	53	7
Cherry strudel	1	460	26	51	50	1	49	5
Chicken & dumpling soup	12 oz	210	7	30	28	2	26	11
Chicken & vegetable stew	12 oz	290	17	53	26	3	23	11
Chicken broccoli alfredo penne	1 oz	60	4	60	3	0	3	2
Chicken broccoli alfredo penne	12 oz	680	43	57	38	2	36	28

	Serving Size	Calories	Fat (g)	Calories from Fat (%)	Total Carbs (g)	Fiber (g)	Net Carbs (g)	Protein (g)
Chicken Caesar asiago wrap	1	610	28	41	61	5	56	34
Chicken Florentine soup	12 oz	250	13	47	25	1	24	8
Chicken gumbo	12 oz	180	8	40	21	2	19	6
Chicken marsala penne	1 oz	35	1	26	4	0	4	2
Chicken noodle soup	12 oz	130	3	21	19	2	17	8
Chicken penne pesto	1 oz	60	3	45	4	0	4	3
Chicken pesto sandwich	1	660	24	33	66	4	62	43
Chicken Provençal	1 oz	25	0	0	4	0	4	2
Chickpea & tomato cucumber salad	1	230	12	47	23	7	16	11
Chocolate cheesecake brownie	1	460	19	37	74	1	73	5
Chocolate cherry tulip	1	410	21	46	54	2	52	5
Chocolate chip brownie	1	510	19	34	74	1	73	6
Chocolate chip cookie	1	280	13	42	40	2	38	3
Chocolate chip muffin	1	580	23	36	83	3	80	9
Chocolate croissant	1	440	22	45	58	3	55	7
Chocolate dipped cranberry almond macaroon	1	300	15	45	36	4	32	4
Chocolate dipped shortbread	1	380	22	52	42	1	41	4
Chocolate orange pecan scone	1	580	28	43	74	3	71	10
Cinnamon crisp bagel	1	410	7	15	77	4	73	11
Cinnamon raisin bagel	1	320	1	3	68	3	65	11
Cinnamon scone	1	530	27	46	60	2	58	9
Cinnamon walnut quinoa	1 oz	45	3	60	4	1	3	2
Clam chowder	12 oz	320	18	51	27	1	26	9
Confetti cookie w/ M&M's	1	280	13	42	39	0	39	3
Corn & green chili bisque	12 oz	260	15	52	27	3	24	6
Corn chowder	12 oz	350	18	46	40	3	37	9
Corn muffin	1	490	17	31	75	3	72	10
Cranberry walnut muffin	1	540	25	42	66	4	62	10
Cream of chicken & wild rice soup	12 oz	240	14	53	22	1	21	6
Creamed spinach	1 oz	30	2	60	2	1	1	1
Crème de fleur	1	500	25	45	57	2	55	11
Crumb cake	1	750	40	48	97	1	96	8
Curried rice & lentil soup	12 oz	170	2	11	30	8	22	8

	Serving Size	Calories	Fat (g)	Calories from Fat (%)	Total Carbs (g)	Fiber (g)	Net Carbs (g)	Protein (g)
Au Bon Pain (cont.)	***	***	*	*	*	*	*	*
Demi chicken sandwich w/ cheddar, on baguette	1	440	15	31	50	3	47	27
Demi chicken sandwich, on baguette	1	370	9	22	49	3	46	22
Demi ham sandwich w/ swiss, on baguette	1	400	10	23	56	3	53	23
Demi ham sandwich, on baguette	1	330	5	14	56	3	53	17
Demi roast beef sandwich w/ brie, on baguette	1	460	18	35	49	3	46	24
Demi roast beef sandwich, on baguette	1	360	8	20	49	3	46	19
Demi tuna sandwich w/ cheddar, on baguette	1	400	14	32	50	3	47	22
Demi tuna sandwich, on baguette	1	320	7	20	49	3	46	17
Demi turkey sandwich w/ swiss, on baguette	1	400	12	27	49	2	47	24
Demi turkey sandwich, on baguette	1	320	6	17	49	2	47	18
Double chocolate chunk muffin	1	620	25	36	86	4	82	11
Egg & bacon bagel sandwich	1	420	8	17	60	3	57	25
Egg & broccoli baked sandwich	1	350	10	26	42	3	39	23
Egg & cheese bagel sandwich	1	450	10	20	61	3	58	26
Egg & cucumber salad	1 oz	40	3	68	1	0	1	2
Egg bagel sandwich	1	360	4	10	60	3	57	21
Egg, bacon & cheese bagel sandwich	1	510	15	26	61	3	58	31
Eggplant & mozzarella sandwich	1	670	30	40	73	6	67	27
Eggplant parmesan	1 oz	50	3	54	4	1	3	2
English toffee cake	1	250	4	14	27	1	26	2
Everything bagel	1	340	5	13	61	3	58	13
Fat free raspberry vinaigrette	2 oz	50	0	0	12	0	12	0
Fire roasted exotic grains & vegetables	1 oz	40	1	23	7	1	6	1

	Serving Size	Calories	Fat (g)	Calories from Fat (%)	Total Carbs (g)	Fiber (g)	Net Carbs (g)	Protein (g)
French Moroccan tomato lentil soup	12 oz	190	2	9	32	10	22	10
French onion soup	12 oz	130	5	35	19	2	17	3
French pecan toast	1 oz	70	4	51	8	0	8	2
Garden salad	1	70	2	26	12	3	9	3
Garden vegetable soup	12 oz	80	2	23	13	3	10	3
Gazpacho	12 oz	90	5	50	11	3	8	2
Grilled chicken Caesar asiago salad	1	300	13	39	18	3	15	28
Ham & cheese croissant	1	400	20	45	38	2	36	15
Ham & swiss half sandwich, on farmhouse roll	1	320	13	37	34	2	32	21
Ham & swiss, on country white bread	1	530	17	29	60	2	58	39
Hazelnut mocha brownie	1	490	22	40	74	3	71	6
Hazelnut vinaigrette dressing	2 oz	270	25	83	11	0	11	1
Hearty cabbage soup	12 oz	110	5	41	14	3	11	5
Honey 9 grain bagel	1	350	4	10	69	6	63	12
Honey pecan cream cheese	2 oz	200	16	72	10	0	10	2
Iced cinnamon roll	1	410	15	33	60	2	58	8
Italian sausage, peppers & onions	1 oz	25	1	36	1	0	1	2
Italian wedding soup	12 oz	170	7	37	19	3	16	8
Jalapeno double cheddar bagel	1	340	10	26	53	2	51	17
Jalapeno mayonnaise	1 oz	50	5	90	1	0	1	2
Jamaican black bean soup	12 oz	250	1	4	43	23	20	16
Jambalaya	1 oz	25	1	36	2	0	2	1
Lemon Danish	1	440	20	41	57	1	56	7
Lemon drop tulip	1	410	19	42	55	1	54	5
Lemon pound cake	1	520	25	43	67	1	66	6
Light ranch dressing	2 oz	120	11	83	3	0	3	2
Lite cream cheese spread	2 oz	120	9	68	5	0	5	4
Lite honey mustard dressing	2 oz	170	9	48	20	0	20	1
Lite olive oil vinaigrette	2 oz	110	10	82	6	0	6	0
Low fat triple berry muffin	1	300	3	9	65	2	63	4
Macaroni & cheese	1 oz	40	3	68	3	0	3	2

	Serving Size	Calories	Fat (g)	Calories from Fat (%)	Total Carbs (g)	Fiber (g)	Net Carbs (g)	Protein (g)
Au Bon Pain *(cont.)*	***	***	*	*	*	*	*	*
Macaroni & cheese	12 oz	500	29	52	36	2	34	20
Mandarin sesame chicken salad	1	310	17	49	29	3	26	20
Marble pound cake	1	490	26	48	59	1	58	6
Mayan chicken harvest rice bowl	1	560	12	19	87	5	82	27
Mayan chicken harvest rice bowl w/ brown rice	1	510	13	23	72	7	65	27
Mayan chicken hot wrap	1	580	13	20	93	6	87	24
Mayonnaise	1 oz	70	7	90	2	0	2	0
Meat lasagna	1 oz	45	2	40	4	0	4	2
Meat lasagna	10.7 oz	470	24	46	41	5	36	22
Meatballs & marinara sauce	1 oz	50	4	72	2	1	1	2
Meatloaf w/ wine sauce	1 oz	50	3	54	2	0	2	2
Mediterranean chicken salad	1	290	16	50	12	3	9	23
Mediterranean pepper soup	12 oz	170	5	26	26	8	18	7
Mediterranean spread	1 oz	120	11	83	2	1	1	2
Mediterranean wrap	1	610	29	43	73	8	65	18
Mini chocolate chip cookie	1	70	3	39	10	0	10	1
Mini oatmeal raisin cookie	1	60	3	45	10	1	9	1
Mint chocolate pound cake	1	530	29	49	64	3	61	7
Mozzarella chicken sandwich	1	680	24	32	67	4	63	48
Mustard	1 tsp	0	0	0	0	0	0	0
Oatmeal raisin cookie	1	230	8	31	36	2	34	3
Oatmeal, med	12 oz	210	4	17	38	5	33	8
Old fashioned tomato soup	12 oz	200	7	32	27	3	24	6
Onion dill bagel	1	280	1	3	57	3	54	11
Orange scone	1	470	23	44	57	1	56	10
Orzo Toscano salad	1 oz	35	1	26	6	1	5	1
Palmier	1	440	23	47	53	1	52	1
Pasta e fagioli soup	12 oz	260	8	28	35	9	26	12
Pecan roll	1	810	41	46	99	3	96	12
Penne marinara	1 oz	30	1	30	55	5	50	1
Pineapple blueberry cobbler	1 oz	45	2	40	8	1	7	1

	Serving Size	Calories	Fat (g)	Calories from Fat (%)	Total Carbs (g)	Fiber (g)	Net Carbs (g)	Protein (g)
Plain bagel	1	280	1	3	56	2	54	11
Plain croissant	1	310	17	49	31	1	30	7
Polenta marinara	1 oz	25	1	36	3	0	3	1
Pomegranate vinaigrette dressing	2 oz	250	22	79	12	0	12	0
Poppy bagel	1	320	4	11	58	4	54	12
Portobello & goat cheese sandwich	1	550	25	41	62	6	56	19
Portobello, egg & cheddar sandwich	1	500	26	47	42	3	39	22
Portuguese kale soup	12 oz	130	5	35	15	4	11	5
Potato bacon salad	1 oz	40	2	45	5	1	4	1
Potato cheese soup	12 oz	260	14	48	24	2	22	7
Potato leek soup	12 oz	300	19	57	28	2	26	5
Prosciutto & egg sandwich, on asiago bagel	1	520	16	28	60	1	59	34
Prosciutto mozzarella sandwich	1	810	41	46	71	4	67	41
Quinoa	1 oz	25	0	0	4	1	3	1
Raisin bran muffin	1	480	11	21	85	10	75	12
Raspberry cheese croissant	1	370	17	41	46	2	44	8
Red beans, Italian sausage & rice soup	12 oz	270	6	20	40	17	23	14
Roast beef & brie half sandwich, on farmhouse roll	1	350	14	36	34	2	32	20
Roast beef & brie sandwich, on country white bread	1	600	21	32	59	3	56	39
Roast beef Caesar sandwich	1	680	27	36	68	3	65	40
Roasted apple cranberry orzo	1 oz	45	1	20	9	1	8	1
Roasted carrots	1 oz	15	0	0	3	1	2	0
Roasted green beans w/ almonds	1 oz	20	1	45	2	1	1	1
Roasted potatoes	1 oz	35	2	51	6	1	5	1
Roasted zucchini & summer squash	1 oz	5	0	0	1	0	1	0
Rocky road brownie	1	490	22	40	74	2	72	6
Sausage w/ peppers & onions	1 oz	50	5	90	1	0	1	2

	Serving Size	Calories	Fat (g)	Calories from Fat (%)	Total Carbs (g)	Fiber (g)	Net Carbs (g)	Protein (g)
Au Bon Pain (cont.)	***	***	*	*	*	*	*	*
Sausage, egg & cheddar sandwich, on asiago bagel	1	810	47	52	58	1	57	38
Scrambled eggs	1 oz	35	3	77	1	0	1	3
Sesame brown rice & orange salad	1 oz	45	3	60	6	0	6	1
Sesame ginger dressing	2 oz	230	20	78	12	0	12	1
Sesame seed bagel	1	330	5	14	59	3	56	12
Shortbread cookie	1	340	20	53	37	1	36	4
Side garden salad	1	50	1	18	8	2	6	2
Smoked salmon & wasabi sandwich, on onion dill bagel	1	430	11	23	64	1	63	23
Southern black-eyed pea soup	12 oz	170	2	11	29	9	20	11
Southwest corn casserole	1 oz	60	4	60	4	0	4	3
Southwest fusilli pasta salad	1 oz	45	3	60	4	0	4	1
Southwest jalapeno muffin	1	560	30	48	64	2	62	8
Southwest panzanella salad	1 oz	50	3	54	7	0	7	1
Southwest tortilla soup	12 oz	190	10	47	23	4	19	4
Southwest tuna wrap	1	750	40	48	66	7	59	39
Southwest vegetable soup	12 oz	170	5	26	37	8	29	8
Spicy tuna sandwich	1	470	16	31	60	11	49	29
Spinach & cheese croissant	1	290	16	50	28	2	26	10
Split pea w/ ham soup	12 oz	250	2	7	41	15	26	18
Steakhouse sandwich, on ciabatta	1	720	30	38	76	4	72	44
Stuffed peppers w/ lentils	1 oz	20	0	0	3	1	2	1
Sundried tomato cream cheese	2 oz	140	11	71	5	1	4	4
Sundried tomato spread	0.5 oz	45	4	80	1	0	1	0
Sweet cheese croissant	1	400	19	43	49	1	48	9
Sweet cheese Danish	1	470	24	46	54	1	53	9
Thai coconut curry soup	12 oz	160	7	39	21	2	19	4
Thai peanut chicken salad	1	240	8	30	19	4	15	22
Thai peanut chicken wrap	1	530	15	25	79	6	73	30
Thai peanut dressing	2 oz	160	8	45	20	0	20	2
Tomato basil bisque	12 oz	210	9	39	27	4	23	7

	Serving Size	Calories	Fat (g)	Calories from Fat (%)	Total Carbs (g)	Fiber (g)	Net Carbs (g)	Protein (g)
Tomato cheddar soup	12 oz	240	16	60	17	2	15	8
Tomato cucumber salad	1 oz	10	0	0	2	0	2	0
Tomato Florentine soup	12 oz	130	3	21	18	2	16	6
Tomato rice soup	12 oz	120	1	8	24	2	22	4
Tomato, green bean & almond salad	1 oz	20	2	90	2	0	2	0
Tuna & cheddar half sandwich, on farmhouse roll	1	360	16	40	35	2	33	19
Tuna & cheddar sandwich, on country white bread	1	610	25	37	63	3	60	37
Tuna garden salad	1	240	12	45	15	4	11	20
Tuna melt	1	690	30	39	71	5	66	42
Tuna salad	1 oz	40	3	68	1	0	1	4
Turkey & strawberry salad	1	110	4	33	10	4	6	11
Turkey & swiss half sandwich, on farmhouse roll	1	320	11	31	34	2	32	22
Turkey & swiss sandwich, on country white	1	530	14	24	60	2	58	42
Turkey club sandwich	1	700	31	40	59	2	57	45
Turkey cobb salad	1	330	19	52	14	4	10	27
Turkey melt	1	810	32	36	79	3	76	47
Tuscan vegetable soup	12 oz	170	5	26	23	3	20	7
Tzatziki	1 oz	15	0	0	2	0	2	1
Vegetable beef barley soup	12 oz	140	3	19	21	4	17	9
Vegetable cream cheese	2 oz	170	16	85	3	0	3	3
Vegetarian chili	12 oz	220	2	8	39	20	19	12
Vegetarian lasagna	1 oz	20	0	0	4	1	3	1
Vegetarian lentil soup	12 oz	170	2	11	31	11	20	9
Vegetarian minestrone soup	12 oz	120	2	15	20	4	16	5
Watermelon & feta salad	1 oz	15	1	60	3	0	3	0
White chocolate macadamia nut cookie	1	300	16	48	36	1	35	3
White chocolate toffee bagel braid	1	350	6	15	63	2	61	11
White rice	1 oz	35	0	0	8	0	8	1
Wild mushroom bisque	12 oz	190	9	43	22	2	20	5

	Serving Size	Calories	Fat (g)	Calories from Fat (%)	Total Carbs (g)	Fiber (g)	Net Carbs (g)	Protein (g)
Baskin Robbins								
(all ice creams 1 sm scoop, unless noted)	***	***	*	*	*	*	*	*
Aloha brownie, light churned	1	150	5	30	26	1	25	3
Butter almond crunch, reduced fat, no sugar added	1	140	7	45	19	3	16	4
Cabana berry banana, reduced fat, no sugar added	1	90	4	40	17	2	15	3
Cake cone	1	25	0	0	5	0	5	0
Cappuccino chip, light churned	1	140	5	32	20	1	19	3
Caramel turtle truffle, reduced fat, no sugar added	1	120	5	38	24	2	22	3
Cherries jubilee	1	150	8	48	19	1	18	3
Chocolate chip cookie dough	1	190	9	43	23	0	23	3
Chocolate chip ice cream	1	170	10	53	17	0	17	3
Chocolate fudge	1	160	10	56	21	0	21	3
Chocolate ice cream	1	160	9	51	21	0	21	3
Chocolate overload, reduced fat, no sugar added	1	120	5	38	23	3	20	4
Gold medal ribbon	1	170	8	42	19	0	19	3
Jamoca almond fudge	1	170	9	48	17	1	16	3
Lemon sorbet	1	80	0	0	21	0	21	0
Mango fruit blast smoothie	16 oz	440	2	4	104	2	102	4
Mango sorbet	1	80	0	0	20	0	20	0
Milk chocolate, light churned	1	130	5	35	20	1	19	4
Mint chocolate chip	1	170	10	53	15	0	15	3
Mint *Oreo*, light churned	1	150	5	30	25	1	24	3
Old fashioned butter pecan	1	170	11	58	20	1	19	3
Orange sherbet freeze	16 oz	370	4	10	82	0	82	3
Oreo cookies 'n cream	1	170	9	48	15	0	15	3
Peach passion banana fruit blast smoothie	16 oz	420	1	2	102	4	98	6
Peach passion fruit blast	16 oz	270	0	0	68	2	66	1
Pineapple coconut, reduced fat, no sugar added	1	100	4	36	18	2	16	3
Pistachio almond	1	180	12	60	22	1	21	4

	Serving Size	Calories	Fat (g)	Calories from Fat (%)	Total Carbs (g)	Fiber (g)	Net Carbs (g)	Protein (g)
Pralines and cream	1	180	9	45	19	0	19	3
Rainbow sherbet	1	100	1.5	14	21	0	21	1
Raspberry chip, light churned	1	140	4	26	24	1	23	3
Reese's Peanut Butter Cup	1	190	11	52	19	0	19	4
Rocky road ice cream	1	180	10	50	22	0	22	3
Strawberry banana fruit blast smoothie	16 oz	390	Tr	0	94	3	91	5
Strawberry Citrus fruit blast	16 oz	240	0	0	61	1	60	1
Strawberry sorbet	1	80	0	0	21	0	21	0
Sugar cone	1	45	Tr	0	9	0	9	1
Vanilla ice cream	1	170	10	53	17	0	17	3
Vanilla yogurt, fat free	1	90	0	0	20	0	20	4
Vanilla, light churned	1	130	5	35	19	1	18	4
Very berry strawberry	1	140	7	45	18	0	18	2
Waffle cone	1	160	4	23	28	0	28	2
Wild mango fruit blast	16 oz	340	1	3	84	2	82	1
World class chocolate	1	180	10	50	19	0	19	3
Blimpie								
(all subs on 6" regular roll, unless otherwise stated)	***	***	*	*	*	*	*	*
Antipasto salad	1	250	14	50	12	4	8	20
Apple turnover	1	340	21	56	35	1	34	4
Bacon, egg & cheese biscuit	1	430	24	50	37	1	36	17
Bacon, egg & cheese bluffin	1	290	14	43	27	2	25	16
Bacon, egg & cheese burrito	1	550	24	39	56	5	51	31
Bacon, egg & cheese croissant	1	370	21	51	30	1	29	14
Bean w/ ham soup	1	140	1	6	23	11	12	8
Beef steak & noodle soup	1	120	3	23	14	0	14	8
Beef stew	1	170	4	21	18	2	16	17
Biscuit, plain	1	260	11	38	34	1	33	6
Blimpie best	1	420	14	30	49	3	46	25
Blimpie best, super stacked	1	520	19	33	52	3	49	37
Blimpie trio, super stacked	1	490	12	22	52	3	49	41
BLT	1	450	22	44	46	3	43	15
BLT, super stacked	1	640	41	58	43	2	41	22

	Serving Size	Calories	Fat (g)	Calories from Fat (%)	Total Carbs (g)	Fiber (g)	Net Carbs (g)	Protein (g)
Blimpie *(cont.)*	***	***	*	*	*	*	*	*
Blue cheese dressing	1.5 oz	230	24	94	2	Tr	2	2
Bluffin, plain	1	30	1	30	25	2	23	5
Breakfast panini, 4"	1	490	14	26	67	2	65	26
Breakfast panini, 6"	1	770	24	28	96	3	93	43
Brownie	1	180	7	35	28	1	27	2
Buffalo chicken ciabatta	1	580	27	42	50	3	47	32
Buffalo chicken salad	1	220	9	37	10	4	6	25
Buttermilk ranch dressing	1.5 oz	230	24	94	2	Tr	2	1
Captain's corn chowder	1	210	7	30	29	4	25	6
Chef salad	1	180	7	35	10	2	8	18
Cherry turnover	1	350	21	54	35	1	34	4
Chicken & dumpling soup	1	170	5	26	19	3	16	11
Chicken Caesar salad	1	190	8	38	6	3	3	25
Chicken Caesar wrap	1	610	29	43	56	4	52	30
Chicken cheddar bacon ranch	1	640	34	48	48	3	45	36
Chicken gumbo	1	90	2	20	13	2	11	6
Chicken noodle soup	1	130	4	28	18	2	16	7
Chicken teriyaki	1	430	9	19	50	1	49	35
Chicken teriyaki, on wheat	1	420	10	21	47	5	42	36
Chicken w/ white & wild rice soup	1	250	10	36	15	4	11	14
Chocolate chunk cookie	1	200	10	45	25	0	25	2
Cinnamon roll	1	450	20	40	60	2	58	9
Club	1	390	10	23	49	3	46	25
Club, on wheat	1	360	11	28	43	6	37	26
Cole slaw	1 svg	160	9	51	20	2	18	1
Cream of broccoli w/ cheese soup	1	190	8	38	15	3	12	6
Cream of potato soup	1	190	9	43	24	3	21	5
Creamy Caesar dressing	1.5 oz	210	21	90	2	Tr	2	1
Creamy Italian dressing	1.5 oz	180	18	90	4	0	4	0
Croissant, plain	1	230	11	43	28	1	27	5
Cuban	1	410	11	24	43	1	42	29
Deli style mustard	0.5 oz	5	0	0	0	0	0	0

	Serving Size	Calories	Fat (g)	Calories from Fat (%)	Total Carbs (g)	Fiber (g)	Net Carbs (g)	Protein (g)
Dijon honey mustard dressing	1.5 oz	180	17	85	8	Tr	8	1
Egg & cheese biscuit	1	390	21	48	37	1	36	14
Egg & cheese bluffin	1	250	10	36	27	2	25	13
Egg & cheese burrito	1	510	20	35	56	5	51	28
Egg & cheese croissant	1	330	18	49	30	1	29	12
Fat free Italian dressing	1.5 oz	25	0	0	5	0	5	0
French dip	1	410	11	24	46	1	45	30
French onion soup	1	80	4	45	11	1	10	2
Garden salad	1	30	0	0	6	3	3	2
Grande chili w/ bean & beef	1	250	9	32	30	18	12	18
Grilled chicken Caesar ciabatta	1	620	24	35	63	3	60	34
Ham & swiss	1	390	10	23	50	3	47	25
Ham & swiss, on wheat	1	370	11	27	44	6	38	26
Ham, egg & cheese biscuit	1	420	21	45	39	1	38	19
Ham, egg & cheese bluffin	1	280	11	35	29	2	27	18
Ham, egg & cheese burrito	1	560	21	34	58	5	53	36
Ham, egg & cheese croissant	1	370	19	46	31	1	30	17
Ham, salami & cheese	1	440	16	33	49	3	46	25
Harvest vegetable soup	1	100	1	9	19	3	16	4
Honey mustard	1 oz	45	1	20	7	1	6	1
Hot pastrami	1	440	16	33	42	1	41	30
Hot pastrami, super stacked	1	570	23	36	43	1	42	46
Italian style wedding soup	1	130	4	28	17	0	17	7
Light buttermilk ranch dressing	1.5 oz	70	4	51	8	Tr	8	1
Light Italian dressing	1.5 oz	20	1	45	2	Tr	2	0
Macaroni salad	1 svg	330	22	60	28	2	26	5
Mayonnaise	1 oz	200	22	99	0	0	0	0
Meatball	1	600	32	48	51	4	47	28
Mediterranean ciabatta	1	450	8	16	65	3	62	26
Minestrone	1	90	3	30	14	4	10	4
New England clam chowder	1	170	3	16	28	2	26	7
Northwest potato salad	1 svg	260	17	59	22	3	19	3
Oatmeal raisin cookie	1	170	7	37	26	1	25	2
Oil blend	0.5 oz	130	14	97	0		0	0

	Serving Size	Calories	Fat (g)	Calories from Fat (%)	Total Carbs (g)	Fiber (g)	Net Carbs (g)	Protein (g)
Blimpie (cont.)	***	***	*	*	*	*	*	*
Pasta fagioli w/ sausage	1	150	5	30	22	4	18	7
Peanut butter cookie	1	200	12	54	20	1	19	3
Peppercorn dressing	1.5 oz	240	26	98	1	0	1	1
Philly steak & onion	1	500	24	43	45	1	44	26
Pilgrim turkey vegetables w/ rice soup	1	110	2	16	19	2	17	4
Potato salad	1 svg	230	12	47	28	3	25	3
Red hot original sauce	1 oz	10	0	0	2	0	2	0
Red wine vinegar	0.5 oz	5	0	0	1	0	1	0
Reuben	1	570	24	38	54	3	51	34
Roast beef & cheddar wrap	1	680	36	48	59	6	53	32
Roast beef & provolone	1	410	11	24	47	3	44	31
Roast beef & provolone, on wheat	1	390	12	28	40	6	34	32
Roast beef, turkey & cheddar	1	570	30	47	48	3	45	27
Roast beef, turkey & cheddar ciabatta	1	590	30	46	51	3	48	28
Sausage, egg & cheese biscuit	1	540	35	58	37	1	36	20
Sausage, egg & cheese bluffin	1	400	24	54	27	2	25	19
Sausage, egg & cheese burrito	1	660	34	46	56	5	51	34
Sausage, egg & cheese croissant	1	520	35	61	30	1	29	18
Seafood	1	330	7	19	56	4	52	13
Seafood gumbo	1	100	2	18	16	2	14	4
Seafood salad	1	120	4	30	17	3	14	6
Sicilian ciabatta	1	640	25	35	68	3	65	33
Southwestern wrap	1	530	22	37	61	4	57	23
Special dressing	0.7 oz	70	7	90	0	Tr	0	0
Special vegetarian	1	590	30	46	66	4	62	17
Spicy brown mustard	0.5 oz	5	0	0	0	Tr	0	0
Split pea w/ ham soup	1	130	2	14	21	6	15	8
Steak & onion wrap	1	770	47	55	62	6	56	28
Sugar cookie	1	330	17	46	41	1	40	3
Thousand Island dressing	1.5 oz	210	20	86	6	0	6	0

	Serving Size	Calories	Fat (g)	Calories from Fat (%)	Total Carbs (g)	Fiber (g)	Net Carbs (g)	Protein (g)
Tomato basil w/ raviolini soup	1	110	1	8	22	0	22	4
Tuna	1	480	21	39	46	3	43	25
Tuna salad	1	270	18	60	7	2	5	18
Turkey & avocado	1	380	9	21	52	4	48	21
Turkey & bacon, super stacked	1	580	24	37	48	2	46	40
Turkey & cranberry	1	350	4	10	58	3	55	20
Turkey & provolone	1	390	10	23	49	3	46	26
Turkey & provolone, on wheat	1	370	10	24	43	6	37	27
Turkey Italiano ciabatta	1	500	11	20	64	3	61	30
Tuscan ciabatta	1	600	23	35	65	3	62	29
Ultimate club ciabatta	1	480	21	39	47	2	45	27
Ultimate club salad	1	290	16	50	10	3	7	25
Veggie supreme	1	550	28	46	48	3	45	29
Vegimax	1	520	20	35	56	5	51	28
Vegimax, on wheat	1	500	21	38	50	8	42	30
White chocolate macadamia nut cookie	1	200	12	54	20	1	19	3
Yankee pot roast soup	1	80	2	23	12	2	10	5
Zesty wrap	1	570	26	41	59	6	53	28
Boston Market	***	***	*	*	*	*	*	*
Apple pie	1 slice	580	30	47	74	3	71	43
Baked beans	1 svg	270	2	7	53	11	42	11
BBQ brisket meal	1	400	20	45	28	0	28	26
BBQ brisket sandwich	1	800	30	34	90	3	87	43
BBQ chicken, half	1	730	30	37	28	1	27	90
BBQ dark chicken	3 pc	430	13	27	28	1	27	52
Beef brisket meal	1	280	20	64	1	0	1	26
Beef gravy	3 oz	350	2	5	4	0	4	1
Boston chicken carver sandwich	1	750	29	35	64	3	61	57
Boston chicken carver sandwich, half	1	375	15	36	32	1	31	28
Boston meatloaf carver sandwich	1	980	46	42	92	4	88	47
Boston turkey carver sandwich	1	700	26	33	65	3	62	50

	Serving Size	Calories	Fat (g)	Calories from Fat (%)	Total Carbs (g)	Fiber (g)	Net Carbs (g)	Protein (g)
Boston Market (cont.)	***	***	*	*	*	*	*	*
Boston turkey carver sandwich, half	1	350	13	33	32	2	30	25
Brisket dip carver sandwich	1	890	51	52	63	3	60	43
Caesar salad dressing	2.5 oz	360	38	95	4	1	3	2
Caesar salad entrée	1	420	38	81	9	2	7	12
Caesar side salad	1	180	17	85	4	1	3	4
Chicken noodle soup	1	250	8	29	23	2	21	22
Chicken tortilla soup	1	410	26	57	30	2	28	17
Chocolate cake	1 svg	580	34	53	67	3	64	5
Chocolate chip fudge brownie	1	320	13	37	49	3	46	5
Cinnamon apples	1 svg	210	3	13	47	3	44	0
Classic chicken salad sandwich	1	800	41	46	65	4	61	40
Coleslaw	1 svg	300	20	60	27	4	23	2
Cornbread	1 svg	180	5	25	31	0	31	2
Creamed spinach	1 svg	280	23	74	12	4	8	9
Crispy country chicken carver sandwich	1	1020	42	37	114	4	110	45
Crispy country chicken w/ country gravy	1	480	23	43	36	1	35	33
Crispy country chicken, add-on	3 oz	220	11	45	16	1	15	16
Dark individual meal	3 pc	390	22	51	1	0	1	51
Dark individual meal, 2 thighs & drumstick	3 pc	490	29	53	0	0	0	60
Dark skinless meal, 2 thighs & drumstick	3 pc	350	15	39	0	0	0	52
Dark skinless meal, thigh & 2 drumsticks	3 pc	290	11	34	0	0	0	45
Fresh steamed vegetables	1 svg	60	2	30	8	3	5	2
Fresh vegetable stuffing	1 svg	190	8	38	25	2	23	3
Fruit salad	1 svg	60	0	0	15	1	14	1
Garlic dill new potatoes	1 svg	140	3	19	24	3	21	3
Green beans	1 svg	60	4	60	7	3	4	2
Lite ranch dressing	1.5 oz	70	4	51	8	0	8	1
Macaroni & cheese	1 svg	300	11	33	35	2	33	11

	Serving Size	Calories	Fat (g)	Calories from Fat (%)	Total Carbs (g)	Fiber (g)	Net Carbs (g)	Protein (g)
Market chopped salad	1	480	40	75	24	7	17	9
Market chopped salad dressing	2.5 oz	360	39	98	2	0	2	0
Mashed potatoes	1 svg	270	11	37	36	4	32	5
Meatloaf meal	1	520	36	62	21	0	21	29
Meatloaf open-faced sandwich	1	670	38	51	48	1	47	34
Pastry top chicken pot pie	1	800	48	54	59	4	55	32
Potato salad	1 svg	390	29	67	26	3	23	3
Poultry gravy	4 oz	50	2	36	7	0	7	0
Roasted sirloin open-faced sandwich	1	410	15	33	32	1	31	35
Roasted sirloin, add-on	3 oz	160	6	34	0	0	0	26
Roasted turkey meal	1	150	3	18	0	0	0	31
Roasted turkey open-faced sandwich	1	330	6	16	43	1	42	26
Roasted turkey, add-on	3 oz	110	2	16	0	0	0	23
Rotisserie chicken open-faced sandwich	1	320	8	23	34	1	33	27
Rotisserie chicken, add-on	5 oz	180	3	15	0	0	0	39
Rotisserie chicken, half	1	610	29	43	1	0	1	89
Smokehouse BBQ chicken sandwich	1	850	29	31	101	4	97	44
Sweet corn	1 svg	170	4	21	37	2	35	6
Sweet potato casserole	1 svg	460	16	31	77	3	74	4
Thigh & drumstick	1	290	17	53	0	0	0	37
White BBQ chicken, quarter	1	430	13	27	28	1	27	52
White rotisserie chicken, no skin, quarter	1	240	4	15	1	0	1	50
White rotisserie chicken, quarter	1	320	12	34	0	0	0	52
Bruegger's								
(all sandwiches on plain bagel, unless otherwise noted)	***	***	*	*	*	*	*	*
Asiago parmesan bagel	1	330	20	55	61	4	57	14
Asian sesame ginger dressing	2 oz	260	21	73	17	0	17	0
Bacon scallion cream cheese	1	140	12	77	5	0	5	3
Balsamic vinaigrette dressing	2 oz	110	9	74	8	0	8	0

	Serving Size	Calories	Fat (g)	Calories from Fat (%)	Total Carbs (g)	Fiber (g)	Net Carbs (g)	Protein (g)
Bruegger's *(cont.)*	***	***	*	*	*	*	*	*
Beef chili	1	190	8	38	18	6	12	10
BLT	1	570	23	36	72	5	67	20
Blueberry bagel	1	320	2	6	67	4	63	11
Blueberry muffin	1	400	17	38	57	2	55	7
Breakfast bagel sandwich w/ ham	1	460	18	35	73	4	69	31
Breakfast bagel sandwich w/ sausage	1	640	30	42	63	4	59	29
Breakfast bagel sandwich, no meat	1	420	18	39	71	4	67	23
Breakfast bagel sandwich w/ bacon	1	460	23	45	65	4	61	28
Butternut squash soup	1	240	17	64	21	1	20	4
Caesar dressing	2 oz	110	9	74	8	0	8	2
Caesar salad w/ chicken & dressing	1	380	20	47	23	2	21	28
Caesar salad w/ dressing	1	270	17	57	22	2	20	9
Caesar salad, no dressing	1	160	8	45	14	2	12	7
Chicken breast sandwich	1	660	11	15	87	5	82	47
Chicken spaetzle soup	1	140	5	32	15	1	14	8
Chicken wild rice soup	1	280	22	71	12	1	11	8
Chocolate chip bagel	1	350	5	13	64	4	60	12
Chocolate chip cookie	1	390	17	39	52	2	50	5
Chocolate chunk brownie	1	330	18	49	40	2	38	4
Chocolate muffin	1	460	24	47	57	3	54	6
Cinnamon raisin bagel	1	330	2	5	69	4	65	11
Cinnamon sugar bagel	1	350	2	5	73	6	67	12
Classic wrap w/ bacon	1	520	45	78	52	4	48	36
Classic wrap w/ ham	1	510	41	72	54	4	50	40
Classic wrap w/ sausage	1	590	53	81	15	4	11	35
Cranberry orange bagel	1	330	2	5	68	4	64	11
Double chocolate cookie	1	390	19	44	51	3	48	5
Everything bagel	1	310	2	6	31	4	27	12
Everything cookie	1	380	18	43	49	2	47	5
Fire roasted tomato soup	1	130	6	42	17	2	15	2

	Serving Size	Calories	Fat (g)	Calories from Fat (%)	Total Carbs (g)	Fiber (g)	Net Carbs (g)	Protein (g)
Fortified multigrain bagel	1	350	4	10	69	6	63	13
Four cheese & tomato panini on hearty white	1	700	35	45	57	3	54	42
Four cheese broccoli soup	1	260	20	69	12	1	11	9
Garden veggie cream cheese	1	130	11	76	5	1	4	3
Garden veggie sandwich	1	400	3	7	82	7	75	16
Garlic bagel	1	320	2	6	65	4	61	12
Ham & swiss panini on honey wheat	1	600	18	27	71	2	69	39
Ham sandwich	1	410	5	11	66	4	62	27
Herby turkey sandwich on sesame bagel	1	600	14	21	80	5	75	43
Honey grain bagel	1	330	3	8	65	5	60	13
Honey walnut cream cheese	1	150	12	72	8	Tr	8	3
Jalapeno bagel	1	320	2	6	64	4	60	12
Jalapeno cream cheese	1	140	13	84	4	0	4	3
Leonardo da veggie sandwich on asiago softwich	1	590	17	26	83	7	76	28
Light garden veggie cream cheese	1	90	6	60	3	0	3	6
Light herb garlic cream cheese	1	100	6	54	4	0	4	6
Light plain cream cheese	1	100	6	54	4	Tr	4	6
Mandarin medley salad w/ balsamic vinaigrette	1	340	17	45	36	4	32	8
Mandarin medley salad w/ chicken & balsamic vinaigrette	1	450	21	42	37		33	26
Mandarin medley salad, no dressing	1	230	8	31	29	4	25	8
Marshmallow chew bar	1	280	6	19	55	0	55	2
New England clam chowder	1	230	14	55	16	Tr	16	23
Olive pimiento cream cheese	1	140	13	84	3	0	3	3
Onion & chive cream cheese	1	140	13	84	3	0	3	3
Onion bagel	1	320	2	6	64	4	60	12
Plain bagel	1	300	2	6	60	4	56	12
Plain cream cheese	1	130	11	76	6	Tr	6	3
Poppy bagel	1	310	3	9	61	4	57	12

	Serving Size	Calories	Fat (g)	Calories from Fat (%)	Total Carbs (g)	Fiber (g)	Net Carbs (g)	Protein (g)
Bruegger's (cont.)	***	***	*	*	*	*	*	*
Primo pesto chicken panini on hearty white	1	700	32	41	56	2	54	49
Pumpernickel bagel	1	330	3	8	67	5	62	12
Ranch dressing	2 oz	190	21	99	2	0	2	0
Rio Grande wrap w/ bacon	1	560	49	79	55	4	51	34
Rio Grande wrap w/ ham	1	630	34	49	55	4	51	31
Rio Grande wrap w/ sausage	1	510	47	83	53	4	49	27
Roast beef sandwich	1	730	39	48	71	5	66	30
Roma roast beef sandwich on hearty white	1	770	44	51	62	3	59	46
Rosemary olive oil bagel	1	350	7	18	64	4	60	12
Sesame bagel	1	310	3	9	61	4	57	13
Sesame salad w/ Asian sesame dressing	1	380	26	62	29	2	27	23
Sesame salad w/ chicken & Asian sesame dressing	1	490	29	53	30	2	28	42
Sesame salad, no dressing	1	120	5	38	12	2	10	4
Seven layer bar	1	650	43	60	58	5	53	10
Smoked salmon cream cheese	1	150	13	78	3	Tr	3	3
Smoked salmon sandwich	1	460	10	20	65	5	60	27
Sourdough bagel	1	310	2	6	63	4	59	12
Spinach & cheddar omelet sandwich	1	500	16	29	64	4	60	24
Spinach & lentil soup	1	110	4	33	16	7	9	7
Spinach, cheddar & bacon omelet, on sesame bagel	1	550	22	36	60	3	57	28
Spinach, cheddar & ham omelet, on sesame bagel	1	540	17	28	65	4	61	30
Spinach, cheddar & sausage omelet, on sesame bagel	1	660	32	44	64	4	60	29
Strawberry cream cheese	1	140	13	84	4	0	4	3
Sundried tomato bagel	1	320	2	6	64	4	60	60
Tarragon chicken salad sandwich on hearty white	1	770	41	48	73	3	70	70
Thai peanut chicken sandwich	1	580	11	17	91	7	84	84
Toffee almond bar	1	400	19	43	53	1	52	52

	Serving Size	Calories	Fat (g)	Calories from Fat (%)	Total Carbs (g)	Fiber (g)	Net Carbs (g)	Protein (g)
Tuna & cheddar melt on honey wheat	1	1020	67	59	61	3	58	58
Tuna salad sandwich	1	620	27	39	73	5	68	68
Turkey chipotle club on honey wheat	1	800	51	57	57	3	54	54
Turkey sandwich	1	510	14	25	70	5	65	65
Turkey Toscana panini on hearty white	1	710	37	47	59	3	56	56
Western omelet sandwich	1	760	56	66	66	4	62	62
White chicken chili	1	240	9	34	26	7	19	19
Whole wheat bagel	1	390	6	14	73	9	64	64
Buffalo Wild Wings	***	***	*	*	*	*	*	*
All-Beef Hamburger Patty	1	410	32	70	0	0	0	30
American cheese slice	1	70	5	64	2	0	2	3
Avocado	1 svg	160	15	84	9	7	2	2
Bacon slices	2	100	8	72	0	0	0	8
Beer-braised mushrooms	1 svg	35	0	0	6	2	4	2
Blue cheese crumbles	1 svg	70	6	77	1	0	1	4
Blue Cheese dressing	1 svg	210	22	94	2	0	2	1
Celery Sticks	1 svg	15	0	0	2	1	1	1
Celery & Carrot Sticks	1 svg	20	0	0	4	1	3	1
Cheddar cheese slice	1	90	7	70	0	0	0	5
Cheddar Jack cheese	1 svg	60	4.5	68	1	0	1	3
Coffee	1	5	0	0	0	0	0	0
Pepper Jack cheese slice	1	80	6	68	0	0	0	4
Pepsi flavor shots (all flavors)	1	0	0	0	0	0	0	0
Queso cheese	1 svg	50	3.5	63	4	0	4	2
Ranch dressing	1 svg	240	25	94	2	0	2	0
Swiss cheese slice	1	50	4	72	0	0	0	4
Traditional Wings only, single (small)	1 svg	650	36	50	0	0	0	80
w/ Blazin' sauce	1 svg	750	44	53	4	1	3	81
w/ Hot sauce	1 svg	720	42	53	4	1	3	81
w/ Medium sauce	1 svg	700	40.5	52	3	1	2	80
w/ Parmesan Garlic sauce	1 svg	840	54	58	4	0	4	82

	Serving Size	Calories	Fat (g)	Calories from Fat (%)	Total Carbs (g)	Fiber (g)	Net Carbs (g)	Protein (g)
Buffalo Wild Wings (cont.)	***	***	*	*	*	*	*	*
w/ Spicy Garlic sauce	1 svg	720	42	53	5	1	4	81
w/ Thai Curry sauce	1 svg	860	57	60	6	1	5	81
w/ Wild sauce	1 svg	720	42	53	4	1	3	80
w/ Buffalo seasoning	1 svg	655	36	49	1	0	1	80
w/ Chipotle BBQ seasoning	1 svg	655	36	49	1	0	1	80
w/ Desert Heat seasoning	1 svg	655	36	49	1	0	1	80
w/ Lemon Pepper seasoning	1 svg	655	36	49	1	0	1	80
Unsweetened Tea	1	0	0	0	1	0	1	0
Yellow mustard	1 svg	5	0	0	0	0	0	0
Burger King	***	***	*	*	*	*	*	*
Bacon cheeseburger - no bun	1	190	14	66	4	0	4	13
Bacon cheeseburger - no bun, ketchup	1	180	14	70	1	0	1	13
Bacon double cheeseburger - no bun	1	280	21	68	4	0	4	21
Bacon double cheeseburger - no bun, ketchup	1	270	21	70	Tr	0	Tr	20
Bacon, egg & cheese biscuit	1	430	25	52	34	1	33	17
Bacon, egg & cheese biscuit - no biscuit	1	150	12	72	1	0	1	9
Bacon, egg & cheese Croissan'wich - no croissant	1	130	9	62	1	0	1	9
Bacon King - no bun, ketchup	1	900	75	75	3	0	3	54
Bacon King Junior - no bun	1	450	37	74	4	0	4	25
Bacon King Junior - no bun, ketchup	1	440	37	76	1	0	1	25
Bacon & Cheese Whopper - no bun, ketchup	1	540	46	77	4	Tr	4	28
Barbecue dipping sauce	1 oz	40	0	0	11	0	11	0
BBQ Bacon Whopper - no bun, sauce	1	540	46	77	4	Tr	4	28
BK Big Fish sandwich	1	640	32	45	66	3	63	23
BK Breakfast Shots, bacon & cheese, 2 pack	1	310	20	58	18	1	17	14

	Serving Size	Calories	Fat (g)	Calories from Fat (%)	Total Carbs (g)	Fiber (g)	Net Carbs (g)	Protein (g)
BK Breakfast Shots, ham & cheese, 2 pack	1	270	16	53	18	1	17	13
BK Breakfast Shots, sausage & cheese, 2 pack	1	420	31	66	18	1	17	18
BK Burger Shots, 2 pack	1	220	10	41	18	1	17	14
BK Burger Shots, 6 pack	1	650	31	43	53	2	51	40
BK chicken fries, 12 pc/svg	1 svg	500	29	52	32	3	29	28
BK chicken fries, 9 pc/svg	1 svg	380	22	52	24	2	22	21
BK chicken fries, 6 pc/svg	1 svg	250	15	54	16	1	15	14
BK Double Stacker	1	620	39	57	32	1	31	34
BK fresh apple fries	1 svg	25	0	0	6	1	5	0
BK Joe coffee, regular or decaf, all sizes	***	0	0	0	0	0	0	0
BK Quad Stacker	1	1010	70	62	34	1	33	64
BK Triple Stacker	1	820	55	60	33	1	32	49
BK veggie burger	1	420	16	34	46	7	39	23
BK veggie burger w/ cheese	1	470	20	38	47	7	40	25
Breakfast Burrito Junior - no tortilla, hash browns	1	200	17	77	2	0	2	10
Breakfast Burrito Junior - no tortilla, hash browns, sauce	1	180	14	70	1	0	1	10
Breakfast syrup	1 svg	80	0	0	21	0	21	0
Buffalo dipping sauce	1 oz	80	8	90	2	0	2	1
Caramel sauce	1 svg	45	Tr	0	10	0	10	0
Cheeseburger	1	340	16	42	31	1	30	18
Cheeseburger - no bun	1	160	11	62	4	0	4	11
Cheeseburger - no bun, ketchup	1	150	11	66	Tr	0	Tr	11
Cheesy Bacon BK wrapper	1	390	24	55	29	2	27	14
Cheesy Tots potatoes, 12 pc/svg	1 svg	440	24	49	41	4	37	14
Cheesy Tots potatoes, 9 pc/svg	1 svg	330	18	49	31	3	28	11
Cheesy Tots potatoes, 6 pc/svg	1 svg	220	12	49	21	2	19	7
Chicken sandwich, original	1	630	39	56	46	3	43	24
Chicken tenders, 4 pc/svg	1 svg	180	11	55	13	0	13	9

	Serving Size	Calories	Fat (g)	Calories from Fat (%)	Total Carbs (g)	Fiber (g)	Net Carbs (g)	Protein (g)
Burger King (cont.)	***	***	*	*	*	*	*	*
Chicken tenders, 5 pc/svg	1 svg	230	13	51	16	0	16	11
Chicken tenders, 6 pc/svg	1 svg	270	16	53	19	0	19	14
Chicken tenders, 8 pc/svg	1 svg	360	21	53	25	0	25	18
Chocolate milkshake, sm	12 fl oz	310	11	32	53	1	52	6
Cini-minis, 4 pc	1 svg	400	18	41	52	2	50	7
Cini-minis, 4 pc, w/ vanilla icing	1 svg	490	18	33	74	2	72	7
Croissan'wich w/ bacon, egg & cheese	1	350	19	49	27	0	27	15
Croissan'wich w/ egg & cheese	1	310	16	46	27	0	27	12
Croissan'wich w/ ham, egg & cheese	1	340	17	45	28	0	28	18
Croissan'wich w/ sausage & cheese	1	380	24	57	26	0	26	14
Croissan'wich w/ sausage, egg & cheese	1	470	31	59	28	0	28	20
Double bacon breakfast sourdough King - no bread	1	280	21	68	3	0	3	19
Double cheeseburger	1	5103	29	5	31	1	30	30
Double cheeseburger - no bun	1	270	19	63	4	0	4	20
Double cheeseburger - no bun, ketchup	1	250	19	68	Tr	0	Tr	20
Double Croissan'wich w/ bacon, egg & cheese	1	430	26	54	28	0	28	20
Double Croissan'wich w/ ham, bacon, egg & cheese	1	430	24	50	29	0	29	23
Double Croissan'wich w/ ham, egg & cheese	1	420	21	45	30	0	30	26
Double Croissan'wich w/ ham, sausage, egg & cheese	1	550	36	59	30	0	30	28
Double Croissan'wich w/ sausage, bacon, egg & cheese	1	560	38	61	29	0	29	25
Double Croissan'wich w/ sausage, egg & cheese	1	690	50	65	30	0	30	30
Double ham breakfast sourdough King - no bread	1	300	19	57	4	0	4	26

	Serving Size	Calories	Fat (g)	Calories from Fat (%)	Total Carbs (g)	Fiber (g)	Net Carbs (g)	Protein (g)
Double hamburger	1	420	22	47	30	1	29	26
Double Quarter Pound King - no bun	1	910	67	66	8	Tr	8	68
Double Quarter Pound King - no bun, ketchup	1	890	67	68	4	0	4	68
Double Quarter Pound King - no bun, ketchup, onions	1	890	67	68	3	0	3	68
Double sausage breakfast sourdough King - no bread	1	560	47	76	3	0	3	30
Double Whopper	1	920	58	57	51	3	48	48
Double Whopper - no bun, ketchup	1	890	71	72	3	Tr	3	60
Double Whopper w/ cheese	1	1010	66	59	53	3	50	53
Dutch apple pie	1	320	13	37	47	1	46	2
Egg & cheese Croissan'wich - no croissant	1	90	7	70	1	0	1	7
French fries, lg	1 svg	580	28	43	74	6	68	6
French fries, med	1 svg	480	23	43	61	5	56	5
French fries, sm	1 svg	340	17	45	44	4	40	4
French fries, value	1 svg	220	11	45	28	2	26	2
French toast sticks, 3 pc/svg	1 svg	230	11	43	29	1	28	3
French toast sticks, 5 pc/svg	1 svg	380	18	43	49	2	47	5
Fully loaded biscuit - no biscuit	1	380	29	69	3	0	3	24
Fully loaded Croissan'wich - no croissant	1	360	28	70	3	0	3	23
Garden side salad w/o dressing	1	60	4	60	3	1	2	4
Garlic parmesan croutons	1 svg	60	2	30	9	0	9	1
Grilled chicken sandwich - no bun	1	270	16	53	1	5	-4	30
Ham omelet sandwich	1	290	12	37	33	1	32	13
Ham, egg & cheese biscuit	1	410	23	50	34	1	33	17
Ham, egg & cheese biscuit - no biscuit	1	130	10	69	1	0	1	9
Ham, egg & cheese Croissan'wich - no croissant	1	130	8	55	2	0	2	12
Hamburger	1	290	12	37	30	1	29	15

	Serving Size	Calories	Fat (g)	Calories from Fat (%)	Total Carbs (g)	Fiber (g)	Net Carbs (g)	Protein (g)
Burger King (cont.)	***	***	*	*	*	*	*	*
Hamburger - no bun	1	120	8	60	3	0	3	9
Hamburger - no bun, ketchup	1	110	8	65	0	0	0	9
Hash browns, med	1	610	39	58	58	8	50	5
Hash browns, sm	1	420	27	58	40	6	34	3
Hash browns, value	1	250	16	58	24	3	21	2
Hershey's sundae pie	1	310	19	55	32	1	31	3
Honey mustard dipping sauce	1 oz	90	6	60	8	0	8	7
Jam, strawberry or grape	1 svg	30	0	0	7	0	7	0
Ken's creamy Caesar dressing	2 oz	210	21	90	4	0	4	3
Ken's honey mustard dressing	2 oz	270	23	77	15	0	15	1
Ken's light Italian dressing	2 oz	120	11	83	5	0	5	0
Ken's ranch dressing	2 oz	190	20	95	2	0	2	1
Ketchup	1 pkt	10	0	0	3	0	3	0
King Croissan'wich w/ double sausage - no croissant	1	490	43	79	2	0	2	23
King Croissan'wich w/ ham & sausage - no croissant	1	340	28	74	3	0	3	19
King Croissan'wich w/ sausage & bacon - no croissant	1	390	33	76	2	0	2	20
Kraft Macaroni & Cheese	1 svg	160	5	28	22	1	21	7
Mayonnaise	1 pkt	80	9	100	1	0	1	0
Mushroom & swiss Steakhouse XT	1	870	49	51	54	4	50	43
Onion rings, lg	1 svg	510	27	48	60	5	55	7
Onion rings, med	1 svg	450	24	48	52	5	47	6
Onion rings, sm	1 svg	310	17	49	36	3	33	4
Onion rings, value	1 svg	150	8	48	17	1	16	2
Oreo BK sundae shake, chocolate, sm	16 fl oz	700	26	33	116	2	114	11
Oreo BK sundae shake, strawberry, sm	16 fl oz	680	25	33	114	1	113	10
Quarter Pound King - no bun	1	350	25	64	7	Tr	7	25
Quarter Pound King - no bun, ketchup	1	330	25	68	3	0	3	24
Quarter Pound King - no bun, ketchup, onions	1	330	25	68	2	0	2	24

	Serving Size	Calories	Fat (g)	Calories from Fat (%)	Total Carbs (g)	Fiber (g)	Net Carbs (g)	Protein (g)
Ranch dipping sauce	1 oz	140	15	96	1	0	1	1
Rodeo King - no bun, BBQ sauce, onion rings	1	1090	89	73	3	0	3	71
Sausage biscuit	1	420	27	58	32	1	31	13
Sausage, egg & cheese biscuit	1	560	37	59	35	1	34	21
Sausage, egg & cheese biscuit - no biscuit	1	280	24	77	1	0	1	14
Sausage, egg & cheese Croissan'wich - no croissant	1	280	24	77	1	0	1	14
Sourdough King, double - no bun	1	740	58	71	8	0	8	47
Sourdough King, single - no bun	1	500	40	72	8	0	8	27
Sourdough King, double - no bun, onions	1	740	58	71	7	0	7	47
Sourdough King, single - no bun, onions	1	500	40	72	7	0	7	27
Sourdough King, double - no bun, sauce	1	610	46	68	2	0	2	46
Sourdough King, single - no bun, sauce	1	370	29	71	2	0	2	27
Sourdough King, double - no bun, onions, sauce	1	610	46	68	1	0	1	46
Sourdough King, single - no bun, onions, sauce	1	370	29	71	1	0	1	27
Spicy Chick'n Crisp sandwich	1	450	30	60	34	2	32	12
Steakhouse burger	1	950	59	56	55	4	51	40
Steakhouse XT	1	970	61	57	55	4	51	42
Strawberry milkshake, sm	12 fl oz	310	11	32	52	0	52	6
Sweet & sour dipping sauce	1 oz	45	0	0	11	0	11	0
Tendercrisp chicken garden salad	1	410	23	50	27	4	23	27
Tendercrisp chicken sandwich	1	800	46	52	68	3	65	32
Tendergrill chicken garden salad	1	210	7	30	8	3	5	29
Tendergrill chicken sandwich	1	490	21	39	51	3	48	26
Three cheese Steakhouse XT	1	1050	71	61	52	3	49	51
Triple Whopper	1	1160	76	59	51	3	48	68

	Serving Size	Calories	Fat (g)	Calories from Fat (%)	Total Carbs (g)	Fiber (g)	Net Carbs (g)	Protein (g)
Burger King (cont.)	***	***	*	*	*	*	*	*
Triple Whopper w/ cheese	1	1250	84	60	52	3	49	73
Vanilla milkshake, sm	12 fl oz	270	11	37	42	0	42	6
Whopper	1	670	40	54	51	3	48	29
Whopper w/ cheese	1	770	48	56	52	3	49	33
Whopper - no bun	1	430	36	75	7	Tr	7	21
Whopper - no bun, ketchup	1	410	36	79	3	Tr	3	20
Whopper - no bun, ketchup, onions	1	410	36	79	2	Tr	2	20
Whopper Junior	1	370	21	51	31	2	29	16
Whopper Junior w/ cheese	1	770	48	56	52	3	49	33
Whopper Junior - no bun	1	190	16	76	4	Tr	4	9
Whopper Junior - no bun, ketchup	1	180	16	80	2	0	2	9
Unsweetened Iced Tea, all sizes	***	0	0	0	0	0	0	0
Zesty onion ring dipping sauce	1 oz	150	15	90	3	1	2	0
Carl's Jr.	***	***	*	*	*	*	*	*
Bacon & egg burrito	1	550	32	52	37	1	36	29
Bacon swiss crispy chicken sandwich	1	750	40	48	62	4	58	36
Big hamburger	1	460	17	33	54	3	51	24
Blue cheese dressing	2 oz	320	34	96	1	0	1	2
Breakfast burger	1	780	41	47	64	3	61	38
Carl's Catch fish sandwich	1	710	37	47	74	4	70	20
Charbroiled BBQ chicken sandwich	1	380	7	17	49	2	47	34
Charbroiled chicken club sandwich	1	560	27	43	44	2	42	39
Charbroiled chicken salad	1	250	9	32	14	4	10	29
Charbroiled chicken salad w/o dressing	1	280	9	29	19	2	17	32
Charbroiled Santa Fe chicken sandwich	1	630	35	50	44	2	42	36
Chicken Stars	4 pc	210	16	69	10	1	9	8
Chicken Stars	6 pc	320	24	68	14	2	12	12
Chicken Stars	9 pc	480	36	68	21	2	19	18

	Serving Size	Calories	Fat (g)	Calories from Fat (%)	Total Carbs (g)	Fiber (g)	Net Carbs (g)	Protein (g)
Chicken strips	3 pc	370	26	63	19	2	17	14
Chicken strips	5 pc	610	43	63	32	3	29	23
Chili cheese fries	1 svg	990	56	51	89	8	81	28
Chili cheeseburger	1	780	41	47	58	4	54	41
Chocolate cake	1 pc	300	12	36	48	1	47	3
Chocolate chip cookie	1	370	19	46	48	2	46	3
Chocolate malt	1	780	34	39	100	1	99	15
Chocolate shake	1	710	33	42	86	1	85	14
CrissCut fries	1 svg	450	29	58	42	4	38	5
Double Western bacon cheeseburger	1	960	52	49	70	3	67	52
Famous Star w/ cheese	1	660	39	53	53	3	50	27
Fish & chips	1 svg	730	39	48	72	6	66	22
French toast dips, no syrup	5 pc	460	21	41	60	3	57	9
Fried zucchini	1 svg	330	18	49	36	2	34	6
Garden side salad w/o dressing	1	140	7	45	15	2	13	6
Gluten Sensitive Famous Star with Cheese	1	430	34	71	10	1	9	21
Gluten Sensitive Guacamole Thickburger - no sauce	1	650	52	72	9	2	7	41
Gluten Sensitive Low Carb Thickburger - no ketchup	1	560	42	68	8	1	7	38
Green burrito taco salad	1	970	58	54	76	17	59	42
Hash brown nuggets	1 svg	350	23	59	32	3	29	3
House dressing	2 oz	220	22	90	3	0	3	1
Jalapeno burger	1	720	46	58	50	3	47	27
Loaded breakfast burrito	1	780	49	57	51	3	48	36
Low Carb It Charbroiled Chicken Club Sandwich	1	370	24	58	8	1	7	30
Low fat balsamic dressing	2 oz	35	2	51	5	0	5	0
Natural cut fries, lg	1	500	24	43	65	5	60	6
Natural cut fries, med	1	460	22	43	60	5	55	5
Natural cut fries, sm	1	320	15	42	42	4	38	4
Onion rings	1 svg	530	28	48	61	3	58	8
Oreo cookie malt	1	790	38	43	95	1	94	17

	Serving Size	Calories	Fat (g)	Calories from Fat (%)	Total Carbs (g)	Fiber (g)	Net Carbs (g)	Protein (g)
Burger King (cont.)	***	***	*	*	*	*	*	*
Oreo cookie shake	1	730	38	47	81	1	80	15
Sourdough breakfast sandwich	1	450	21	42	38	1	37	29
Spicy chicken sandwich	1	420	27	58	33	2	31	12
Steak & egg burrito	1	650	36	50	43	1	42	41
Strawberry malt	1	770	34	40	99	0	99	15
Strawberry shake	1	700	33	42	85	0	85	14
Strawberry swirl cheesecake	1 pc	290	16	50	32	0	32	6
Sunrise croissant sandwich	1	590	44	67	27	1	26	20
Super Star w/ cheese	1	920	58	57	54	3	51	47
The Bacon Cheese Six Dollar Burger	1	950	62	59	49	3	46	51
The Guacamole Six Dollar Burger	1	1040	70	61	53	4	49	49
The Jalapeno Six Dollar Burger	1	930	61	59	52	3	49	45
The Low Carb Six Dollar Burger	1	570	43	68	7	1	6	38
The Original Six Dollar Burger	1	890	54	55	58	3	55	45
The Western Bacon Six Dollar Burger	1	1020	53	47	81	3	78	53
Thousand Island dressing	2 oz	240	23	86	7	0	7	0
Vanilla malt	1	780	34	39	101	0	101	15
Vanilla shake	1	710	33	42	86	0	86	14
Western bacon cheeseburger	1	710	33	42	69	3	66	32
Checkers	***	***	*	*	*	*	*	*
All beef hot dog	1	280	17	55	23	2	21	11
Bacon Buford	1	680	46	61	31	3	28	34
Bacon cheddar burger	1	370	19	46	29	1	28	20
Bacon cheddar fries	1	560	37	59	44	5	39	11
Bacon double bacon	1	710	43	55	43	3	40	38
Bacon double cheeseburger	1	650	42	58	32	4	28	35
Bacon Philly cheesesteak burger	1	560	30	48	42	2	40	31
Bacon ranch fries	1	640	43	60	50	5	45	12
Bacon swiss Buford	1	660	45	61	28	4	24	35

	Serving Size	Calories	Fat (g)	Calories from Fat (%)	Total Carbs (g)	Fiber (g)	Net Carbs (g)	Protein (g)
Banana shake, med	1	440	12	25	71	0	71	11
Big Buford	1	570	36	57	31	3	28	31
BLT	1	380	16	38	47	4	43	13
Checkerburger	1	390	22	51	32	3	29	16
Checkerburger w/ cheese	1	420	24	51	33	3	30	18
Cheese double cheese	1	510	31	55	31	3	28	29
Chili cheese dog	1	390	23	53	28	3	25	17
Chili cheese fries	1	550	34	56	48	6	42	13
Chili cheeseburger	1	320	15	42	30	3	27	18
Chili dog	1	410	25	55	27	3	24	19
Chocolate shake, med	1	430	12	25	72	0	72	9
Cinnamon apple pie	1	240	12	45	31	2	29	3
Crispy chicken breast sandwich	1	610	29	43	61	4	57	26
Crispy chicken club sandwich	1	740	41	50	60	4	56	34
Crispy fish sandwich	1	430	19	40	51	4	47	14
Deep Sea Double	1	640	31	44	63	5	58	25
Double chili cheeseburger	1	460	26	51	30	3	27	27
Double decker	1	480	28	53	31	3	28	27
Frank's RedHot chicken sandwich	1	340	16	42	34	2	32	16
Fries, lg	1	590	38	58	57	6	51	7
Fries, med	1	420	27	58	40	4	36	5
Fries, sm	1	300	19	57	28	3	25	3
Fully loaded bacon cheddar ranch fries	1	640	44	62	51	6	45	11
Grilled chicken club sandwich	1	450	17	34	33	3	30	40
Grilled chicken sandwich	1	370	9	22	40	3	37	31
Half pound double Champ	1	740	52	63	30	3	27	39
Half pound double Champ w/ cheese	1	790	54	62	34	4	30	42
Homestyle chicken strip sandwich	1	670	41	55	50	4	46	27
Homestyle chicken strips meal	2 pc	670	37	50	58	5	53	27
Homestyle chicken strips meal	3 pc	890	49	50	77	7	70	36
Philly cheesesteak burger	1	500	26	47	38	3	35	29

	Serving Size	Calories	Fat (g)	Calories from Fat (%)	Total Carbs (g)	Fiber (g)	Net Carbs (g)	Protein (g)
Checkers (cont.)	***	***	*	*	*	*	*	*
Quarter pound bacon cheese Champ	1	630	41	59	35	5	30	29
Quarter pound Champ	1	490	30	55	32	4	28	22
Quarter pound Champ w/ cheese	1	580	39	61	33	4	29	24
Rallyburger	1	390	22	51	32	3	29	16
Rallyburger w/ cheese	1	420	24	51	33	3	30	18
Screamin' chicken strip sandwich	1	650	41	57	45	3	42	25
Screamin' chicken strips meal	2 pc	570	38	60	59	6	53	23
Screamin' chicken strips meal	3 pc	970	55	51	82	8	74	36
Spicy chicken sandwich	1	550	37	61	39	3	36	17
Strawberry shake, med	1	440	13	27	71	0	71	9
Triple cheeseburger	1	690	43	56	33	4	29	43
Vanilla shake, med	1	410	13	29	64	0	64	10
Cheesecake Factory	***	***	*	*	*	*	*	*
Insufficient information	***	***	*	*	*	*	*	*
Chick-Fil-A	***	***	*	*	*	*	*	*
Insufficient information	***	***	*	*	*	*	*	*
Chili's	***	***	*	*	*	*	*	*
Insufficient information	***	***	*	*	*	*	*	*
Avocado slices	1 svg	80	7	79	4	3	1	1
Applewood smoked bacon	1 svg	70	6	77	0	0	0	5
Bone-in buffalo wings (party platter)	1	73	4.5	55	0.5	Tr	0.5	8
Caesar salad (low-carb), no croutons	1 svg	190	17	81	7	1	6	3
Chili's premium blend coffee	***	0	0	0	0	0	0	0
Fresco salad (low-carb), sub the honey-lime vinaigrette	1 svg	70	5	64	4	1	3	2
House salad (low-carb), no croutons	1 svg	80	3.5	39	8	1	7	3
Salad Dressings (low-carb)	***	***	*	*	*	*	*	*
Ancho chile ranch	1 svg	170	17	90	3	0	3	1
Avocado ranch	1 svg	140	14	90	3	1	2	1

	Serving Size	Calories	Fat (g)	Calories from Fat (%)	Total Carbs (g)	Fiber (g)	Net Carbs (g)	Protein (g)
Bleu cheese	1 svg	270	29	97	1	0	1	1
Caesar	1 svg	220	23	94	2	0	2	2
Citrus balsamic vinaigrette	1 svg	250	25	90	5	0	5	0
Ranch	1 svg	170	18	95	2	0	2	1
Santa Fe	1 svg	210	22	94	2	0	2	1
Sides & extras	***	***	*	*	*	*	*	*
Steamed broccoli	1 svg	40	0	0	8	4	4	3
Avocado slices	1 svg	80	7	79	4	3	1	1
American cheese	1 svg	70	6	77	1	0	1	4
Cheddar cheese	1 svg	80	7	79	0	0	0	5
Pepperjack cheese	1 svg	80	6	68	1	0	1	5
Swiss cheese	1 svg	80	7	79	0	0	0	6
Fresh guacamole, small side	1 svg	130	11	76	7	5	2	2
Pickles	1 svg	5	0	0	0	0	0	0
Salsa (1.5 oz)	1 svg	10	0	0	3	1	2	0
Sour cream	1 svg	60	6	90	2	0	2	1
Wing sauce (1.5 oz)	1 svg	35	3	77	2	1	1	0
Chinese Restaurant - see *Panda Express Chinese Food*	***	***	*	*	*	*	*	*
Chipotle Mexican Grill	***	***	*	*	*	*	*	*
Barbacoa	1 svg	170	7	37	2	1	1	24
Black beans	1 svg	120	1	8	23	11	12	7
Carnitas	1 svg	210	12	51	0	0	0	23
Cheese	1 svg	110	8	65	1	0	1	6
Chicken	1 svg	180	7	35	0	0	0	32
Chipotle honey vinaigrette	1 svg	220	16	65	18	1	17	1
Chips	1 svg	570	27	43	73	8	65	8
Chorizo	1 svg	300	18	54	2	1	1	32
Cilantro-lime rice	1 svg	130	3	21	23	0	23	2
Corn salsa	1 svg	80	2	23	15	3	12	3
Crispy taco shell	1	60	2	30	9	1	8	Tr
Fajita vegetables	1 svg	20	0	0	5	1	4	1
Flour tortilla, burrito	1	290	9	28	44	2	42	7
Flour tortilla, taco	1	90	3	30	13	Tr	13	2

	Serving Size	Calories	Fat (g)	Calories from Fat (%)	Total Carbs (g)	Fiber (g)	Net Carbs (g)	Protein (g)
Chipotle Mexican Grill (cont.)	***	***	*	*	*	*	*	*
Guacamole	1 svg	230	22	86	8	6	2	2
Pinto beans	1 svg	120	1	8	22	10	12	7
Queso	1 svg	120	8	60	4	0.5	3.5	6
Tomatillo-green chili salsa	1 svg	5	0	0	4	0	4	0
Tomatillo-red chili salsa	1 svg	5	0	0	4	1	3	0
Romaine lettuce, salad	1 svg	10	0	0	2	1	1	1
Romaine lettuce, taco	1 svg	5	0	0	1	1	0	0
Sofritas	1 svg	150	10	60	9	3	6	8
Sour cream	1 svg	110	9	74	2	0	2	2
Steak	1 svg	150	6	36	1	1	0	21
Tomato salsa	1 svg	25	0	0	4	1	3	0
Church's Chicken	***	***	*	*	*	*	*	*
Apple pie	1	260	11	38	39	1	38	2
BBQ sauce	1 pkg	30	0	0	7	0	7	0
Bigger better chicken sandwich w/ cheese	1	510	27	48	46	4	42	20
Cajun rice	1 svg	130	7	48	16	Tr	16	1
Cole slaw	1 svg	150	10	60	15	2	13	1
Collard greens	1 svg	25	0	0	5	2	3	2
Corn on the cob	1 svg	140	3	19	24	9	15	4
Country fried steak sandwich	1	490	32	59	38	2	36	13
Country fried steak w/ white gravy	2 pc	610	43	63	31	2	29	24
Country fried steak w/ white gravy	1 pc	470	28	54	36	1	35	21
Creamy jalapeno sauce	1 pkg	100	11	99	1	0	1	0
Crunchy tenders	1 pc	120	6	45	6	Tr	6	12
Edward's double lemon pie	1	300	14	42	39	0	39	5
Edward's strawberry cream cheese pie	1	280	15	48	32	2	30	4
French fries	1 svg	290	14	43	38	4	34	3
Honey	1 pkg	25	0	0	7	0	7	0
Honey butter biscuits	1	240	12	45	28	1	27	3
Honey mustard sauce	1 pkg	110	11	90	4	0	4	0

	Serving Size	Calories	Fat (g)	Calories from Fat (%)	Total Carbs (g)	Fiber (g)	Net Carbs (g)	Protein (g)
Hot sauce	1 pkg	20	0	0	0	0	0	0
Jalapeno bombers	4 pc	240	10	38	29	3	26	8
Ketchup	1 pkg	20	0	0	5	0	5	0
Macaroni & cheese	1 svg	210	11	47	23	1	22	8
Mashed potatoes & gravy	1 svg	70	2	26	12	1	11	2
Okra	1 svg	350	22	57	36	5	31	3
Original breast	1	200	11	50	3	1	2	22
Original leg	1	110	6	49	3	0	3	10
Original thigh	1	330	23	63	8	1	7	21
Original wing	1	300	19	57	7	3	4	27
Purple pepper sauce	1 pkg	45	0	0	12	0	12	0
Ranch sauce	1 pkg	130	13	90	1	0	1	0
Spicy breast	1	320	20	56	12	2	10	21
Spicy crunchy tenders	1 pc	140	7	45	7	4	3	11
Spicy fish fillet	1 pc	160	9	51	13	1	12	7
Spicy fish sandwich	1	320	20	56	25	2	23	10
Spicy leg	1	180	11	55	8	1	7	12
Spicy thigh	1	480	35	66	20	2	18	22
Spicy wing	1	430	27	57	17	2	15	29
Sweet & sour sauce	1 pkg	30	0	0	8	0	8	0
Sweet corn nuggets	1 svg	600	29	44	72	5	67	7
Whole jalapeno peppers	2	10	0	0	2	1	1	0
Cracker Barrel	***	***	*	*	*	*	*	*
10 oz rib eye steak	1	650	47	65	1	1	0	52
Blue cheese dressing	1 svg	250	26	94	2	0	2	2
Boiled cabbage	1 svg	90	5	50	8	4	4	2
Buttermilk Caesar dressing	1 svg	230	4	16	2	0	2	2
Buttermilk ranch dressing	1 svg	190	3	14	2	0	2	Tr
Coffee	1	0	0	0	0	0	0	0
Cottage cheese	1 svg	150	6	36	7	0	7	17
Country green beans	1 svg	60	3	45	7	3	4	1
Fresh steamed broccoli	1 svg	40	0	0	6	4	2	4
Eggs (any way)	2	150	10	60	2	0	2	14
Grilled catfish fillet	1	130	5	35	Tr	Tr	Tr	19

	Serving Size	Calories	Fat (g)	Calories from Fat (%)	Total Carbs (g)	Fiber (g)	Net Carbs (g)	Protein (g)
Cracker Barrel (cont.)	***	***	*	*	*	*	*	*
Grilled chicken tenderloins	6	230	6	23	7	2	5	37
Grilled country pork chops	2	490	25	46	0	2	-2	70
Grilled Southwest sausage	1	510	43	76	8	2	6	20
Grilled Southwest sausage link	1	210	17	73	4	1	3	10
Half pound hamburger steak	1	440	33	68	0	0	0	33
Hickory smoked country ham	1	270	13	43	6	1	5	33
Lemon pepper grilled rainbow trout fillets	2	330	14	38	6	Tr	6	43
Mixed green side salad	1	15	0	0	3	2	1	1
Plain latte, hot	1	140	5	32	13	0	13	9
Plain latte, iced	1	90	3.5	35	8	0	8	6
Pork chops	2	490	25	46	0	2	-2	70
Ranch dip	1 svg	190	20	95	2	0	2	Tr
Sirloin steak	1	320	11	31	Tr	Tr	Tr	54
Smoked sausage patties	2	240	19	71	2	0	2	13
Spicy grilled catfish fillets	2	260	11	38	2	1	1	38
Sugar cured ham	1	180	7	35	4	Tr	4	24
Tartar sauce	1 svg	140	14	90	2	0	2	0
Thick sliced bacon	3	210	17	73	0	0	0	14
Turkey sausage patties	2	110	6	49	1	0	1	13
Turnip greens	1 svg	100	4	36	6	4	2	10
Unsweetened iced tea	1	0	0	0	Tr	0	Tr	0
Dairy Queen								
(all listings medium size, unless noted)	***	***	*	*	*	*	*	*
All beef cheese dog	1	290	19	59	19	1	18	12
All beef chili cheese dog	1	430	22	46	39	2	37	18
All beef chili cheese foot-long dog	1	840	54	58	52	2	50	37
All beef chili dog	1	290	17	53	24	1	23	11
All beef foot-long hot dog	1	560	35	56	39	2	37	20
All beef hot dog	1	250	14	50	21	1	20	9
Banana cream pie Blizzard	1	780	30	35	115	1	114	14

	Serving Size	Calories	Fat (g)	Calories from Fat (%)	Total Carbs (g)	Fiber (g)	Net Carbs (g)	Protein (g)
Banana malt	1	740	20	24	120	2	118	21
Banana shake, med	1	620	19	28	96	2	94	19
Banana split	1	520	13	23	94	3	91	9
Banana split Blizzard	1	570	16	25	93	1	92	13
Banana sundae	1	330	10	27	53	1	52	8
Buster bar	1	480	31	58	45	2	43	11
Butterfinger Blizzard	1	740	26	32	114	0	114	16
Butterscotch Dilly bar	1	210	11	47	24	0	24	3
Butterscotch dipped cone	1	490	23	42	59	0	59	9
Cappuccino Heath Blizzard	1	870	38	39	122	1	121	15
Caramel malt	1	960	24	23	163	0	163	22
Caramel shake	1	850	23	24	140	0	140	20
Caramel sundae	1	430	11	23	75	0	75	9
Cherry ChesseQuake Blizzard	1	690	28	37	92	0	92	15
Cherry Dilly bar	1	210	12	51	24	0	24	3
Cherry dipped cone	1	480	24	45	59	0	59	9
Cherry malt	1	800	22	25	130	0	130	20
Cherry shake	1	690	21	27	106	0	106	18
Cherry Starkiss bar	1	80	0	0	21	0	21	0
Cherry sundae	1	350	10	26	58	0	58	8
Chicken strip basket w/ country gravy	4 pc	1360	63	42	103	8	95	39
Chicken strip basket w/ country gravy	6 pc	1640	74	41	121	10	111	54
Choco cherry love Blizzard	1	730	33	41	94	1	93	14
Chocolate chip Blizzard	1	880	50	51	96	2	94	14
Chocolate coated waffle cone w/ soft serve	1	540	21	35	77	1	76	10
Chocolate cone	1	340	10	26	54	0	54	9
Chocolate covered strawberry waffle bowl sundae	1	790	40	46	99	2	97	10
Chocolate Dilly bar	1	240	15	56	24	1	23	4
Chocolate Dilly bar, mint	1	240	15	56	24	1	23	4
Chocolate dipped cone	1	470	22	42	60	1	59	9
Chocolate extreme Blizzard	1	980	44	40	130	3	127	17

	Serving Size	Calories	Fat (g)	Calories from Fat (%)	Total Carbs (g)	Fiber (g)	Net Carbs (g)	Protein (g)
Dairy Queen (cont.)	***	***	*	*	*	*	*	*
Chocolate malt	1	900	22	22	154	0	154	20
Chocolate shake	1	790	21	24	130	0	130	18
Chocolate sundae	1	400	10	23	70	0	70	8
Classic Grillburger	1	470	21	40	42	2	40	24
Cookie dough Blizzard	1	1010	40	36	148	1	147	18
Crispy chicken salad	1	460	19	37	31	6	25	29
Crispy chicken sandwich	1	560	28	45	48	3	45	20
Crispy chicken sandwich w/ cheese	1	610	32	47	48	3	45	22
Crispy chicken wrap	1	290	16	50	17	2	15	11
Crispy Flame Thrower chicken sandwich	1	860	55	58	51	3	48	30
Crispy Flame Thrower chicken wrap	1	310	19	55	17	2	15	11
Dilly bar, no sugar added	1	190	13	62	24	5	19	3
DQ frozen heart cake	1 pc	290	11	34	42	1	41	6
DQ frozen log cake	1 pc	310	12	35	44	1	43	6
DQ frozen round cake, 10"	1 pc	500	19	34	72	1	71	11
DQ frozen round cake, 8"	1 pc	410	15	33	59	1	58	9
DQ frozen sheet cake	1 pc	320	12	34	47	1	46	6
DQ fudge bar, no sugar added	1	50	0	0	13	6	7	4
DQ sandwich	1	190	5	24	31	1	30	4
DQ vanilla orange bar, no sugar added	1	60	0	0	18	6	12	2
Fab fudge waffle bowl sundae	1	750	30	36	108	1	107	10
French fries, lg	1	500	21	38	70	5	65	6
French fries, reg	1	310	13	38	43	3	40	2
French silk pie Blizzard	1	920	44	43	117	2	115	15
Fudge brownie temptation waffle bowl sundae	1	970	49	45	120	3	117	14
Georgie Mud Fudge Blizzard	1	1010	54	48	114	4	110	19
Grilled chicken salad	1	280	11	35	14	4	10	31
Grilled chicken sandwich	1	370	16	39	32	1	31	24
Grilled chicken wrap	1	200	12	54	9	1	8	12

	Serving Size	Calories	Fat (g)	Calories from Fat (%)	Total Carbs (g)	Fiber (g)	Net Carbs (g)	Protein (g)
Grilled Flame Thrower chicken sandwich	1	590	36	55	34	1	33	34
Half pound classic Grillburger w/ cheese	1	910	54	53	42	2	40	52
Half pound Flame Thrower Grillburger	1	1060	75	64	41	2	39	54
Half pound Grillburger	1	720	40	50	42	2	40	42
Half pound Grillburger w/ cheese	1	870	51	53	42	2	40	51
Hawaiian Blizzard	1	600	21	32	92	3	89	13
Heath Dilly bar	1	220	13	53	25	0	25	3
Heath Blizzard	1	920	41	40	126	1	125	16
Hot fudge malt	1	979	31	28	146	0	146	22
Hot fudge shake	1	850	30	32	123	0	123	20
Hot fudge sundae	1	440	14	29	66	0	66	9
Iron grilled chicken quesadilla basket	1	1070	50	42	117	5	112	34
Iron grilled classic club sandwich	1	580	29	45	43	2	41	32
Iron grilled supreme BLT sandwich	1	590	33	50	42	2	40	26
Iron grilled turkey sandwich	1	530	25	42	42	2	40	29
Iron grilled veggie quesadilla basket	1	1020	46	41	114	9	105	26
M&Ms chocolate candy Blizzard	1	840	29	31	127	1	126	16
Marshmallow malt	1	900	22	22	157	0	157	20
Marshmallow shake	1	780	21	24	133	0	133	18
Marshmallow sundae	1	410	10	22	72	0	72	8
Mint Oreo Blizzard	1	740	25	30	116	1	115	14
Mocha chip Blizzard	1	810	37	41	107	3	104	15
Nut & fudge waffle bowl sundae	1	880	47	48	99	4	95	17
Onion rings	1 svg	360	16	40	47	2	45	6
Oreo brownie CheeseQuake	1	760	27	32	117	2	115	11
Oreo CheeseQuake Blizzard	1	820	35	38	108	1	107	16
Oreo cookies Blizzard	1	680	25	33	100	1	99	14

	Serving Size	Calories	Fat (g)	Calories from Fat (%)	Total Carbs (g)	Fiber (g)	Net Carbs (g)	Protein (g)
Dairy Queen (cont.)	***	***	*	*	*	*	*	*
Original bacon double cheeseburger	1	730	41	51	35	1	34	41
Original cheeseburger	1	400	18	41	34	1	33	19
Original double cheeseburger	1	640	34	48	34	1	33	34
Original double hamburger	1	540	26	43	33	1	32	29
Original hamburger	1	350	14	36	33	1	32	17
Peanut Buster parfait	1	700	30	39	94	2	92	16
Peanut butter Butterfinger Blizzard	1	1050	54	46	122	5	117	20
Pineapple malt	1	750	20	24	123	1	122	20
Pineapple shake	1	650	21	29	99	1	98	18
Pineapple sundae	1	340	10	26	54	0	54	8
Popcorn shrimp basket	1	990	49	45	115	8	107	18
Quarter pound bacon cheddar Grillburger	1	650	35	48	41	2	39	36
Quarter pound classic Grillburger w/ cheese	1	560	28	45	42	2	40	30
Quarter pound Flame Thrower Grillburger	1	780	52	60	41	2	39	34
Reese's Peanut Butter Cups Blizzard	1	760	31	37	101	2	99	18
Side salad	1	45	0	0	11	3	8	2
Snicker's Blizzard	1	850	33	35	123	2	121	18
Stars & Stripes Starkiss bar	1	80	0	0	21	0	21	0
Strawberry CheeseQuake Blizzard	1	690	28	37	92	0	92	15
Strawberry malt	1	770	20	23	128	1	127	21
Strawberry shake	1	650	21	29	97	1	96	18
Strawberry sundae	1	350	10	26	56	0	56	8
Tropical Blizzard	1	750	40	48	87	5	82	15
Turtle pecan cluster Blizzard	1	1050	54	46	127	3	124	17
Turtle waffle bowl sundae	1	810	34	38	116	2	114	12
Vanilla cone	1	330	10	27	53	0	53	9
Waffle cone w/ soft serve	1	420	13	28	67	0	67	10
Denny's	***	***	*	*	*	*	*	*
All American Slam	1	820	69	76	5	1	4	42

	Serving Size	Calories	Fat (g)	Calories from Fat (%)	Total Carbs (g)	Fiber (g)	Net Carbs (g)	Protein (g)
Appetizer sampler	1	1380	71	46	139	6	133	53
Apple crisp a la mode	1	750	21	25	134	4	130	7
Apple pie	1 pc	510	23	41	72	3	69	4
Applesauce	1 svg	60	0	0	15	1	14	0
Bacon	2	100	8	72	1	0	1	7
Bacon cheddar burger	1	1100	72	59	55	6	49	61
Bacon, lettuce & tomato sandwich	1	570	37	58	36	2	34	20
Bagel & cream cheese	1	430	12	25	48	2	46	11
Baja salad w/ chicken	1	330	16	44	14	4	10	35
Baja salad w/ shrimp	1	280	17	55	12	3	9	21
Banana	1	110	0	0	29	4	25	1
Belgian waffle platter	1	650	50	69	31	2	29	20
Biscuit	1	210	11	47	25	0	25	3
Biscuits & sausage gravy	1	580	34	53	57	0	57	9
Black & bleu salad	1	270	16	53	6	1	5	24
Boca burger	1	500	15	27	62	10	52	30
Breaded chicken sandwich w/ honey mustard dressing	1	1190	65	49	104	5	99	44
Breaded shrimp	6 pc	190	8	38	20	2	18	9
Broccoli & cheddar soup	1	370	29	71	16	4	12	10
Butter roll	2	260	9	31	38	1	37	5
Buttermilk pancakes	3	510	6	11	102	3	99	12
Cheesecake	1 pc	640	41	58	58	0	58	9
Cheesecake, no sugar added	1 pc	290	23	71	23	0	23	6
Cheese three pack appetizer	1	1940	125	58	164	8	156	54
Chicken deluxe salad, chicken strip	1	590	29	44	44	4	40	42
Chicken noodle soup	1	170	4	21	19	1	18	12
Chicken ranch melt	1	920	42	41	79	4	75	53
Chicken sausage patty	1	110	9	74	0	0	0	7
Chicken strips dinner	1	560	24	39	41	0	41	45
Chicken strips w/ buffalo sauce	1	730	32	39	53	1	52	57
Chicken wings w/ buffalo sauce	1	300	21	63	5	2	3	20

	Serving Size	Calories	Fat (g)	Calories from Fat (%)	Total Carbs (g)	Fiber (g)	Net Carbs (g)	Protein (g)
Denny's (cont.)	***	***	*	*	*	*	*	*
Cinnamon apples	1 svg	90	0	0	20	1	19	0
Clam chowder	1	270	17	57	24	2	22	5
Classic cheeseburger	1	930	58	56	56	5	51	49
Classic cheeseburger w/o cheese	1	770	45	53	56	5	51	39
Club sandwich	1	660	34	46	55	4	51	29
Coconut cream pie	1 pc	630	39	56	65	1	64	6
Coleslaw	1 svg	260	22	76	15	3	12	2
Corn	1 svg	130	3	21	26	1	25	4
Cottage cheese	1 svg	70	2	26	5	0	5	9
Country fried potatoes	1 svg	390	28	65	30	10	20	3
Country fried steak w/ gravy	1	1000	65	59	54	6	48	51
Country fried steak & eggs	1	660	42	57	29	3	26	39
Cranberry pecan salad w/ chicken	1	250	8	29	11	1	10	32
Cranberry pecan salad w/ shrimp	1	190	9	43	9	1	8	18
Dippable veggies w/ ranch dressing	1	280	25	80	11	1	10	2
Double cheeseburger	1	1540	116	68	33	5	28	92
Eggs, fried	2	190	16	76	1	0	1	11
Eggs, hard or soft boiled	2	130	8	55	1	0	1	11
Eggs, scrambled	2	220	17	70	1	0	1	14
Egg whites	2	80	1	11	1	0	1	13
English muffin w/ margarine	1	180	3	15	25	1	24	4
English muffin w/o margarine	1	130	1	7	25	1	24	5
English muffin, gluten free - see Gluten-free English muffin	***	***	*	*	*	*	*	*
Fabulous French toast platter	1	1010	52	46	93	5	88	43
Fit-fare Boca burger	1	410	8	18	60	17	43	25
Fit-fare chicken sandwich w/ fruit	1	490	7	13	67	5	62	38
Fit-fare grilled chicken w/ vegetables & tomatoes	1	380	10	24	12	2	10	57

	Serving Size	Calories	Fat (g)	Calories from Fat (%)	Total Carbs (g)	Fiber (g)	Net Carbs (g)	Protein (g)
Fit-fare grilled chicken breast salad	1	290	10	31	15	4	11	36
Fit-fare grilled tilapia	1	600	11	17	66	3	63	58
French fries	1 svg	450	23	46	57	6	51	6
French silk pie	1	770	57	67	59	2	57	6
French toast Slam	1	940	53	51	68	4	64	47
Fried shrimp w/ buffalo sauce	1	380	17	40	37	4	33	17
Garden salad w/o dressing	1	110	7	57	7	2	5	7
Garlic dinner bread	2 pc	170	9	48	210	1	209	4
Grand Slam burrito	1	1160	62	48	106	6	100	43
Grand Slamwich	1	1030	66	58	68	3	65	37
Granola w/ 8 oz milk	1	690	12	16	131	9	122	20
Gluten-free English muffin w/ margarine	1	210	6	26	36	1	35	4
Gluten-free English muffin w/o margarine	1	180	1.5	8	36	1	35	4
Grapes	1 svg	55	0	0	29	4	25	1
Green beans, canned	1 svg	45	1	20	7	3	4	2
Green beans, frozen	1 svg	45	2	40	4	2	2	1
Grilled chicken	1	290	10	31	15	4	11	36
Grilled chicken dinner	1	280	4	13	4	0	4	55
Grilled chicken sandwich w/ honey mustard dressing	1	970	58	54	69	4	65	39
Grilled chicken sizzlin' skillet dinner	1	770	34	40	72	5	67	41
Grilled ham slice	3 oz	90	3	30	1	0	1	15
Grilled honey ham slice	1	110	5	41	1	0	1	14
Grilled shrimp skewer	1	90	4	40	0	0	0	14
Grits	1 svg	260	5	17	47	1	46	5
Half Moons Over My Hammy	1	390	21	48	25	24	1	23
Ham & cheddar omelette	1	590	44	67	4	4	0	40
Hash browns	1 svg	210	12	51	26	24	2	2
Hash browns w/ cheese	1 svg	310	19	55	26	24	2	8
Hash browns w/ onions, cheese & gravy	1 svg	480	22	41	60	58	2	10
Heartland scramble	1	1150	66	52	97	90	7	40

	Serving Size	Calories	Fat (g)	Calories from Fat (%)	Total Carbs (g)	Fiber (g)	Net Carbs (g)	Protein (g)
Denny's (cont.)	***	***	*	*	*	*	*	*
Hearty breakfast sausage	1	350	31	80	5	0	5	14
Hershey's chocolate cake	1 pc	580	28	43	75	73	2	6
Homestyle meatloaf w/ gravy	1	600	46	69	14	14	0	33
Hot fudge brownie a la mode	1	830	37	40	122	118	4	9
Lemon pepper tilapia	1	640	27	38	41	39	2	55
Lumberjack Slam	1	850	46	49	60	57	3	45
Mashed potatoes	1 svg	170	7	37	76	75	1	2
Meat lover's scramble	1	1130	66	53	80	74	6	51
Milkshake, chocolate or vanilla	12 fl oz	560	26	42	76	76	0	11
Moons Over My Hammy	1	780	42	48	50	48	2	46
Mozzarella cheese sticks	1 svg	750	40	48	195	194	1	16
Mushroom swiss burger	1	900	54	54	59	53	6	47
Mushroom swiss chopped steak	1	930	75	73	18	1	17	46
Oatmeal w/ 8 oz milk	1	270	7	23	37	4	33	14
Omelette, Build Your Own, egg white, plain	7 oz	110	1.5	12	1	0	1	20
Omelette, Build Your Own, plain	7 oz	340	26	69	2	0	2	21
Omelette, Build Your Own, add-ins	***	***	*	*	*	*	*	*
American cheese	1 slice	80	7	79	1	0	1	4
Avocado, fresh	1 svg	45	4	80	2	2	0	1
Bacon	2 slices	100	8	72	1	0	1	7
Caramelized onions	1 oz	70	7	90	2	1	1	0
Cheddar cheese	1 oz	80	6	68	0	0	0	5
Chorizo sausage	3 oz	330	27	74	4	0	4	17
Feta cheese	1 oz	80	5	56	2	0	2	7
Fire-roasted bell peppers & onions	2 oz	70	6	77	4	1	3	0
Ham	3 oz	90	3	30	1	0	1	15
Italian cheese blend	1 oz	70	6	77	0	0	0	5
Jalapenos	1 oz	5	0	0	1	0	1	0
Pepper Jack queso	2 oz	100	7	63	3	0	3	5
Pico de gallo	2 oz	15	0	0	3	1	2	1

	Serving Size	Calories	Fat (g)	Calories from Fat (%)	Total Carbs (g)	Fiber (g)	Net Carbs (g)	Protein (g)
Sausage	1.5 oz	180	18	90	1	0	1	6
Sautéed mushrooms	1 oz	50	6	108	1	0	1	1
Spinach, fresh	0.5 oz	5	0	0	0	0	0	0
Swiss cheese	1 slice	80	6	68	0	0	0	6
Tomatoes	2 oz	10	0	0	2	1	1	0
Onion rings	1 svg	520	36	62	48	3	45	6
Pancake puppies	6 ea	390	12	28	67	2	65	6
Pancakes	3	510	6	11	102	3	99	12
Prime rib sizzlin' breakfast skillet	1	850	40	42	77	6	71	41
Prime rib sizzlin' skillet dinner	1	900	42	42	77	5	72	49
Sausage links	2	160	15	84	1	1	0	5
Seasonal fruit	1 svg	70	0	0	18	3	15	1
Seasoned fries	1 svg	510	33	58	48	5	43	6
Slamburger	1	750	60	72	13	2	11	41
Smokin' Q three pack appetizer	1	1870	106	51	179	9	170	62
Smothered cheese fries	1 svg	870	52	54	75	7	68	27
Southwestern sizzlin' skillet	1	990	61	55	71	6	65	35
Spicy buffalo chicken melt	1	940	46	44	81	4	77	46
Super bird sandwich	1	560	27	43	43	2	41	38
Super grand Slamwich	1	1320	89	61	71	4	67	53
Sweet & tangy BBQ chicken strips	1	820	30	33	83	2	81	58
Sweet & tangy BBQ chicken wings	1	420	19	41	41	1	40	21
Sweet & tangy BBQ shrimp	1	460	14	27	66	4	62	18
T-bone steak	1	740	56	68	0	0	0	59
T-bone steak & breaded shrimp	1	920	64	63	20	2	18	68
T-bone steak & eggs	1	780	36	42	4	0	4	110
T-bone steak & shrimp skewer	1	830	60	65	0	0	0	72
Toast w/ margarine	1 slice	130	7	48	16	1	15	3
Tomato slices	3	10	0	0	2	1	1	1
Top sirloin steak	1	220	6	25	1	0	1	41
Top sirloin steak & breaded shrimp	1	440	15	31	23	2	21	52

	Serving Size	Calories	Fat (g)	Calories from Fat (%)	Total Carbs (g)	Fiber (g)	Net Carbs (g)	Protein (g)
Denny's (cont.)	***	***	*	*	*	*	*	*
Top sirloin steak & eggs	1	420	21	45	1	0	1	54
Top sirloin steak & shrimp skewers	1	310	9	26	1	0	1	55
Turkey bacon	2	60	3.5	53	1	0	1	7
Two egg breakfast	1	200	15	68	1	0	1	13
Ultimate omelette	1	670	54	73	8	2	6	36
Vegetable beef soup	1	120	1	8	18	3	15	10
Vegetable rice pilaf	1 svg	200	3	14	37	1	36	4
Veggie cheese omelette	1	500	37	67	10	2	8	29
Western burger	1	1300	82	57	83	6	77	58
Wheat pancakes	2	310	2	6	64	8	56	10
Yogurt, low fat	6 oz	160	2	11	30	0	30	6
Zesty nachos	1	1150	49	38	138	11	127	46
Domino's Pizza	***	***	*	*	*	*	*	*
Crusts, Plain (⅛ of 12" pizza)	***	***	*	*	*	*	*	*
Hand tossed	1 slice	120	2	15	22	1	21	4
Thin crust	1 slice	80	4	45	12	1	11	2
Deep dish	1 slice	160	5	28	24	3	21	4
Feast Pizza Toppings (⅛ of 12" pizza)	***	***	*	*	*	*	*	*
America's favorite	1 slice	120	10	75	4	1	3	6
Bacon cheeseburger	1 slice	140	11	71	3	1	2	8
Barbecue	1 slice	130	8	55	8	0	8	7
Deluxe	1 slice	100	8	72	4	1	3	5
Extravaganza	1 slice	150	12	72	5	1	4	9
Hawaiian	1 slice	90	6	60	5	1	4	6
Meatzza	1 slice	150	11	66	4	1	3	9
Pepperoni	1 slice	130	11	76	4	1	3	7
Philly cheesesteak	1 slice	100	7	63	1	0	1	7
Vegi	1 slice	80	6	68	4	1	3	5
Side Orders & Condiments	***	***	*	*	*	*	*	*
Barbeque buffalo wings	2 pc	230	14	55	6	0	6	17
Blue cheese dipping sauce	1 svg	210	22	94	2	0	2	1

	Serving Size	Calories	Fat (g)	Calories from Fat (%)	Total Carbs (g)	Fiber (g)	Net Carbs (g)	Protein (g)
Blue cheese dressing	1 pkg	230	24	94	2	0	2	2
Breadsticks	1 pc	110	6	49	11	0	11	2
Buffalo chicken kickers	2 pc	100	5	45	7	1	6	9
Buttermilk ranch dressing	1 pkg	220	24	98	2	0	2	1
Cheesy bread	1 pc	120	6	45	11	0	11	4
Cinna Stix	1 pc	120	6	45	14	1	13	2
Creamy Caesar dressing	1 pkg	210	22	94	2	0	2	1
Croutons	1 pkg	45	2	40	6	0	6	1
Garden fresh salad w/o dressing	1 svg	70	4	51	5	2	3	4
Garlic dipping sauce	1 svg	250	28	100	0	0	0	0
Golden Italian dressing	1 pkg	220	23	94	2	0	2	0
Grilled chicken Caesar salad w/o dressing	1 svg	100	5	45	6	2	4	10
Hot buffalo wings	2 pc	200	14	63	2	0	2	16
Hot dipping sauce	1 svg	50	5	90	3	0	3	0
Italian dipping sauce	1 svg	25	0	0	5	1	4	1
Light Italian dressing	1 pkg	20	1	45	2	0	2	0
Marinara dipping sauce	1 svg	25	0	0	5	1	4	1
Parmesan peppercorn dipping sauce	1 svg	190	21	99	2	0	2	0
Ranch dipping sauce	1 svg	190	21	99	2	0	2	0
Sweet icing	1 svg	250	3	11	57	0	57	0
Dunkin' Donuts	***	***	*	*	*	*	*	*
Bagels	***	***	*	*	*	*	*	*
Cinnamon raisin	1	370	4	10	72	3	69	13
Everything	1	360	5	13	74	3	71	15
Garlic	1	350	4	10	76	4	72	15
Onion	1	340	4	11	65	3	62	12
Plain	1	330	3	8	71	3	0	14
Poppyseed	1	370	6	15	73	3	70	15
Salt	1	330	3	8	71	3	0	14
Sesame	1	370	7	17	72	3	69	16
Multigrain	1	400	9	20	65	10	55	18
Wheat	1	350	4	10	66	5	61	13

	Serving Size	Calories	Fat (g)	Calories from Fat (%)	Total Carbs (g)	Fiber (g)	Net Carbs (g)	Protein (g)
Dunkin' Donuts *(cont.)*	***	***	*	*	*	*	*	*
Cream Cheese	***	***	*	*	*	*	*	*
Plain	1 pkt	150	15	90	3	0	3	3
Reduced fat	1 pkt	100	8	72	5	0	5	4
Reduced fat blueberry	1 pkt	150	9	54	15	0	15	2
Reduced fat onion & chive	1 pkt	130	11	76	6	0	6	3
Reduced fat smoked salmon	1 pkt	140	11	71	6	0	6	4
Reduced fat strawberry	1 pkt	150	10	60	15	0	15	2
Reduced fat veggie	1 pkt	120	10	75	6	0	6	2
Cookies	***	***	*	*	*	*	*	*
Chocolate chunk	1	540	23	38	80	3	77	7
Oatmeal raisin	1	480	14	26	83	5	78	8
Danish	***	***	*	*	*	*	*	*
Apple cheese	1	330	16	44	41	1	40	4
Cheese	1	330	17	46	39	1	38	5
Strawberry cheese	1	320	16	45	40	1	39	4
Donuts	***	***	*	*	*	*	*	*
Apple crumb	1	460	14	27	80	2	78	4
Apple & spice	1	240	11	41	32	1	31	3
Bavarian kreme	1	250	12	43	31	1	30	3
Black raspberry	1	210	8	34	32	1	31	3
Blueberry cake	1	330	18	49	38	1	37	3
Blueberry crumb	1	470	14	27	84	2	82	4
Boston kreme	1	280	12	39	38	1	37	3
Chocolate coconut cake	1	400	22	50	49	2	47	3
Chocolate frosted	1	230	10	39	32	1	31	3
Chocolate frosted cake	1	340	19	50	38	1	37	3
Chocolate glazed cake	1	280	15	48	33	1	32	3
Chocolate kreme filled	1	310	16	46	37	1	36	4
Cinnamon cake	1	290	18	56	30	1	29	3
Double chocolate cake	1	290	16	50	34	1	33	3
French cruller	1	250	20	72	18	0	18	2
Glazed cake	1	320	18	51	37	1	36	3
Glazed	1	220	9	37	31	1	30	3

	Serving Size	Calories	Fat (g)	Calories from Fat (%)	Total Carbs (g)	Fiber (g)	Net Carbs (g)	Protein (g)
Jelly filled	1	260	11	38	36	1	35	3
Maple frosted	1	230	10	39	33	1	32	3
Marble frosted	1	230	10	39	32	1	31	3
Old fashioned cake	1	280	18	58	27	1	26	3
Powdered cake	1	300	18	54	30	1	29	3
Strawberry	1	210	8	34	32	1	31	3
Strawberry frosted	1	230	10	39	33	1	32	3
Sugar raised	1	190	9	43	22	1	21	3
Vanilla kreme filled	1	320	17	48	37	1	36	3
Whole white glazed cake	1	310	19	55	32	1	31	4
Donut, Fancies	***	***	*	*	*	*	*	*
Apple fritter	1	400	15	34	63	2	61	5
Bow tie donut	1	310	15	44	39	1	38	4
Chocolate frosted coffee roll	1	380	19	45	50	2	48	5
Chocolate iced Bismarck	1	350	14	36	53	1	52	4
Coffee roll	1	370	18	44	49	2	47	5
Éclair	1	350	14	36	53	1	52	4
Glazed fritter	1	400	15	34	63	2	61	5
Maple frosted coffee roll	1	380	18	43	50	2	48	5
Vanilla frosted coffee roll	1	380	18	43	50	2	48	5
Donut, Munchkins	***	***	*	*	*	*	*	*
Cinnamon cake	1	60	3	45	6	0	6	1
Glazed	1	50	3	54	7	0	7	1
Glazed cake	1	60	3	45	8	0	8	1
Glazed chocolate cake	1	60	3	45	8	0	8	1
Jelly filled	1	60	3	45	8	0	8	1
Plain cake	1	50	3	54	5	0	5	1
Powdered cake	1	60	4	60	6	0	6	1
Sugar raised	1	40	3	68	5	0	5	1
Donut, Sticks	***	***	*	*	*	*	*	*
Cinnamon cake	1	310	20	58	30	1	29	3
Glazed cake	1	340	20	53	38	1	37	3
Glazed chocolate cake	1	390	25	58	40	2	38	3
Jelly	1	400	20	45	54	1	53	3

	Serving Size	Calories	Fat (g)	Calories from Fat (%)	Total Carbs (g)	Fiber (g)	Net Carbs (g)	Protein (g)
Dunkin' Donuts (cont.)	***	***	*	*	*	*	*	*
Plain cake	1	300	20	60	26	1	25	3
Powdered cake	1	320	20	56	31	1	30	3
Muffins	***	***	*	*	*	*	*	*
Blueberry	1	510	16	28	87	3	84	6
Chocolate chip	1	630	23	33	98	5	93	8
Coffee cake	1	620	25	36	93	2	91	7
Corn	1	510	17	30	84	2	82	6
Honey bran raisin	1	500	14	25	86	9	77	7
Reduced fat blueberry	1	450	10	20	86	3	83	6
Other Misc. Items	***	***	*	*	*	*	*	*
Biscuit, plain	1	280	14	45	32	1	31	5
Brownie	1	430	23	48	56	1	55	3
Cinnamon twist	1	210	11	47	25	1	24	3
Croissant, plain	1	310	16	46	35	1	34	7
English muffin	1	160	2	11	31	2	29	6
Sandwiches, Breakfast Type	***	***	*	*	*	*	*	*
Bagel w/ egg, bacon, cheese	1	530	18	31	76	3	73	26
Bagel w/ egg, ham, cheese	1	520	17	29	75	3	72	28
Bagel w/ egg, sausage, cheese	1	660	29	40	76	3	73	30
Biscuit w/ egg & cheese	1	430	26	54	36	1	35	13
Biscuit w/ sausage, egg, cheese	1	600	40	60	37	1	36	20
Croissant w/ egg, ham, cheese	1	510	30	53	39	1	38	21
English muffin w/ egg, cheese	1	320	13	37	34	2	32	14
English muffin w/ egg, bacon, cheese	1	360	16	40	35	2	33	18
English muffin w/ egg, ham, cheese	1	350	15	39	35	2	33	21
Beverages	***	***	*	*	*	*	*	*
Cappuccino	10 fl oz	80	4	45	7	0	7	4
Cappuccino w/ sugar	10 fl oz	140	4	26	24	0	24	4
Coffee, sm	10 fl oz	5	0	0	1	0	1	0

	Serving Size	Calories	Fat (g)	Calories from Fat (%)	Total Carbs (g)	Fiber (g)	Net Carbs (g)	Protein (g)
Coffee, med	14 fl oz	10	0	0	1	0	1	1
Coffee, lg	20 fl oz	10	0	0	2	0	2	1
Coffee, xl	24 fl oz	15	0	0	2	0	2	1
Coffee w/ cream, sm	10 fl oz	60	6	90	2	0	2	1
Coffee w/ cream, med	14 fl oz	90	9	90	3	0	3	2
Coffee w/ cream, lg	20 fl oz	120	11	83	4	0	4	2
Coffee w/ cream, xl	24 fl oz	160	14	79	5	0	5	3
Coffee w/ cream & sugar	10 fl oz	120	6	45	19	0	19	1
Coffee w/ milk	10 fl oz	25	1	36	2	0	2	1
Coffee w/ milk & sugar	10 fl oz	80	1	11	20	0	20	1
Coffee w/ skim milk	10 fl oz	15	0	0	3	0	3	2
Coffee w/ skim milk & sugar	10 fl oz	70	0	0	20	0	20	2
Coffee w/ sugar	10 fl oz	60	0	0	18	0	18	0
Coffee coolatta w/ cream	16 fl oz	330	23	63	28	0	28	3
Coffee coolatta w/ milk	16 fl oz	170	4	21	29	0	29	4
Coffee coolatta w/ skim milk	16 fl oz	140	0	0	30	0	30	4
Cold brew coffee, sm	16 fl oz	10	0	0	2	0	2	1
Cold brew coffee, med	24 fl oz	15	0	0	2	0	2	1
Cold brew coffee, lg	32 fl oz	20	0	0	3	0	3	1
Cold brew coffee w/ cream, sm	16 fl oz	70	6	77	2	0	2	1
Cold brew coffee w/ cream, med	24 fl oz	100	9	81	4	0	4	2
Cold brew coffee w/ cream, lg	32 fl oz	140	12	77	6	0	6	3
Cold brew coffee w/ cream & sugar, sm	16 fl oz	130	6	42	20	0	20	1
Cold brew coffee w/ cream & sugar, med	24 fl oz	200	9	41	30	0	30	2
Cold brew coffee w/ cream & sugar, lg	32 fl oz	270	12	40	40	0	40	3
Coolatta, grape	16 fl oz	240	0	0	59	0	59	0
Coolatta, orange mango	16 fl oz	220	0	0	52	0	52	1
Coolatta, strawberry fruit	16 fl oz	330	0	0	72	0	72	0
Coolatta, vanilla bean	16 fl oz	430	6	13	90	0	90	3
Coolatta, watermelon	16 fl oz	250	0	0	60	0	60	0

	Serving Size	Calories	Fat (g)	Calories from Fat (%)	Total Carbs (g)	Fiber (g)	Net Carbs (g)	Protein (g)
Dunkin' Donuts (cont.)	***	***	*	*	*	*	*	*
Dunkaccino	16 fl oz	230	11	43	35	1	34	2
Espresso	1.75 fl oz	0	0	0	0	0	0	0
Espresso w/ sugar	1.75 fl oz	30	0	0	7	0	7	0
Hot Americano, sm	10 fl oz	5	0	0	1	0	1	0
Hot Americano, med	14 fl oz	10	0	0	2	0	2	0
Hot Americano, lg	20 fl oz	10	0	0	2	0	2	0
Hot chocolate	10 fl oz	210	7	30	39	20	19	2
Latte, plain	10 fl oz	120	6	45	10	0	10	6
Latte w/ sugar	10 fl oz	170	6	32	27	0	27	6
Latte w/ caramel swirl	10 fl oz	220	6	25	35	0	35	8
Latte w/ mocha swirl	10 fl oz	220	6	25	35	1	34	7
Iced Americano, sm	16 fl oz	5	0	0	1	0	1	0
Iced Americano, med	24 fl oz	10	0	0	2	0	2	0
Iced Americano, lg	32 fl oz	10	0	0	2	0	2	0
Iced coffee	16 fl oz	10	0	0	2	0	2	1
Iced coffee w/ cream	16 fl oz	70	6	77	3	0	3	1
Iced coffee w/ cream & sugar	16 fl oz	120	6	45	20	0	20	1
Iced coffee w/ milk	16 fl oz	30	1	30	3	0	3	2
Iced coffee w/ milk & sugar	16 fl oz	90	1	10	21	0	21	2
Iced coffee w/ skim milk	16 fl oz	20	0	0	3	0	3	2
Iced coffee w/ skim milk & sugar	16 fl oz	80	0	0	21	0	21	2
Iced coffee w/ sugar	16 fl oz	70	0	0	19	0	19	1
Iced latte	16 fl oz	120	6	45	10	0	10	6
Iced latte w/ sugar	16 fl oz	170	6	32	27	0	27	6
Iced latte w/ caramel swirl	16 fl oz	220	6	25	35	0	35	8
Iced latte w/ mocha swirl	16 fl oz	220	6	25	35	1	34	7
Vanilla chai	14 fl oz	330	9	25	53	0	53	11
Tea, plain, w/o milk or sugar	***	***	*	*	*	*	*	*
Decaffeinated	10 fl oz	0	0	0	0	0	0	0
Earl Grey	10 fl oz	0	0	0	0	0	0	0
English breakfast	10 fl oz	0	0	0	0	0	0	0
Green	10 fl oz	0	0	0	0	0	0	0

	Serving Size	Calories	Fat (g)	Calories from Fat (%)	Total Carbs (g)	Fiber (g)	Net Carbs (g)	Protein (g)
Tea w/ milk, no sugar	10 fl oz	20	1	45	1	0	1	1
Tea w/ milk & sugar	10 fl oz	80	1	11	19	0	19	1
Tea w/ skim milk, no sugar	10 fl oz	10	0	0	2	0	2	1
Tea w/ skim milk & sugar	10 fl oz	70	0	0	19	0	19	1
Einstein Bros Bagels	***	***	*	*	*	*	*	*
Apple cream cheese bagel	1	550	17	28	89	4	85	11
Asiago cheese bagel	1	330	5	14	59	2	57	15
Asiago cheese bagel pretzel	1	300	7	21	52	2	50	11
Bacon & spinach panini	1	860	51	53	66	6	60	27
Bagel croutons	1 oz	100	4	36	15	1	14	2
Blueberry bagel	1	290	2	6	64	3	61	9
Blueberry muffin	1	480	22	41	65	2	63	6
Blueberry reduced fat whipped cream cheese	2 Tbsp	70	5	64	6	0	6	1
Braided challah roll	1	220	4	16	41	1	40	8
Bros bistro salad	1	820	68	75	38	7	31	14
Bros bistro salad w/ chicken	1	940	71	68	39	7	32	36
Caesar dressing	2 Tbsp	150	16	96	1	0	1	1
Caesar salad	1	690	63	82	18	4	14	18
Caesar salad w/ chicken	1	820	66	72	20	4	16	42
California chicken wrap	1	630	28	40	63	8	55	33
Candied walnuts	1.5 oz	260	22	76	9	3	6	4
Cheese pizza bagel	1	420	12	26	63	3	60	23
Cheesy garlic & herb pizza bagel	1	500	19	34	65	2	63	24
Chicken chipotle salad	1	710	41	52	54	10	44	34
Chicken noodle soup	1 cup	120	4	30	14	1	13	5
Chile lime dressing	2 Tbsp	60	4	60	5	0	5	1
Chipotle salad	1	590	38	58	53	10	43	13
Chipotle turkey wrap	1	730	37	46	70	9	61	34
Chocolate chip bagel	1	290	3	9	60	3	57	10
Chocolate chip coffee cake	1	760	34	40	110	2	108	6
Chocolate mudslide cookie	1	320	17	48	46	1	45	4
Ciabatta bread	1	290	3	9	60	2	58	10
Cinnamon raisin swirl bagel	1	290	1	3	64	3	61	10

	Serving Size	Calories	Fat (g)	Calories from Fat (%)	Total Carbs (g)	Fiber (g)	Net Carbs (g)	Protein (g)
Einstein Bros Bagels *(cont.)*	***	***	*	*	*	*	*	*
Cinnamon stix	1	370	21	51	41	2	39	5
Cinnamon sugar bagel pretzel	1	320	5	14	66	3	63	8
Cinnamon sugar bagel, Chicago style	1	310	3	9	66	3	63	10
Cinnamon walnut strudel	1	630	42	60	56	4	52	9
Club mex sandwich, on challah	1	750	49	59	46	2	44	36
Cole slaw	1 svg	230	21	82	12	3	9	2
Corn crab chowder	1 cup	280	18	58	18	1	17	8
Cranberry bagel	1	290	1	3	64	3	61	9
Deli bacon sandwich	1	830	52	56	52	4	48	39
Deli chicken salad sandwich	1	460	18	35	47	4	43	28
Deli ham sandwich	1	5210	26	4	48	4	44	26
Deli pastrami sandwich	1	630	33	47	53	5	48	34
Deli tuna salad sandwich	1	440	15	31	50	4	46	29
Deli turkey & swiss sandwich	1	690	41	53	49	4	45	36
Dutch apple bagel	1	340	7	19	66	2	64	8
Egg bagel	1	300	6	18	52	2	50	12
Egg way sandwich w/ bacon	1	580	24	37	59	2	57	33
Egg way sandwich w/ black forest ham	1	570	21	33	62	2	60	37
Egg way sandwich w/ sausage	1	600	24	36	63	2	61	38
Egg way sandwich, original	1	530	20	34	62	2	60	30
Egg way sandwich, spinach, mushroom & swiss omelette	1	540	20	33	65	3	62	29
Elvis' favorite bagel	1	700	30	39	98	8	90	24
Everything bagel	1	270	2	7	56	2	54	10
Fruit & yogurt parfait	1	230	2	8	42	4	38	12
Fruit salad, side	1	140	0	0	36	3	33	2
Fudge brownie	1	510	25	44	74	2	72	6
Garden vegetable reduced fat whipped cream cheese	2 Tbsp	60	5	75	3	0	3	1
Garlic dip'd bagel	1	290	3	9	60	2	58	10
Garlic herb reduced fat whipped cream cheese	2 Tbsp	60	5	75	3	0	3	1

	Serving Size	Calories	Fat (g)	Calories from Fat (%)	Total Carbs (g)	Fiber (g)	Net Carbs (g)	Protein (g)
Good grains bagel	1	290	3	9	62	4	58	10
Green chile bagel	1	370	8	19	62	2	60	16
Grilled chicken, bacon & swiss sandwich	1	750	46	55	45	2	43	40
Ham deli melt	1	510	16	28	62	3	59	36
Heavenly chocolate chunk cookie	1	360	18	45	48	2	46	4
Honey almond reduced fat whipped cream cheese	2 Tbsp	70	5	64	6	0	6	1
Honey whole wheat bagel	1	270	1	3	61	3	58	9
Iced sugar cookie	1	480	15	28	76	1	75	4
Italian chicken panini	1	800	40	45	66	5	61	35
Italian wedding soup	1 cup	160	6	34	15	2	13	11
Jalapeno salsa reduced fat whipped cream cheese	2 Tbsp	60	5	75	3	0	3	1
Kettle classic natural potato chips	1 oz	150	9	54	15	1	14	2
Lemon pound cake	1	440	16	33	69	1	68	7
Lox & bagels	1	520	21	36	66	3	63	25
Marshmallow crispy treat	1	220	4	16	48	0	48	3
Mini chocolate mudslide cookie	1	160	8	45	23	1	22	2
Mini heavenly chocolate chunk cookie	1	180	9	45	24	1	23	2
Mini iced sugar cookie	1	230	7	27	39	1	38	2
Mini oatmeal raisin cookie	1	160	5	28	27	1	26	2
Mixed berry coffee cake	1	710	29	37	110	2	108	5
Multigrain bread	1 slice	130	3	21	23	2	21	5
Oatmeal raisin cookie	1	320	11	31	54	2	52	5
Onion & chive whipped cream cheese	2 Tbsp	70	6	77	3	0	3	1
Onion bagel	1	270	2	7	59	2	57	9
Onion dip'd bagel	1	270	1	3	59	2	57	9
Original asiago bagel dog	1	490	21	39	56	2	54	22
Original asiago bagel dog w/ cheddar cheese	1	560	27	43	56	2	54	26
Original bagel dog	1	470	20	38	56	2	54	20

	Serving Size	Calories	Fat (g)	Calories from Fat (%)	Total Carbs (g)	Fiber (g)	Net Carbs (g)	Protein (g)
Einstein Bros Bagels (cont.)	***	***	*	*	*	*	*	*
Original bagel dog w/ cheddar cheese	1	550	26	43	56	2	54	25
Pastrami deli melt	1	540	17	28	64	3	61	38
Pepperoni pizza bagel	1	470	16	31	63	3	60	24
Plain bagel	1	260	1	3	56	2	54	9
Plain bagel pretzel	1	270	5	17	52	2	50	8
Plain reduced fat whipped cream cheese	2 Tbsp	60	5	75	2	0	2	1
Plain whipped cream cheese	2 Tbsp	70	7	90	1	0	1	1
Poppy dip'd bagel	1	280	3	10	56	2	54	10
Potato bagel	1	260	1	3	58	2	56	9
Power bagel, fruit & nut	1	380	6	14	72	5	67	13
Pumpernickel bagel	1	250	2	7	55	3	52	9
Rachel, overstuffed	1	1030	68	59	53	2	51	54
Rachel, regular	1	910	64	63	51	2	49	36
Raspberry vinaigrette dressing	2 Tbsp	160	14	79	8	0	8	0
Reuben, overstuffed	1	760	42	50	49	3	46	51
Reuben, regular	1	650	38	53	47	3	44	34
Roasted turkey & swiss sandwich	1	690	41	53	49	4	45	35
Salt bagel pretzel	1	270	5	17	52	2	50	8
Sant Fe wrap	1	720	37	46	60	7	53	37
Sausage ranchero panini	1	680	29	38	64	4	60	32
Seafood minestrone	1 cup	130	5	35	16	2	14	8
Sesame dip'd bagel	1	280	3	10	56	2	54	10
Six cheese bagel	1	350	6	15	60	2	58	16
Smoked salmon whipped cream cheese	2 Tbsp	60	6	90	2	0	2	1
Spicy Elmo wrap	1	720	41	51	56	6	50	34
Spinach & mushroom pizza bagel	1	580	25	39	70	4	66	26
Spinach Florentine bagel	1	360	8	20	61	2	59	16
Strawberry cream cheese bagel	1	480	12	23	82	3	79	11
Strawberry reduced fat whipped cream cheese	2 Tbsp	70	5	64	5	0	5	1

	Serving Size	Calories	Fat (g)	Calories from Fat (%)	Total Carbs (g)	Fiber (g)	Net Carbs (g)	Protein (g)
Strawberry white chocolate muffin	1	550	25	41	78	1	77	7
Sundried tomato bagel	1	270	2	7	58	3	55	10
Sundried tomato basil reduced fat whipped cream cheese	2 Tbsp	60	5	75	2	0	2	1
Tasty turkey sandwich, on asiago bagel	1	580	20	31	69	3	66	37
Traditional potato salad	½ cup	360	29	73	20	2	18	3
Tuna salad deli melt	1	590	23	35	64	3	61	38
Turkey chili	1 cup	220	7	29	24	5	19	20
Turkey club panini	1	790	41	47	66	6	60	34
Turkey deli melt	1	510	15	26	62	3	59	38
Turkey Rachel, overstuffed	1	1100	74	61	54	2	52	59
Turkey Rachel, regular	1	870	62	64	49	1	48	38
Turkey Reuben, overstuffed	1	680	37	49	45	3	42	54
Turkey Reuben, regular	1	610	36	53	45	3	42	36
Veg out sandwich, on sesame seed bagel	1	440	14	29	66	4	62	17
Vegetable breakfast panini	1	730	36	44	68	4	64	26
Vegetarian broccoli cheese soup	1 cup	290	20	62	16	2	14	14
Veggie deli melt	1	640	29	41	76	5	71	24
El Pollo Loco	***	***	*	*	*	*	*	*
Avocado salsa	1 svg	40	4	90	2	1	1	0
BBQ black beans	1 svg	200	3	14	36	4	32	7
BRC burrito	1	440	12	25	68	6	62	15
Caramel flan	1	260	12	42	34	0	34	5
Cheese quesadilla	1	420	23	49	35	2	33	19
Chicken Caesar bowl	1	490	22	40	44	2	42	28
Chicken Caesar salad, no dressing	1	230	7	27	18	3	15	25
Chicken soft taco	1	260	12	42	18	2	16	16
Chicken taquito w/ avocado salsa	1	230	12	47	20	2	18	10
Chicken tortilla soup, lg	1	450	20	40	37	5	32	34
Chicken tortilla soup, reg	1	210	9	39	18	2	16	16

	Serving Size	Calories	Fat (g)	Calories from Fat (%)	Total Carbs (g)	Fiber (g)	Net Carbs (g)	Protein (g)
El Pollo Loco (cont.)	***	***	*	*	*	*	*	*
Chicken tortilla soup, reg, no tortilla strips	1	140	6	39	88	2	86	15
Chicken tortilla soup, sm	1	160	8	45	14	2	12	10
Chicken tostada salad, no dressing	1	840	42	45	74	7	67	40
Chicken tostada salad, no dressing, no shell	1	410	13	29	39	5	34	33
Chips & guacamole	1 svg	250	14	50	26	4	22	3
Churros	2	300	18	54	32	2	30	3
Classic chicken burrito	1	550	17	28	69	6	63	31
Cole slaw	1 svg	130	10	69	9	2	7	1
Corn cobbette	1	90	Tr	0	19	2	17	2
Corn tortilla, 6"	2	120	2	15	24	2	22	2
Creamy cilantro dressing, lg	1 svg	440	46	94	3	0	3	3
Creamy cilantro dressing, light	1 pkt	70	5	64	6	0	6	1
Creamy cilantro dressing, reg	1 svg	190	20	95	1	0	1	1
Crunchy chicken taco	1	190	8	38	16	2	14	12
Flame grilled chicken breast	1	220	9	37	0	0	0	36
Flame grilled chicken breast, skinless	1	180	4	20	0	0	0	35
Flame grilled chicken leg	1	90	4	40	0	0	0	12
Flame grilled chicken thigh	1	220	15	61	0	0	0	21
Flame grilled chicken wing	1	90	5	50	0	0	0	11
Flame grilled chopped chicken breast meat	1	100	2	18	0	0	0	21
Flour tortilla, 6.5"	2	210	7	30	30	2	28	5
French fries	1 svg	330	17	46	42	4	38	4
Fresh vegetables w/ margarine	1 svg	60	3	45	8	3	5	2
Fresh vegetables w/o margarine	1 svg	35	0	0	8	3	5	2
Garden salad, sm, no dressing	1	70	4	51	8	2	6	2
Garden salad, sm, no dressing, no tortilla strips	1	35	2	51	4	1	3	2
Gravy	1 oz	10	0	0	2	0	2	0
Grilled chicken nachos	1	810	40	44	70	10	60	39

	Serving Size	Calories	Fat (g)	Calories from Fat (%)	Total Carbs (g)	Fiber (g)	Net Carbs (g)	Protein (g)
Grilled chicken tortilla roll, no sauce	1	390	16	37	37	3	34	26
Guacamole	1 svg	70	6	77	3	2	1	1
Horchata	20 fl oz	60	2	30	9	0	9	0
House salsa	1 svg	10	0	0	2	0	2	0
Jalapeno hot sauce	1 pkt	5	0	0	1	0	1	0
Ketchup	1 pkt	10	0	0	2	0	2	0
Light Italian dressing	1 pkt	20	1	45	2	0	2	0
Loco salad w/ creamy cilantro dressing	1	170	14	74	7	1	6	3
Macaroni & cheese	1 svg	280	17	55	28	0	28	11
Mashed potatoes	1 svg	110	2	16	23	2	21	2
Pico de gallo	1 svg	15	1	60	2	0	2	0
Pinto beans	1 svg	200	4	18	29	8	21	11
Queso sauce	1 svg	80	6	68	3	0	3	2
Ranch dressing	1 pkt	230	24	94	2	0	2	1
Refried beans w/ cheese	1 svg	270	7	23	36	10	26	14
Salsa de arbol	1 svg	10	0	0	2	0	2	0
Skinless breast meal	1	280	8	26	12	4	8	39
Sour cream	1 svg	80	7	79	1	0	1	1
Spanish rice	1 svg	220	2	8	45	1	44	4
Taco al carbon	1	150	5	30	17	1	16	11
The Original Pollo Bowl	1	690	10	13	106	12	94	40
Thousand Island dressing	1 pkt	220	21	86	6	0	6	0
Tortilla chips	1 svg	170	8	42	23	2	21	2
Twice grilled burrito	1	840	39	42	56	6	50	66
Ultimate grilled burrito	1	710	23	29	86	8	78	39
Ultimate pollo bowl	1	1050	34	29	110	13	97	71
Vanilla soft serve, cone, regular	1	320	8	23	53	0	53	8
Vanilla soft serve, cup	5 oz	300	8	24	48	0	48	8
Fatburger	***	***	*	*	*	*	*	*
American cheese, add-on	1	70	5	64	1	0	1	5
American cheese, Kingburger add-on	1	150	11	66	1	0	1	9

	Serving Size	Calories	Fat (g)	Calories from Fat (%)	Total Carbs (g)	Fiber (g)	Net Carbs (g)	Protein (g)
Fatburger *(cont.)*	***	***	*	*	*	*	*	*
Baby Fat	1	400	21	47	37	2	35	17
Bacon & egg sandwich	1	350	16	41	37	1	36	18
Bacon, add-on	1	80	7	79	0	0	0	7
Big fat float	1	390	12	28	73	0	73	3
Cheddar cheese, add-on	1	110	9	74	1	0	1	7
Chili cheese fat fries	1 svg	590	33	50	53	6	47	21
Chili cheese hot dog	1	480	27	51	35	2	33	24
Chili cheese skinny fries	1 svg	600	30	45	64	5	59	19
Chili cup	1	200	11	50	10	2	8	16
Chili cup w/ cheese & onions	1	320	20	56	12	2	10	23
Chili fat fries	1 svg	480	24	45	52	6	46	14
Chili skinny fries	1 svg	490	21	39	63	5	58	12
Chili, add-on	1	50	3	54	2	1	1	4
Chocolate shake	1	910	45	45	115	2	113	14
Cookies & cream shake	1	1180	59	45	163	2	161	18
Crispy chicken sandwich	1	560	27	43	53	2	51	26
Egg, add-on	1	90	7	70	0	0	0	6
Fat fries	1 svg	380	18	43	47	5	42	6
Fat salad wedge w/ chicken, no dressing	1	210	6	26	8	2	6	33
Fat salad wedge, no dressing	1	60	4	60	5	2	3	5
Fatburger	1	590	31	47	46	2	44	33
Fatburger, w/o bun	1	410	29	64	10	2	8	28
Fish sandwich	1	560	31	50	55	2	53	20
Grilled chicken sandwich	1	430	14	29	42	2	40	33
Grilled onions	1 svg	120	14	100	1	0	1	0
Hot dog	1	320	15	42	32	1	31	13
Kingburger	1	850	41	43	69	4	65	50
Lettuce	1 svg	5	0	0	1	0	1	0
Maui-banana shake	1	940	44	42	126	1	125	13
Mayonnaise	1 svg	90	10	100	1	0	1	0
Mustard	1 svg	5	0	0	0	0	0	0
Onion rings	1 svg	540	29	48	64	4	60	7
Onions	1 svg	5	0	0	1	0	1	0

	Serving Size	Calories	Fat (g)	Calories from Fat (%)	Total Carbs (g)	Fiber (g)	Net Carbs (g)	Protein (g)
Peanut butter shake	1	950	53	50	114	1	113	14
Pickles	1 svg	5	0	0	1	0	1	0
Pickles, Kingburger	1 svg	5	0	0	1	0	1	0
Relish	1 svg	20	0	0	5	0	5	0
Sausage & egg sandwich	1	780	53	61	47	1	46	27
Skinny fries	1 svg	390	15	35	58	4	54	4
Spicy chicken sandwich	1	520	21	36	58	2	56	26
Strawberry shake	1	880	44	45	111	1	110	14
Tomato	1 svg	5	0	0	1	0	1	0
Tomato, Kingburger	1 svg	5	0	0	2	0	2	0
Turkeyburger	1	480	21	39	50	3	47	26
Vanilla shake	1	890	44	44	113	0	113	13
Veggieburger	1	510	20	35	60	11	49	33
Wing sauce	1 svg	50	4	72	6	0	6	0
Friendly's	***	***	*	*	*	*	*	*
All American burger	1	860	54	57	55	4	51	39
All American burger, side bacon	1	70	6	77	0	0	0	6
All American burger, side cheese	1	90	7	70	1	0	1	4
Apple juice, lg	1	210	0	0	53	0	53	0
Apple juice, sm	1	120	0	0	32	0	32	0
Apple slices	1 svg	100	0	0	26	5	21	1
Applesauce	1 svg	110	0	0	27	1	26	0
Bacon	2 pc	70	6	77	0	0	0	6
Bacon	3 pc	110	8	65	0	0	0	8
Bacon	4 pc	140	11	71	0	0	0	11
Bacon cheese supermelt, w/o potatoes	1	680	39	52	52	3	49	33
Bacon cheeseburger	1	940	61	58	55	3	52	43
Bagel	1	350	11	28	55	5	50	10
Bagel w/ cream cheese	1	440	19	39	57	5	52	11
Balsamic vinaigrette dressing	1 svg	180	15	75	9	0	9	0
Balsamic vinaigrette dressing, side salad	1 svg	90	8	80	5	0	5	0

	Serving Size	Calories	Fat (g)	Calories from Fat (%)	Total Carbs (g)	Fiber (g)	Net Carbs (g)	Protein (g)
Friendly's (cont.)	***	***	*	*	*	*	*	*
Banana	1	40	0	0	9	0	9	0
Banana smoothie	1	520	4	7	104	1	103	17
Barq's float	1	580	19	29	98	0	98	6
BBQ chicken platter	1	1010	42	37	75	2	73	79
BBQ chicken, 2+2	1	590	26	40	46	2	44	41
BBQ sauce	1 svg	90	0	0	20	0	20	0
Birthday cake, Friend-z	1	690	29	38	100	0	100	9
Black raspberry ice cream	1 scoop	120	5	38	15	0	15	2
Bleu cheese dressing, side salad	1 svg	240	24	90	2	0	2	3
Blue cheese dressing	1 svg	470	48	92	3	0	3	6
Blueberry muffin	1	610	36	53	64	1	63	7
Broccoli	1 svg	90	6	60	6	4	2	3
Broccoli cheddar soup	1 cup	170	12	64	10	1	9	6
Broccoli cheddar soup	1 bowl	340	24	64	20	2	18	12
Buffalo chicken	1	1200	95	71	45	5	40	41
Buffalo chicken sandwich	1	940	61	58	69	6	63	30
Buffalo chicken wrap	1	1180	80	61	75	5	70	38
Butter crunch ice cream	1 scoop	130	6	42	16	0	16	2
Butter pecan ice cream	1 scoop	130	8	55	13	0	13	2
Butterfinger pieces topping	1 svg	120	5	38	18	1	17	1
Butterfinger sundae	1	830	36	39	117	2	115	9
Cake cone	1	30	0	0	7	0	7	1
Caramel fudge brownie sundae	1	1410	66	42	186	2	184	19
Caramel topping	1 svg	130	2	14	27	0	27	1
Cereal, *Froot Loops*	1 svg	250	3	11	46	1	45	8
Cereal, *Raisin Bran Crunch*	1 svg	370	3	7	77	6	71	11
Cheddar jack chicken	1	640	34	48	5	1	4	78
Cheddar jack chicken, 2+2	1	320	17	48	3	1	2	39
Cherry	1	10	0	0	2	0	2	0
Chicken Caesar salad, w/ dressing	1	1030	84	73	32	3	29	47
Chicken deluxe sandwich, side bacon	1	70	6	77	0	0	0	6

	Serving Size	Calories	Fat (g)	Calories from Fat (%)	Total Carbs (g)	Fiber (g)	Net Carbs (g)	Protein (g)
Chicken deluxe sandwich, side cheese	1	90	7	70	1	0	1	4
Chicken fajita quesadilla	1	1220	77	57	65	7	58	67
Chicken parm supermelt	1	830	43	47	73	4	69	43
Chicken quesadilla	1	1020	67	59	56	4	52	29
Chicken quesadilla, half size	1	570	35	55	29	3	26	33
Chicken strips basket	6 pc	650	38	53	39	3	36	39
Chicken strips basket	5 pc	540	32	53	32	3	29	32
Chocolate almond chip ice cream	1 scoop	120	7	53	11	0	11	2
Chocolate chip cookie dough ice cream	1 scoop	130	7	48	17	0	17	2
Chocolate chip ice cream	1 scoop	130	7	48	15	0	15	2
Chocolate ice cream	1 scoop	110	6	49	10	0	10	2
Chocolate soft serve	4 oz	170	6	32	24	0	24	4
Chocolate soft serve	8 oz	340	12	32	49	0	49	9
Chocolate sprinkles	1 svg	120	5	38	19	0	19	0
Chocolate syrup topping	1 svg	100	0	0	23	1	22	1
Chunky chicken noodle soup	1 cup	260	9	31	27	2	25	19
Chunky chicken noodle soup	1 bowl	510	17	30	54	3	51	38
Clamboat basket	1	990	54	49	104	6	98	24
Cocktail sauce	1 svg	30	0	0	8	0	8	1
Coffee ice cream	1 scoop	110	6	49	13	0	13	2
Cole slaw	1 svg	160	12	68	13	2	11	1
Colossal burger	1	1490	104	63	56	4	52	82
Cookies 'n cream ice cream	1 scoop	130	6	42	16	0	16	2
Corn	1 svg	160	7	39	20	4	16	4
Country club chicken sandwich	1	940	57	55	71	6	65	40
Cranberry juice, lg	1	250	0	0	62	0	62	0
Cranberry juice, sm	1	150	0	0	37	0	37	0
Cranberry muffin	1	630	40	57	59	2	57	8
Crispy chicken Caesar wrap	1	1180	80	61	75	5	70	40
Crispy chicken salad	1	710	42	53	45	6	39	37
Crispy chicken tender deluxe sandwich	1	800	46	52	72	6	66	28

	Serving Size	Calories	Fat (g)	Calories from Fat (%)	Total Carbs (g)	Fiber (g)	Net Carbs (g)	Protein (g)
Friendly's (cont.)	***	***	*	*	*	*	*	*
Crispy chicken wrap	1	800	40	45	84	6	78	27
Crushed *Heath* topping	1 svg	170	10	53	19	0	19	1
Crushed *Oreo* topping	1 svg	60	2	30	9	0	9	1
Deluxe cheeseburger "set-up"	1	850	61	65	35	3	32	40
Double thick milkshake, chocolate	1	700	32	41	85	1	84	21
Double thick milkshake, coffee	1	770	32	37	107	0	107	15
Double thick milkshake, strawberry	1	740	27	33	110	0	110	16
Double thick milkshake, vanilla	1	770	32	37	106	0	106	15
Eggbeaters, scrambled	1	50	3	54	1	0	1	8
Eggbeaters, scrambled	2	100	5	45	1	0	1	16
Eggbeaters, scrambled	3	160	8	45	2	0	2	24
Eggs, poached	1	70	5	64	0	0	0	6
Eggs, poached	2	140	10	64	1	0	1	13
Eggs, poached	3	210	15	64	1	0	1	19
Eggs, scrambled	1	110	8	65	1	0	1	7
Eggs, scrambled	2	220	16	65	3	0	3	14
Eggs, scrambled	3	320	25	70	4	0	4	21
Eggs, sunny-side up	1	90	7	70	0	0	0	6
Eggs, sunny-side up	2	180	14	70	1	0	1	13
Eggs, sunny-side up	3	270	21	70	1	0	1	19
English muffin	1	310	11	32	45	2	43	8
Fat free Italian dressing, side salad	1 svg	30	0	0	8	0	8	0
Fishamajig	1	640	37	52	51	3	48	26
Forbidden chocolate ice cream	1 scoop	130	7	48	14	0	14	3
Forbidden fudge brownie	1	940	41	39	131	4	127	13
Four cheese & bacon omelette, w/o potatoes or toast	1	670	50	67	8	0	8	46
French toast	3 pc	760	20	24	128	3	125	16
Fribble shake, *Butterfinger*	1	990	33	30	155	2	153	19
Fribble shake, chocolate	1	590	17	26	94	1	93	19
Fribble shake, coffee	1	630	19	27	102	0	102	16

	Serving Size	Calories	Fat (g)	Calories from Fat (%)	Total Carbs (g)	Fiber (g)	Net Carbs (g)	Protein (g)
Fribble shake, strawberry	1	610	19	28	93	0	93	16
Fribble shake, vanilla	1	620	19	28	100	0	100	16
Fried shrimp, 2+2	1	330	17	46	32	2	30	12
Friendly frank	1	410	30	66	25	1	24	11
Friendly's BLT	1	680	45	60	51	3	48	20
Friend-z *Butterfinger*	1	820	32	35	122	3	119	11
Friend-z *Heath*	1	680	34	45	88	0	88	9
Friend-z *Kit Kat*	1	690	31	40	93	1	92	11
Friend-z *M&M's*	1	560	23	37	80	2	78	10
Friend-z *Oreo*	1	580	23	36	84	2	82	9
Friend-z *Reese's Peanut Butter Cup*	1	860	45	47	96	4	92	20
Friend-z strawberry shortcake	1	470	17	33	72	1	71	8
Friend-z strawberry/banana	1	430	14	29	69	1	68	8
Fruit & sherbet happy ending sundae	1	240	5	19	47	0	47	2
Fudge topping, no sugar added	1 svg	90	0	0	25	2	23	1
Garden omelette, w/o potatoes or toast	1	860	55	58	52	5	47	40
Garden vegetables	1 svg	110	6	49	13	4	9	3
Garlic bread	1 svg	130	6	42	18	0	18	3
Giant crowd pleaser	1	2480	118	43	317	4	313	41
Golden fries	1 svg	300	13	39	44	4	40	3
Grape jelly	1 svg	60	0	0	15	0	15	0
Grapefruit juice, lg	1	190	0	0	45	0	45	4
Grapefruit juice, sm	1	120	0	0	27	0	27	2
Grilled cheese	1	460	23	45	48	2	46	16
Grilled chicken deluxe sandwich	1	640	32	45	54	5	49	38
Grilled flounder	1	520	32	55	28	2	26	29
Grilled flounder, 2+2	1	260	16	55	15	2	13	15
Grilled ham & cheese	1	510	23	41	49	2	47	28
Gummy bear topping	1 svg	90	0	0	21	0	21	1
Ham & cheese omelette, w/o potatoes or toast	1	580	43	67	9	0	9	50

	Serving Size	Calories	Fat (g)	Calories from Fat (%)	Total Carbs (g)	Fiber (g)	Net Carbs (g)	Protein (g)
Friendly's (cont.)	***	***	*	*	*	*	*	*
Ham & cheese supermelt, w/o potatoes	1	660	35	48	53	3	50	34
Hickory smoked ham	1 pc	100	4	36	2	0	2	14
Homefries	1 svg	290	12	37	41	4	37	5
Homestyle clam chowder	1 cup	240	17	64	13	1	12	10
Homestyle clam chowder	1 bowl	490	35	64	26	1	25	20
Homestyle mashed potatoes	1 svg	240	12	45	29	2	27	4
Homestyle meatloaf	1	850	49	52	45	1	44	54
Honey BBQ chicken strips	6 pc	1020	38	34	133	3	130	39
Honey BBQ chicken strips	5 pc	910	32	32	126	3	123	32
Honey BBQ chicken supermelt	1	1080	62	52	86	4	82	47
Honey BBQ sauce	1 svg	180	15	75	12	0	12	0
Honey mustard chicken sandwich	1	850	49	52	74	6	68	33
Honey mustard dressing	1 svg	360	30	75	24	0	24	0
Honey mustard dressing, side salad	1 svg	180	15	75	12	0	12	0
Hot fudge topping	1 svg	120	4	30	19	0	19	2
Hunka chunka fudge ice cream	1 scoop	180	11	55	17	1	16	3
Italian dressing	1 svg	410	42	92	6	0	6	0
Italian dressing, side salad	1 svg	210	21	90	3	0	3	0
Jim dandy	1	1090	47	39	156	2	154	14
Jumbo fronions & waffle fries	1	1270	76	54	134	8	126	12
Kick's buffalo chicken salad	1	770	50	58	48	6	42	31
Kick's buffalo chicken strips	6 pc	910	65	64	42	3	39	39
Kick's buffalo chicken strips	5 pc	810	59	66	35	3	32	32
Kit Kat bar topping	1 svg	80	4	45	11	0	11	1
Kit Kat sundae	1	740	37	45	91	1	90	10
Loaded waffle fries	1	1660	112	61	123	9	114	32
Loaded jumbo fronions & waffle fries	1	1600	110	62	129	8	121	23
M&M's topping	1 svg	100	5	45	15	1	14	1
Malt powder, add-on	1 svg	90	2	20	15	0	15	2
Mandarin oranges	1 svg	80	0	0	20	0	20	0

	Serving Size	Calories	Fat (g)	Calories from Fat (%)	Total Carbs (g)	Fiber (g)	Net Carbs (g)	Protein (g)
Maple walnut ice cream	1 scoop	130	8	55	13	0	13	2
Marshmallow topping	1 svg	100	0	0	24	0	24	0
Minestrone soup	1 cup	60	1	15	11	2	9	3
Minestrone soup	1 bowl	120	2	15	23	5	18	6
Mini mozzarella cheese sticks	1	680	40	53	55	4	51	24
Mint chocolate ice cream	1 scoop	130	7	48	15	0	15	2
Mocha mud crunch ice cream	1 scoop	160	9	51	18	1	17	2
Munchie mania	1	1670	108	58	123	8	115	52
Mushroom swiss bacon burger	1	1240	87	63	61	3	58	59
New England fish 'n chips	1	660	44	60	45	3	42	21
Non-fat red raspberry swirl yogurt	1 scoop	90	0	0	19	0	19	3
Non-fat vanilla yogurt	1 scoop	80	0	0	17	0	17	3
Nuts over caramel ice cream	1 scoop	150	8	48	18	0	18	2
Orange juice, lg	1	210	0	0	49	0	49	4
Orange juice, sm	1	130	0	0	29	0	29	2
Orange marmalade	1 svg	40	0	0	10	0	10	0
Orange sherbet ice cream	1 scoop	80	1	11	17	0	17	1
Orange slammer	1	600	4	6	138	0	138	3
Oreo freeze	1	770	25	29	120	2	118	18
Oriental chicken salad	1	500	21	38	41	5	36	37
Pancake syrup	1 svg	240	0	0	58	0	58	0
Pancakes	3	930	17	16	175	5	170	14
Pancakes	2	500	17	31	77	3	74	9
Peanut butter cup ice cream	1 scoop	150	9	54	16	1	15	3
Peanut butter cup topping	1 svg	90	5	50	10	1	9	2
Peanut butter topping	1 svg	210	17	73	7	3	4	7
Pineapple smoothie	1	590	4	6	122	1	121	16
Pistachio ice cream	1 scoop	130	7	48	14	0	14	3
Popcorn chicken	1	610	30	44	46	3	43	38
Rainbow sprinkles	1 svg	120	5	38	18	0	18	0
Ranch dressing	1 svg	330	33	90	3	0	3	3
Ranch dressing, side salad	1 svg	160	17	96	2	0	2	2
Reese's Peanut Butter Cup sundae	1	890	52	53	90	7	83	17

	Serving Size	Calories	Fat (g)	Calories from Fat (%)	Total Carbs (g)	Fiber (g)	Net Carbs (g)	Protein (g)
Friendly's (cont.)	***	***	*	*	*	*	*	*
Reese's Pieces sundae	1	640	71	100	152	4	148	23
Reese's Pieces topping	1 svg	130	6	42	15	1	14	3
Reuben supermelt	1	800	42	47	57	2	55	50
Rice	1 svg	210	3	13	41	0	41	3
Roasted sliced almond topping	1 svg	110	10	82	3	2	1	4
Royal banana split	1	880	35	36	132	2	130	10
Saltine crackers	1 pkt	30	1	30	4	0	4	1
Sausage	2	200	19	86	0	0	0	6
Sausage	3	300	29	87	1	0	1	9
Sausage	4	390	38	88	1	0	1	12
Sausage mushroom swiss supermelt, w/o potatoes	1	910	58	57	56	4	52	42
Sesame oriental dressing	1 svg	270	14	47	36	0	36	0
Sesame oriental dressing, side salad	1 svg	130	7	48	18	0	18	0
Shrimp basket	1	570	35	55	42	4	38	21
Side Caesar salad, w/ dressing	1	410	36	79	15	1	14	9
Side salad	1	60	1	15	10	2	8	2
Sirloin steak	1	510	28	49	19	1	18	46
Sirloin steak, 2+2	1	490	20	37	31	5	26	46
Sirloin steak tips	1	490	20	37	31	5	26	46
Sirloin steak tips, 2+2	1	490	20	37	31	5	26	46
Slider munchie mania, chicken	1	1990	127	57	161	14	147	52
Slider munchie mania, mini cheeseburger	1	1740	109	56	141	12	129	49
Southwest BBQ steak	1	760	42	50	37	2	35	57
Southwest BBQ steak, 2+2	1	750	42	50	37	1	36	57
Spanish rice	1 svg	330	15	41	41	0	41	7
Strawberry banana smoothie	1	520	4	7	105	2	103	17
Strawberry ice cream	1 scoop	110	5	41	14	0	14	2
Strawberry shortcake sundae	1	580	27	42	79	2	77	8
Strawberry topping	1 svg	190	0	0	48	4	44	1
Sugar cone	1	50	0	0	11	0	11	1

	Serving Size	Calories	Fat (g)	Calories from Fat (%)	Total Carbs (g)	Fiber (g)	Net Carbs (g)	Protein (g)
Super sizzlin' bacon, w/o eggs & toast	1	440	23	47	43	4	39	16
Super sizzlin' combo, w/o eggs & toast	1	570	37	58	43	4	39	16
Super sizzlin' ham, w/o eggs & toast	1	450	18	36	45	4	41	26
Super sizzlin' sausage, w/o eggs & toast	1	690	50	65	43	4	39	17
Swiss chocolate topping	1 svg	100	0	0	25	0	25	0
Swiss patty melt	1	1030	64	56	62	4	58	52
Tartar sauce	1 svg	230	23	90	6	0	6	0
Thousand Island dressing	1 svg	390	36	83	15	0	15	0
Thousand Island dressing, side salad	1 svg	190	18	85	8	0	8	0
Toast, rye	1	340	12	32	48	2	46	10
Toast, wheat	1	200	10	45	22	2	20	5
Toast, white	1	200	10	45	23	2	21	4
Tomato juice, lg	1	90	0	0	19	4	15	4
Tomato juice, sm	1	60	0	0	11	2	9	2
Towering fronions	1	1430	90	57	140	7	133	14
Tri-tip steak	1 pc	350	19	49	0	0	0	44
Tuna roll	1	580	43	67	25	2	23	24
Tuna supermelt	1	810	52	58	50	3	47	35
Turkey burger	1	1140	78	62	61	3	58	50
Turkey club supermelt	1	670	33	44	54	3	51	42
Twist soft serve	4 oz	170	7	37	25	0	25	4
Twist soft serve	8 oz	350	13	33	50	0	50	8
Ultimate bacon cheeseburger	1	1050	69	59	55	3	52	52
Ultimate cookies & cream	1	690	33	43	86	1	85	11
Vanilla ice cream	1 scoop	120	6	45	14	0	14	2
Vanilla ice cream, no sugar added	1 scoop	100	7	63	11	3	8	2
Vanilla soft serve	4 oz	180	7	35	25	0	25	3
Vanilla soft serve	8 oz	360	14	35	51	0	51	7
Vegetable fajita quesadilla	1	1210	82	61	77	12	65	43

	Serving Size	Calories	Fat (g)	Calories from Fat (%)	Total Carbs (g)	Fiber (g)	Net Carbs (g)	Protein (g)
Friendly's (cont.)	***	***	*	*	*	*	*	*
Vienna mocha chunk ice cream	1 scoop	140	8	51	16	0	16	2
Waffle cone	1	90	1	10	20	1	19	2
Waffle fries	1 svg	590	33	50	67	5	62	7
Walnut topping	1 svg	100	10	90	2	0	2	0
Watermelon sherbet	1 scoop	80	1	11	17	0	17	1
Watermelon slammer	1	450	4	8	100	0	100	3
Western BBQ burger	1	1230	77	56	86	4	82	51
Western omelette, w/o potatoes or toast	1	610	45	66	12	1	11	45
Whipped topping	1 svg	80	6	68	5	0	5	1
Golden Corral	***	***	*	*	*	*	*	*
Beef	***	***	*	*	*	*	*	*
Bacon Wrapped Sirloin Filet	109 g	190	12	57	1	0	1	20
Barbacoa	3 oz	270	23	77	0	0	0	18
BBQ Beef (not ribs)	3 oz	120	5	38	0	0	0	18
Beef Liver and Onions	4 oz	210	11	47	8	2	6	20
Carne Guisada	½ cup	140	6	39	4	1	3	17
Chuck Tips	3 oz	140	5	32	0	0	0	21
Garlic Herb Butter Sirloin	3 oz	140	9	58	1	0	1	14
Garlic Parmesan Sirloin	3 oz	130	5	35	1	0	1	20
Grilled Chopped Steaks	111 g	290	20	62	2	0	2	25
Honey Teriyaki Carved Sirloin	3 pc	130	4	28	2	0	2	22
Lemon Rosemary Sirloin	3 oz	180	12	60	1	0	1	18
Prime Rib	3 oz	280	22	71	1	0	1	18
Portobello Mushroom Carved Sirloin	3 oz	150	10	60	0	0	0	16
Ribeye	3 oz	170	9	48	0	0	0	23
Roast Beef (beef flat)	3 oz	180	10	50	1	0	1	22
Roast Beef (inside round)	3 oz	110	3	25	0	0	0	19
Salisbury Steak	85 g (3 oz)	70	8	100	7	0	7	8
Sirloin Steak	3 oz	130	8	55	1	0	1	14

	Serving Size	Calories	Fat (g)	Calories from Fat (%)	Total Carbs (g)	Fiber (g)	Net Carbs (g)	Protein (g)
Sirloin Steak Strips	3 oz	130	8	55	1	0	1	14
Sirloin Tips	3 oz	170	8	42	0	0	0	23
Smoked Beef Short Ribs	3 oz	340	27	71	0	0	0	25
Smoked Brisket	3 oz	230	17	67	0	0	0	21
Smoked Texas BBQ Beef	3 oz	250	17	61	0	0	0	25
Smothered Chopped Steaks	167 g	290	18	56	4	0	4	27
Steak Fajitas	3 oz	110	6	49	2	0	2	12
Taco Meat	¼ cup	110	8	65	2	1	1	7
Teriyaki Sirloin	3 oz	200	13	59	3	0	3	17
Beverages	***	***	*	*	*	*	*	*
Coffee	8 fl oz	0	0	0	0	0	0	0
Hot Tea	8 fl oz	0	0	0	1	0	1	0
Breakfast	***	***	*	*	*	*	*	*
Bacon	3	60	4.5	68	0	0	0	4
Chorizo and Eggs	½ cup	200	16	72	2	0	2	13
Crabmeat, Surimi (fake crab)	1 Tbsp	25	1	36	2	0	2	1
Down Home Fried Bacon	2	130	10	69	4	1	3	4
Made-to-Order Eggs	1	130	11	76	1	0	1	6
Omelet (variety unspecified)	1	270	23	77	3	0	3	12
Sausage Links	1	120	11	83	1	0	1	5
Scrambled Eggs	½ cup	180	14	70	2	0	2	11
Sugar-Free Syrup	2 Tbsp	15	0	0	6	0	6	0
Chicken	***	***	*	*	*	*	*	*
Baked BBQ Chicken Legs	1	140	7	45	5	0	5	16
BBQ Chicken Breast (baked bone-in)	1	350	12	31	5	1	4	55
BBQ Chicken Legs	1	150	7	42	4	0	4	18
BBQ Chicken Thighs (baked bone-in)	1	350	24	62	6	1	5	28
BBQ Chicken Wings	3	180	2	10	3	0	3	15
Bourbon Street Chicken	3 oz	170	9	48	4	1	3	19
Bourbon Street Chicken Wings (bone-in)	3	190	12	57	3	0	3	16

	Serving Size	Calories	Fat (g)	Calories from Fat (%)	Total Carbs (g)	Fiber (g)	Net Carbs (g)	Protein (g)
Golden Corral (cont.)	***	***	*	*	*	*	*	*
Buffalo Wings with *Frank's RedHot* Sauce (bone-in)	3	180	12	60	0	0	0	16
Carved Turkey Breast	3 oz	110	6	49	2	0	2	15
Carved Turkey Dark Meat	3 oz	180	9	45	0	0	0	23
Carved Turkey White Meat	3 oz	170	7	37	0	0	0	24
Chicken Fajitas	3 oz	80	3	34	3	0	3	10
Chicken Lemonata	105 g	140	6	39	4	1	3	15
Chicken Machaca	3 oz	120	6	45	2	1	1	15
Chicken Strips	3 oz	60	1	15	0	0	0	11
Golden Roasted Chicken (dark meat)	3 oz	160	9	51	0	0	0	19
Golden Roasted Chicken (white meat)	3 oz	140	6	39	0	0	0	22
Honey Sesame Glazed Wings (bone-in)	3	200	13	59	4	0	4	16
Hot Buffalo Chicken Legs	1	150	7	42	2	1	1	18
Hot Buffalo Chicken Wings (bone-in)	3	180	12	60	1	1	0	16
Mild Buffalo Chicken Legs	1	150	7	42	2	1	1	18
Mild Buffalo Chicken Wings (bone-in)	3	180	12	60	1	1	0	16
Pulled Chicken in Poultry Gravy	3 oz	80	1.5	17	3	0	3	14
Rotisserie Chicken	170 g	310	15	44	1	1	0	43
Smoked BBQ Turkey Breast	3 oz	120	4	30	3	0	3	19
Smoked BBQ Wings (bone-in)	3	180	11	55	2	0	2	17
Smoked Chicken (dark meat)	3 oz	170	11	58	0	0	0	18
Smoked Chicken (white meat)	3 oz	150	6	36	0	0	0	23
Smothered Grilled Chicken	141 g	200	10	45	2	0	2	27
Spicy Garlic Chicken Legs	1	140	7	45	1	1	0	18
Spicy Garlic Wings (bone-in)	3	180	12	60	1	0	1	16
Spicy Ranch Chicken Breast	1	280	15	48	3	1	2	33

	Serving Size	Calories	Fat (g)	Calories from Fat (%)	Total Carbs (g)	Fiber (g)	Net Carbs (g)	Protein (g)
Sweet Buffalo Chicken Thighs	1	400	26	59	6	1	5	36
Teriyaki Honey Pineapple Chicken Wings (bone-in)	3	190	12	57	5	0	5	16
Turkey Sausage	1	90	2.5	25	0	0	0	8
Turkey Slices with Poultry Gravy	3 oz	90	4.5	45	2	0	2	11
Fish	***	***	*	*	*	*	*	*
Baked Fish	85 g (3 oz)	150	8	48	1	0	1	20
Baked Fish w/ Lemon Herb Sauce	3 oz	150	13	78	1	0	1	7
Baked Fish w/ Piccata Sauce	3 oz	150	10	60	2	1	1	14
Baked Florentine Fish	86 g	170	12	64	1	1	0	14
Carved Salmon	3 oz	130	6	42	1	1	0	15
Fried, Breaded Fish	1	90	5	50	4	1	3	8
Honey Chipotle Grilled Shrimp Skewer	2	140	6	39	4	0	4	16
Salmon Lemonata	3 oz	140	10	64	2	1	1	8
Shrimp Fajitas	3 oz	70	3.5	45	3	1	2	7
Shrimp Topped Baked Fish w/ Lemon Herb Butter Sauce	3 oz	120	9	68	1	0	1	8
Smokey Garlic Grilled Shrimp Skewer	2	160	10	56	9	1	8	11
Pork	***	***	*	*	*	*	*	*
Baby Back Pork Ribs	1	190	13	62	3	0	3	15
BBQ Pork	3 oz	170	8	42	5	1	4	18
BBQ Pork Ribs	3 oz	220	12	49	5	0	5	23
BBQ Pork Ribs, boneless	1	120	7	53	3	0	3	10
Cajun Double Smoked Sausage	1	240	21	79	2	1	1	12
Country Rope Sausage	1	180	15	75	0	0	0	12
Fatback	3	180	17	85	1	0	1	6
Grilled BBQ Pork	3 oz	230	15	59	3	0	3	21
Grilled BBQ Pork Loin	3 oz	140	7	45	3	0	3	18
Grilled BBQ Pork Steaks	3 oz	210	13	56	5	0	5	17

	Serving Size	Calories	Fat (g)	Calories from Fat (%)	Total Carbs (g)	Fiber (g)	Net Carbs (g)	Protein (g)
Golden Corral (cont.)	***	***	*	*	*	*	*	*
Grilled Cajun Sausage w/ Apples	3 oz	210	18	77	5	1	4	6
Grilled Ham Steaks	2	110	4.5	37	5	0	5	11
Grilled Teriyaki Pineapple Pork Loin	3 oz	150	6	36	5	0	5	18
Grilled Teriyaki Pork	3 oz	240	15	56	5	0	5	21
Grilled Teriyaki Pork Loin	3 oz	150	6	36	5	0	5	18
Grilled Teriyaki Pork Steaks	3 oz	210	13	56	6	0	6	17
Italian Sausage	3 oz	200	15	68	0	0	0	14
Italian Sausage w/ Onions and Peppers	3 oz	190	16	76	2	0	2	9
Pork Fillets	1	250	17	61	1	0	1	22
Pork Loin	3 oz	140	7	45	1	1	0	17
Pork Loin with Poultry Gravy	3 oz	150	7	42	3	1	2	17
Pork Machaca	3 oz	170	10	53	2	1	1	18
Pork Pot Roast (w/ sauce)	3 oz	200	12	54	5	1	4	17
Sausage Crumbles	1 oz	120	11	83	1	0	1	4
Sausage Patties	1	80	7	79	0	0	0	5
Sliced Ham	3 oz	120	4.5	34	3	0	3	15
Smoked BBQ Pork	3 oz	210	12	51	0	0	0	25
Smoked Cajun Sausage	3 oz	320	30	84	0	0	0	11
Smoked Pitt Ham	3 oz	110	6	49	1	0	1	14
Smoked Pork Spare Ribs (2 bones w/ rib meat)	1	870	76	79	1	0	1	46
Smoked Sausage	1	220	19	78	3	0	3	6
Smoked Sausage w/ Onions and Peppers	3 oz	220	19	78	4	0	4	8
Smokehouse Baby Back Ribs (2 rib bones w/ meat)	1	300	17	51	3	1	2	33
Split Smoked Sausage	1	240	21	79	1	0	1	11
Salad Bar	***	***	*	*	*	*	*	*
Artichoke Hearts	¼ cup	10	0	0	2	1	1	1
Baby Carrots	5	20	0	0	4	1	3	0
Bacon Bits	2 Tbsp	50	3.5	63	0	0	0	5

	Serving Size	Calories	Fat (g)	Calories from Fat (%)	Total Carbs (g)	Fiber (g)	Net Carbs (g)	Protein (g)
Balsamic Vinegar	1 Tbsp	15	0	0	3	0	3	0
Beets	¼ cup	20	0	0	4	1	3	1
Black Olives	10	40	4	90	2	0	2	0
BLT Salad	1 cup	80	6	68	4	1	3	3
Blue Cheese Dressing	2 Tbsp	150	16	96	1	0	1	1
Caesar Dressing	2 Tbsp	150	15	90	2	0	2	1
Carrots	¼ cup	10	0	0	3	1	2	0
Cauliflower	¼ cup	5	0	0	1	1	0	1
Celery Sticks	1	5	0	0	1	0	1	0
Cheddar Cheese	2 Tbsp	60	4.5	68	0	0	0	4
Cherry Peppers	3	10	0	0	2	0	2	0
Cherry Tomatoes	5	15	0	0	3	1	2	1
Chicken Salad (not Southern Style)	½ cup	250	22	79	3	0	3	10
Chopped Peanuts	2 Tbsp	110	9	74	4	2	2	4
Coleslaw	½ cup	110	9	74	6	1	5	1
Cottage Cheese	½ cup	90	2.5	25	5	0	5	12
Cucumbers	¼ cup	5	0	0	1	0	1	0
Deviled Eggs	1	70	5	64	1	0	1	3
Diced Eggs	¼ cup	50	3.5	63	0	0	0	4
Diced Ham	3 oz	110	4	33	4	0	4	14
Diced Onions	¼ cup	15	0	0	4	1	3	0
Diced Tomatoes	¼ cup	10	0	0	2	1	1	0
Dill Pickle Spears	1	0	0	0	0	0	0	0
Dried Onions	2 Tbsp	45	3.5	70	3	0	3	0
Egg Salad	½ cup	200	17	77	3	0	3	8
Green Olives	10	50	4	72	0	0	0	1
Green Peppers	3	5	0	0	1	1	0	0
Guacamole	¼ cup	70	7	90	5	3	2	1
Iceberg Lettuce	1 cup	10	0	0	2	1	1	1
Lettuce	1 cup	10	0	0	2	1	1	1
Lettuce Wedge	1 wedge	10	0	0	2	1	1	1
Lite Olive Oil Vinaigrette	2 Tbsp	70	6	77	3	0	3	0
Marinated Mushroom Salad	½ cup	80	6	68	5	0	5	1

	Serving Size	Calories	Fat (g)	Calories from Fat (%)	Total Carbs (g)	Fiber (g)	Net Carbs (g)	Protein (g)
Golden Corral (cont.)	***	***	*	*	*	*	*	*
Marinated Vegetable Salad	½ cup	35	2	51	3	1	2	1
Mozzarella Cheese	2 Tbsp	110	8	65	1	0	1	7
Mushrooms	¼ cup	5	0	0	1	0	1	0
Onions	3	5	0	0	1	0	1	0
Parmesan	2 Tbsp	45	4	80	0	0	0	3
Pecan Pieces (plain, not praline)	2 Tbsp	90	10	100	2	1	1	1
Pepper jack Cheese	5 cubes (47 g)	170	13	69	0	0	0	12
Pepperoncini	3	10	0	0	2	1	1	0
Pepperoni	5	50	4.5	81	0	0	0	2
Pico de Gallo	¼ cup	15	0	0	3	1	2	1
Ranch Dressing (full fat)	2 Tbsp	110	12	98	2	0	2	1
Red Grapes	10	15	0	0	4	0	4	0
Red Wine Vinegar	1 Tbsp	5	0	0	0	0	0	0
Roasted Peppers	½ cup	90	8	80	5	1	4	1
Romaine Lettuce	1 cup	10	0	0	2	1	1	1
Shrimp (salad topping)	¼ cup	20	0	0	0	0	0	5
Sliced Almonds	2 Tbsp	70	6	77	2	1	1	2
Sliced Jalapenos	¼ cup	10	0	0	2	0	2	0
Soy Nuts	2 Tbsp	50	2.5	45	4	1	3	5
Spinach	1 cup	15	0	0	2	1	1	1
Spring Lettuce Mix	1 cup	5	0	0	1	0	1	0
Squash	5 rounds (49 g)	10	0	0	2	1	1	1
Sriracha Ranch Dressing	2 Tbsp	110	12	98	2	0	2	1
Strawberries	5	20	0	0	5	1	4	0
Strawberry Spinach Salad	1 cup	40	2.5	56	5	2	3	2
Summer Salad	½ cup	70	5	64	5	1	4	1
Sunflower Seeds	2 Tbsp	90	8	80	4	1	3	3
Tomato and Onion Salad	½ cup	40	2	45	5	1	4	1
Tomato Wedges	5	15	0	0	3	1	2	1
Tuna Salad	½ cup	190	12	57	4	0	4	16
Water Chestnuts	¼ cup	20	0	0	5	1	4	1

	Serving Size	Calories	Fat (g)	Calories from Fat (%)	Total Carbs (g)	Fiber (g)	Net Carbs (g)	Protein (g)
Whole Eggs	1	80	5	56	1	0	1	6
Zucchini	5 rounds (49 g)	10	0	0	2	0	2	1
Sauces & Condiments	***	***	*	*	*	*	*	*
Alfredo Sauce	¼ cup	150	14	84	3	0	3	3
Au Jus Gravy	2 oz	30	2.5	75	2	0	2	0
Brown Gravy	2 oz	20	0.5	23	4	0	4	0
Cheese Sauce	¼ cup	100	8	72	3	0	3	3
Horseradish Sauce	2 Tbsp	100	10	90	2	0	2	1
Italian Red Sauce	¼ cup	45	3	60	3	1	2	1
Jelly, Reduced Sugar	1 pkt	10	0	0	3	0	3	0
Margarine	1 Tbsp	100	11	99	0	0	0	0
Mushroom Gravy	2 oz	20	0.5	23	4	0	4	1
Olive Oil	1 Tbsp	120	14	100	0	0	0	0
Queso Cheese Sauce	¼ cup	70	6	77	3	0	3	2
Salsa	2 Tbsp	10	0	0	2	0	2	0
Tartar Sauce	2 Tbsp	150	16	96	1	0	1	0
Vegetable Oil	1 Tbsp	120	14	100	0	0	0	0
Whipped Margarine	1 Tbsp	70	8	100	0	0	0	0
White Gravy	2 oz	40	2.5	56	5	0	5	0
White Queso Cheese Sauce	¼ cup	80	7	79	2	0	2	2
Veggies & Sides	***	***	*	*	*	*	*	*
Asparagus, Steamed	4	80	7	79	2	1	1	2
Broccoli, Steamed	½ cup	25	0	0	6	3	3	2
Brussels Sprouts	½ cup	80	6	68	4	3	1	3
Brussels Sprouts w/ Lemon Herb Butter Sauce	½ cup	100	8	72	4	2	2	2
Cabbage	½ cup	60	5	75	4	2	2	1
Cabbage, Kettle Cooked	½ cup	45	2.5	50	4	1	3	2
Cauliflower, Steamed	½ cup	20	0	0	3	2	1	1
Collard Greens, Seasoned (not Kettle Cooked)	½ cup	35	1	26	4	2	2	1
Diced Sautéed Green Peppers	¼ cup	50	5	90	2	1	1	0
Diced Sautéed Onions	¼ cup	70	6	77	5	1	4	1

	Serving Size	Calories	Fat (g)	Calories from Fat (%)	Total Carbs (g)	Fiber (g)	Net Carbs (g)	Protein (g)
Golden Corral *(cont.)*	***	***	*	*	*	*	*	*
Green Beans	½ cup	35	1.5	39	4	2	2	1
Green Beans, Fresh	½ cup	70	6	77	3	1	2	1
Green Chilies	2 Tbsp	10	0	0	2	0	2	0
Italian Vegetable Medley	½ cup	60	5	75	4	1	3	1
Okra and Tomato Stew	½ cup	60	2.5	38	7	2	5	1
Onions and Peppers, Sautéed	¼ cup	30	1.5	45	4	1	3	1
Sauerkraut	2 Tbsp	15	0	0	4	3	1	1
Sautéed Mushrooms	½ cup	60	5	75	3	0	3	2
Savory Dill Vegetables	½ cup	80	5	56	7	2	5	2
Skillet Vegetables	½ cup	90	8	80	5	1	4	1
Spinach	½ cup	50	3	54	5	3	2	4
Squash Medley	½ cup	45	3	60	4	1	3	1
Squash, Yellow, Sautéed	½ cup	60	5	75	4	1	3	1
Stewed Tomatoes	½ cup	30	0	0	6	2	4	1
Turnip Greens	½ cup	60	3	45	4	2	2	2
Turnip Greens, Kettle Cooked	½ cup	70	3	39	8	3	5	3
Vegetable Trio	½ cup	30	0	0	6	2	4	2
Vegetable Trio w/ Lemon Butter Herb Sauce	½ cup	60	5	75	5	2	3	1
Zucchini, Sautéed	½ cup	60	5	75	3	1	2	1
Hardee's	***	***	*	*	*	*	*	*
⅓-lb Bacon Cheese Thickburger - no bun	1	550	45	74	6	1	5	35
Apple turnover	1	290	15	47	36	1	35	2
Bacon cheese Thickburger	1	850	57	60	49	3	46	38
Bacon, egg & cheese biscuit	1	530	36	61	36	0	36	15
BBQ chicken sandwich	1	400	6	14	62	5	57	27
Big chicken fillet sandwich	1	710	38	48	62	5	57	33
Big country breakfast platter w/ bacon	1	910	48	47	91	4	87	27
Big roast beef sandwich	1	400	21	47	28	1	27	25
Biscuit 'n' gravy	1	530	33	56	48	1	47	9
Breaded pork chop biscuit	1	640	39	55	46	1	45	25

	Serving Size	Calories	Fat (g)	Calories from Fat (%)	Total Carbs (g)	Fiber (g)	Net Carbs (g)	Protein (g)
Charbroiled chicken club sandwich	1	630	32	46	54	4	50	32
Cheeseburger	1	620	33	48	51	3	48	35
Chicken fillet biscuit	1	600	34	51	50	1	49	24
Chicken strips	3 pc	370	26	63	19	2	17	14
Chicken strips	5 pc	610	43	63	32	3	29	23
Chocolate cake	1 svg	300	12	36	56	2	54	4
Chocolate chip cookie	1	290	11	34	44	0	44	4
Chocolate chip cookie, fresh baked	1	250	14	50	30	1	29	2
Cinnamon 'n' raisin biscuit	1	300	15	45	40	1	39	3
Cole slaw, sm	1 svg	170	10	53	20	2	18	1
Country ham biscuit	1	440	26	53	36	0	36	14
Country potatoes, med	1	290	12	37	39	4	35	6
Country steak biscuit	1	630	43	61	45	0	45	16
Crispy curls, med	1	410	20	44	52	4	48	5
Double bacon cheese Thickburger	1	1200	84	63	50	3	47	65
Double cheeseburger	1	530	32	54	34	1	33	27
Double Thickburger	1	1150	78	61	53	2	51	62
Fish supreme sandwich	1	630	38	54	51	3	48	22
French fries, lg	1	470	21	40	65	5	60	5
French fries, med	1	430	19	40	60	4	56	5
French fries, sm	1	320	14	39	45	3	42	4
Fried chicken breast	1	370	15	36	29	0	29	29
Fried chicken leg	1	170	7	37	15	0	15	13
Fried chicken thigh	1	330	15	41	30	0	30	19
Fried chicken wing	1	200	8	36	23	0	23	10
Frisco breakfast sandwich	1	400	18	41	27	2	25	23
Gluten Sensitive Low Carb Breakfast Bowl	1	660	52	71	10	2	8	38
Gluten Sensitive Side Salad	1	120	7	53	7	2	5	7
Grits	1 svg	110	5	41	16	1	15	2
Ham, egg & cheese biscuit	1	540	33	55	36	0	36	23
Hand scooped malt	1	780	35	40	98	0	98	17

	Serving Size	Calories	Fat (g)	Calories from Fat (%)	Total Carbs (g)	Fiber (g)	Net Carbs (g)	Protein (g)
Hardee's	***	***	*	*	*	*	*	*
Hand scooped shake	1	705	33	42	86	0	86	14
Hot ham 'n' cheese sandwich	1	460	20	39	40	2	38	36
Jelly biscuit	1	520	34	59	44	0	44	5
Jumbo chili dog	1	400	26	59	25	1	24	16
Little Thick cheeseburger	1	450	23	46	38	3	35	24
Little Thickburger	1	570	39	62	35	3	32	24
Loaded biscuit 'n' gravy breakfast bowl	1	740	52	63	49	1	48	20
Loaded breakfast burrito	1	760	49	58	39	1	38	39
Loaded omelet biscuit	1	610	42	62	36	0	36	20
Low carb breakfast bowl	1	620	50	73	6	2	4	36
Low Carb lt Charbroiled Chicken Club Sandwich	1	340	22	58	13	1	12	24
Low Carb lt ⅓-lb Thickburger - no ketchup	1	430	36	75	0	1	-1	22
Low carb Thickburger	1	420	32	69	5	2	3	30
Made from scratch biscuit	1	370	23	56	35	0	35	5
Mashed potatoes, sm	1 svg	90	2	20	17	0	17	1
Monster biscuit	1	770	55	64	37	0	37	29
Monster Thickburger	1	1320	95	65	46	2	44	70
Mushroom & swiss Thickburger	1	650	36	50	47	3	44	39
Original Thickburger	1	770	48	56	53	4	49	35
Pancakes	3	300	5	15	55	2	53	8
Peach cobbler, sm	1 svg	290	7	22	56	1	55	1
Pork chop 'n' gravy biscuit	1	680	42	56	48	1	47	26
Regular roast beef sandwich	1	310	15	44	28	1	27	17
Sausage & egg biscuit	1	590	42	64	36	0	36	16
Sausage biscuit	1	530	38	65	36	0	36	11
Side salad, w/o dressing	1	120	7	53	7	2	5	7
Single scoop ice cream bowl	1	235	13	50	27	0	27	5
Single scoop ice cream cone	1	285	13	41	37	0	37	6
Six Dollar Thickburger	1	930	59	57	57	4	53	46
Small cheeseburger	1	350	19	49	32	1	31	16

	Serving Size	Calories	Fat (g)	Calories from Fat (%)	Total Carbs (g)	Fiber (g)	Net Carbs (g)	Protein (g)
Small hamburger	1	310	15	44	32	1	31	14
Smoked sausage biscuit	1	620	46	67	37	0	37	14
Spicy chicken sandwich	1	440	21	43	41	3	38	11
Sunrise croissant w/ ham	1	400	23	52	27	1	26	21
Trim It Charbroiled BBQ Chicken Sandwich - no BBQ	1	150	3.5	21	14	1	13	18
Trim It Low Carb ¼-lb Little Thickburger - no ketchup	1	220	15	61	5	3	2	15
IHOP	***	***	*	*	*	*	*	
Bacon	2	80	6	68	1	0	1	7
Fried eggs	2	170	12	64	1	0	1	13
Hard or soft boiled eggs	2	160	11	62	1	0	1	13
Poached eggs	2	130	8	55	1	0	1	11
Sausage	2	180	17	85	1	0	1	6
Southwest scramble - no sides	1	650	51	71	13	5	8	38
In-N-Out Burger	***	***	*	*	*	*	*	*
Cheeseburger w/ onion, ketchup & mustard	1	400	18	41	41	3	38	22
Cheeseburger w/ onion, spread	1	480	27	51	39	3	36	22
Cheeseburger w/ onion, protein style (lettuce, no bun)	1	330	25	68	11	3	8	18
Chocolate shake	15 oz	690	36	47	83	0	83	9
Double-Double w/ onion, ketchup & mustard	1	590	32	49	41	3	38	37
Double-Double w/ onion, spread	1	670	41	55	39	3	36	37
Double-Double w/ onion, protein style (lettuce, no bun)	1	520	39	68	11	3	8	33
French fries	1 svg	400	18	41	54	2	52	7
Hamburger w/ onion, ketchup & mustard	1	310	10	29	41	3	38	16
Hamburger w/ onion, spread	1	390	19	44	39	3	36	16
Hamburger w/ onion, protein style (lettuce, no bun)	1	240	17	64	11	3	8	13
Lemonade	16 oz	180	0	0	40	0	40	0

	Serving Size	Calories	Fat (g)	Calories from Fat (%)	Total Carbs (g)	Fiber (g)	Net Carbs (g)	Protein (g)
In-N-Out Burger (cont.)	***	***	*	*	*	*	*	*
Minute Maid Light Lemonade	16 oz	10	0	0	1	0	1	0
Strawberry shake	15 oz	690	33	43	91	0	91	9
Vanilla shake	15 oz	680	37	49	78	0	78	9
Jack-In-The-Box	***	***	*	*	*	*	*	*
Asian chicken salad w/ crispy chicken	1	340	13	34	38	8	30	21
Asian chicken salad w/ grilled chicken	1	180	2	10	22	6	16	22
Asian sesame dressing	1 svg	190	14	66	16	0	16	1
Bacon, egg & cheese biscuit	1	440	25	51	37	2	35	15
Bacon ranch dressing	1 svg	260	26	90	3	0	3	2
Beef taco	1	190	11	52	17	2	15	6
Breakfast Jack	1	290	12	37	29	1	28	16
Breakfast sandwich, sourdough	1	440	24	49	37	2	35	19
Burger, sirloin - mini	1	750	29	35	77	3	74	42
Burger, sirloin, swiss & grilled onions	1	930	59	57	60	4	56	42
Burger, sirloin, swiss & grilled onions, w/ bacon	1	990	64	58	61	4	57	47
Cheeseburger, big	1	650	40	55	50	2	48	24
Cheeseburger, junior bacon	1	400	23	52	30	1	29	18
Cheeseburger, sirloin	1	950	60	57	61	4	57	41
Cheeseburger, sirloin, w/ bacon	1	1010	65	58	62	4	58	46
Cheeseburger, ultimate	1	920	63	62	52	2	50	38
Cheeseburger, ultimate, w/ bacon	1	980	67	62	52	2	50	43
Cheesecake	1 pc	310	16	46	34	0	34	7
Chicken breast strips (4), crispy	1 svg	500	25	45	36	3	33	35
Chicken breast strips (4), grilled	1 svg	180	19	95	3	0	3	37
Chicken club salad w/ crispy chicken	1	480	27	51	28	6	22	33
Chicken club salad w/ grilled chicken	1	320	16	45	12	4	8	34

	Serving Size	Calories	Fat (g)	Calories from Fat (%)	Total Carbs (g)	Fiber (g)	Net Carbs (g)	Protein (g)
Chicken fajita pita, whole grain, no sauce	1	320	11	31	33	4	29	24
Chicken sandwich	1	400	21	47	38	2	36	15
Chicken sandwich, w/ bacon	1	440	24	49	38	2	36	19
Chocolate overload cake	1 svg	300	7	21	57	2	55	4
Chorizo sausage burrito	1	700	38	49	59	6	53	28
Creamy southwest dressing	1 svg	470	23	44	44	9	35	30
Denver breakfast burrito	1	720	53	66	36	5	31	26
Egg roll	1	130	6	42	15	2	13	5
Egg rolls	3	400	19	43	44	6	38	14
Extreme sausage sandwich	1	670	47	63	32	2	30	28
Fish & chips, sm	1	630	35	50	61	5	56	19
French fries, curly, lg	1	570	32	51	63	7	56	8
French fries, curly, reg	1	420	24	51	46	5	41	6
French fries, curly, sm	1	280	15	48	30	3	27	4
French toast sticks	1 svg	430	18	38	58	2	56	8
Fruit cup	1	50	0	0	14	1	13	1
Gourmet seasoned croutons	1 svg	100	5	45	11	0	11	2
Gourmet seasoned croutons (side)	1 svg	50	3	54	5	2	3	3
Hamburger	1	280	12	39	29	1	28	14
Hamburger deluxe	1	340	18	48	31	2	29	14
Hamburger deluxe, w/ cheese	1	430	25	52	33	2	31	19
Hamburger, w/ cheese	1	320	15	42	30	1	29	16
Hash browns	5	230	16	63	20	2	18	2
Hearty breakfast burrito	1	780	61	70	34	4	30	27
Homestyle ranch chicken club	1	720	33	41	74	3	71	33
Jack's spicy chicken	1	550	24	39	59	4	55	24
Jack's spicy chicken, w/ cheese	1	630	30	43	61	4	57	29
Jalapenos, stuffed	3 pc	230	13	51	22	2	20	7
Jalapenos, stuffed	7 pc	530	30	51	51	4	47	15
Jumbo Jack	1	580	33	51	51	2	49	20
Jumbo Jack - no bun	1	230	19	74	2	1	1	12
Jumbo Jack - no sauce	1	470	23	44	47	2	45	20

	Serving Size	Calories	Fat (g)	Calories from Fat (%)	Total Carbs (g)	Fiber (g)	Net Carbs (g)	Protein (g)
Jack-In-The-Box (cont.)	***	***	*	*	*	*	*	*
Jumbo Jack, w/ cheese	1	670	40	54	53	2	51	24
Lite ranch dressing	1 svg	150	15	90	3	0	3	1
Low fat balsamic dressing	1 svg	35	2	51	5	0	5	0
Meaty breakfast burrito	1	630	39	56	41	4	37	34
Mini churros	10 pc	650	35	48	76	4	72	6
Mini churros	5 pc	320	17	48	39	2	37	3
Mozzarella cheese sticks	3 pc	240	14	53	20	1	19	10
Mozzarella cheese sticks	6 pc	480	27	51	39	2	37	20
Natural cut fries, lg	1	620	32	46	75	8	67	9
Natural cut fries, med	1	460	24	47	55	6	49	6
Natural cut fries, sm	1	290	15	47	35	4	31	4
Onion rings	8 ea	500	30	54	51	3	48	6
Potato wedges, bacon & cheddar	1 svg	760	52	62	53	4	49	21
Ranch dressing	1 svg	310	33	96	3	0	3	1
Roasted slivered almonds	1 svg	110	9	74	4	2	2	4
Sausage croissant	1	580	38	59	37	1	36	21
Sausage, egg & cheese biscuit	1	590	39	59	38	2	36	20
Shake, chocolate, lg	1	1430	69	43	179	2	177	24
Shake, chocolate, reg	1	750	36	43	95	1	94	12
Shake, *Oreo* cookie, lg	1	1450	75	47	166	2	164	24
Shake, *Oreo* cookie, reg	1	760	40	47	67	1	66	12
Shake, strawberry, lg	1	1400	68	44	170	1	169	23
Shake, strawberry, reg	1	730	35	43	90	0	90	11
Shake, vanilla, lg	1	1290	68	47	141	1	140	23
Shake, vanilla, reg	1	650	35	48	70	0	70	11
Side salad	1	100	5	45	11	0	11	2
Smoothie, mango, reg	1	290	0	0	72	0	72	2
Smoothie, pomegranate berry, reg	1	280	0	0	69	0	69	2
Smoothie, strawberry, reg	1	280	0	0	69	1	68	2
Smoothie, strawberry banana, reg	1	290	0	0	73	1	72	2

	Serving Size	Calories	Fat (g)	Calories from Fat (%)	Total Carbs (g)	Fiber (g)	Net Carbs (g)	Protein (g)
Sourdough grilled chicken club	1	530	28	48	34	3	31	36
Sourdough grilled chicken club - no bun	1	230	10	39	5	1	4	30
Sourdough Jack	1	680	46	61	41	2	39	26
Sourdough steak melt	1	650	40	55	34	3	31	37
Southwest chicken salad w/ crispy chicken	1	310	12	35	28	7	21	31
Southwest chicken salad w/ grilled chicken	1	100	5	45	11	0	11	2
Spicy corn sticks	1 svg	220	22	90	3	0	3	1
Steak & egg burrito	1	450	25	50	36	1	35	19
Supreme croissant	1	450	25	50	36	1	35	19
Teriyaki bowl, chicken	1	580	5	8	106	4	102	26
Teriyaki bowl, steak	1	650	10	14	106	4	102	30
Ultimate breakfast sandwich	1	570	26	41	48	2	46	34
Wonton strips	1 svg	110	6	49	13	2	11	2
Jason's Deli	***	***	*	*	*	*	*	*
American potato salad	8 oz	420	29	62	32	4	28	6
Amy's turkey-o sandwich	1	560	27	43	71	7	64	33
Baklava	1	380	16	38	50	2	48	6
Beefeater po'boy	1	790	38	43	41	1	40	64
Big chef salad	1	550	28	46	25	7	18	53
Bird to the wise, w/ mayo	1	1490	113	68	49	0	49	71
Bird to the wise, no dressing	1	1390	102	66	49	0	49	71
BLT	1	800	49	55	68	10	58	30
Broccoli cheese soup	12 oz	450	30	60	27	2	25	19
Bronx baker potato	1	860	26	27	132	14	118	28
Caesar salad w/ bread	1	1220	93	69	68	6	62	30
Caesar salad, side	1	660	43	59	53	6	47	16
Café wrap	1	780	50	58	38	4	34	49
California club sandwich	1	830	57	62	42	2	40	39
Cantina wrapini	1	690	35	46	57	17	40	55
Carrot cake	1	510	28	49	63	4	59	6
Chicken pasta primo, w/ bread	1	990	61	55	68	5	63	50

	Serving Size	Calories	Fat (g)	Calories from Fat (%)	Total Carbs (g)	Fiber (g)	Net Carbs (g)	Protein (g)
Jason's Deli (cont.)	***	***	*	*	*	*	*	*
Cheesecake, fruit topped	1	570	34	54	61	1	60	8
Cheesecake, plain	1	520	31	54	54	1	53	9
Cheesecake, strawberry	1	530	31	53	56	1	55	5
Cheesecake, triple chocolate	1	550	32	52	58	2	56	8
Cheesecake, turtle	1	500	30	54	50	2	48	8
Chicago club sandwich	1	780	50	58	46	7	39	46
Chicken Caesar salad, w/ bread	1	1400	99	64	72	6	66	61
Chicken club wrapini	1	780	46	53	42	4	38	56
Chicken noodle soup	12 oz	210	8	34	24	2	22	12
Chicken panini	1	840	48	51	49	2	47	53
Chicken pasta alfredo, w/ bread	1	1200	80	60	68	3	65	58
Chicken pot pie, w/ pastry	12 oz	450	23	46	45	3	42	17
Chocolate chip cookie	1	330	18	49	40	Tr	40	4
Chocolate soft serve dessert	1	170	5	26	25	0	25	5
Chocolate topping, for ice cream	1 oz	100	1	9	22	1	21	1
Ciabatta bing sandwich	1	520	19	33	60	11	49	30
Ciabatta garden sandwich	1	420	19	41	50	7	43	16
Clam chowder	12 oz	300	20	60	21	1	20	10
Club lite	1	510	16	28	50	6	44	43
Club royale sandwich	1	850	51	54	44	2	42	53
Cranberry walnut cookie	1	310	16	46	39	3	36	5
Creamy fruit dip	1	60	3	45	8	0	8	1
Creamy Irish potato soup	12 oz	460	33	65	33	2	31	8
Deli club sandwich	1	880	44	45	70	9	61	58
Deli cowboy po'boy	1	830	47	51	66	2	64	70
Dill pickle spear	1 oz	5	0	0	1	1	0	0
Fire roasted tortilla soup	12 oz	320	16	45	35	5	30	9
Fresh fruit cup	1	230	8	31	41	3	38	3
Fresh fruit cup, no dip	1	90	0	0	23	3	20	1
Fresh fruit plate	1	390	9	21	78	8	70	7
Fresh fruit plate, no dip	1	240	1	4	61	8	53	5

	Serving Size	Calories	Fat (g)	Calories from Fat (%)	Total Carbs (g)	Fiber (g)	Net Carbs (g)	Protein (g)
Fudge nut brownie	1	420	24	51	51	3	48	6
Garlic olive oil focaccia bread, for Caesar salad	1	400	27	61	37	2	35	7
Garlic olive oil focaccia bread, side	2 pc	400	27	61	37	2	35	7
Grilled portobello wrapini	1	670	47	63	45	7	38	24
Guacamole	4 oz	170	15	79	10	7	3	2
Ham muffaletta, ½	1	870	41	42	71	7	64	52
Ham muffaletta, ¼	1	440	21	43	36	3	33	26
Ham muffaletta, whole	1	1750	83	43	142	13	129	105
Ham panini	1	470	20	38	46	2	44	24
Hamit down sandwich	1	460	11	22	49	2	47	40
Homemade salsa	4 oz	30	0	0	7	2	5	1
Honey mustard coleslaw	8 oz	190	9	43	25	4	21	4
House chips	1 oz	230	15	59	22	1	21	3
Ice cream cone	1	20	0	0	4	0	4	0
Italian pasta salad	8 oz	720	25	31	106	6	100	20
JB's bagelini	1	620	35	51	50	5	45	28
Low fat fruit & yogurt parfait cup	1	230	3	12	43	2	41	9
Macadamia white chip cookie	1	340	18	48	39	Tr	39	4
Marinated chicken breast salad	1	580	30	47	32	10	22	52
Mario's Big Cheesy sandwich	1	700	42	54	58	15	43	33
Meatabella po'boy	1	1070	65	55	62	3	59	52
Mediterranean wrap	1	310	10	29	43	6	37	14
Miami panini	1	570	21	33	44	2	42	49
Nutty mixed up salad	1	920	45	44	93	9	84	36
Nutty mixed up salad w/o chicken	1	740	40	49	87	9	78	10
Nutty mixed up salad w/o chicken & dressing	1	460	12	23	77	8	69	10
Nutty mixed up salad w/o dressing	1	640	18	25	80	8	72	41
Oatmeal cookie	1	270	7	23	48	2	46	4
Organic blue corn tortilla chips	1 oz	210	11	47	26	3	23	3
Pasta alfredo, w/ bread	1	1020	74	65	65	3	62	28

	Serving Size	Calories	Fat (g)	Calories from Fat (%)	Total Carbs (g)	Fiber (g)	Net Carbs (g)	Protein (g)
Jason's Deli (cont.)	***	***	*	*	*	*	*	*
Pasta primo, w/ bread	1	800	54	61	64	5	59	18
Pastrami melt po'boy	1	1230	94	69	44	1	43	50
Peanut butter cookie	1	340	20	53	34	2	32	7
Penne pasta, w/ meatballs, w/ bread	1	1110	74	60	74	5	69	40
Philly chic sandwich	1	610	25	37	52	5	47	47
Pizza adobe	1	740	41	50	49	3	46	48
Pizza blue	1	850	65	69	35	10	25	37
Plain Jane potato	1	1610	80	45	180	17	163	41
Plain Jane potato (lighter)	1	920	40	39	119	11	108	23
Poblano corn chowder	12 oz	340	19	50	38	34	4	8
Pollo Mexicano potato	1	1760	81	41	200	184	16	65
Portobello garden pasta w/ chicken, w/ bread	1	1120	69	55	76	64	12	57
Portobello garden pasta w/ mushrooms, w/ bread	1	950	63	60	74	12	62	26
Pot roast melt po'boy	1	770	32	37	47	4	43	67
Pulled pork sandwich, onion bun	1	660	22	30	74	2	72	43
Pulled pork sandwich, wheat bun	1	710	23	29	83	2	81	44
Ranchero wrap	1	890	49	50	62	13	49	61
Red beans & rice w/ sausage	12 oz	280	6	19	56	23	33	19
Reuben the Great sandwich	1	860	32	33	56	9	47	75
Roasted red pepper hummus	4 oz	240	14	53	28	8	20	8
Santa Fe chicken sandwich	1	760	38	45	52	7	45	57
Seafood gumbo	12 oz	300	10	30	37	3	34	16
Sergeant Pepper po'boy	1	900	43	43	52	4	48	66
Smokey Jack melt	1	590	25	38	53	5	48	42
Smokey Jack panini	1	790	42	48	52	3	49	50
Spinach veggie wrap	1	360	17	43	40	6	34	16
Spud au broc	1	1540	56	33	203	17	186	68
Steamed veggies	1	60	0	0	13	5	8	4
Strawberry short cake	1	410	15	33	63	1	62	6
SW chicken chili, plain	12 oz	270	9	30	27	7	20	25

	Serving Size	Calories	Fat (g)	Calories from Fat (%)	Total Carbs (g)	Fiber (g)	Net Carbs (g)	Protein (g)
Taco salad w/ chili	1	1970	111	51	189	27	162	55
Taco salad w/ SW chicken chili	1	1910	105	49	193	28	165	49
Texas chili	12 oz	400	20	45	20	6	14	35
Texas style spud w/ beef	1	1640	75	41	189	13	176	46
Texas style spud w/ pork	1	1550	68	39	191	13	178	48
The Italian Cruz po'boy	1	650	35	48	50	4	46	32
The New York Yankee sandwich, no dressing	1	1190	69	52	47	2	45	92
The VJ sandwich, no dressing	1	890	57	58	37	2	35	58
The VJ sandwich, w/ mayo	1	990	68	62	37	2	35	58
The VJ sandwich, w/ mustard	1	910	57	56	37	2	35	58
Three bean salad	8 oz	400	14	32	41	12	29	22
Tomato basil soup	12 oz	320	25	70	22	4	18	3
Tuna & roasted tomato wrap	1	560	27	43	59	11	48	22
Tuna melt	1	960	62	58	47	6	41	54
Tuna pasta salad	8 oz	590	27	41	67	4	63	23
Turkey muffaletta, ½	1	780	32	37	73	7	66	52
Turkey muffaletta, ¼	1	390	16	37	37	3	34	26
Turkey muffaletta, whole	1	1560	64	37	146	13	133	103
Turkey Reuben sandwich	1	510	13	23	53	6	47	44
Turkey wrap	1	360	14	35	40	5	35	22
Twisted turkey salad, w/ dressing	1	1020	68	60	48	13	35	52
Twisted turkey salad, w/o dressing	1	860	60	63	28	13	15	52
Uptown turkey melt	1	400	16	36	28	3	25	38
Vanilla soft serve dessert	1	160	5	28	24	0	24	3
Vegetarian French onion soup, w/ bread & cheese	12 oz	270	19	63	17	1	16	9
Vegetarian vegetable pasta soup	12 oz	130	3	21	23	4	19	3
Kentucky Fried Chicken								
(all salads listed w/o dressing & croutons)	***	***	*	*	*	*	*	*
BBQ baked beans	1 svg	200	2	9	39	9	30	8

	Serving Size	Calories	Fat (g)	Calories from Fat (%)	Total Carbs (g)	Fiber (g)	Net Carbs (g)	Protein (g)
Kentucky Fried Chicken (cont.)	***	***	*	*	*	*	*	*
Biscuit	1	180	8	40	23	1	22	4
Boneless fiery buffalo wings	1	80	4	45	6	1	5	5
Boneless HBBQ wings	1	80	4	45	7	1	6	5
Caesar side salad	1	40	2	45	2	1	1	3
Chicken little	1	190	10	47	20	1	19	6
Chicken pot pie, w/ pastry	1	690	40	52	57	3	54	27
Cole slaw	1 svg	180	10	50	22	3	19	1
Corn on the cob, 3"	1	70	Tr	0	16	2	14	2
Corn on the cob, 5.5"	1	140	1	6	33	4	29	5
Country fried steak w/ gravy	1	390	26	60	23	2	21	16
Creamy ranch dipping sauce	1 svg	140	15	96	1	0	1	0
Crispy chicken BLT salad	1	340	19	50	14	3	11	30
Crispy chicken Caesar salad	1	320	19	53	12	3	9	28
Crispy strips	2	250	15	54	8	1	7	22
Crispy strips	3	380	22	52	12	1	11	33
Crispy twister w/ crispy strip	1	580	30	47	49	3	46	28
Crispy twister w/ original recipe strip	1	540	26	43	48	4	44	28
Double crunch sandwich w/ crispy strip	1	510	27	48	36	1	35	27
Double crunch sandwich w/ original recipe strip	1	470	23	44	35	2	33	27
Extra crispy chicken, breast	1	490	31	57	17	0	17	38
Extra crispy chicken, drumstick	1	150	9	54	6	0	6	11
Extra crispy chicken, thigh	1	370	27	66	12	0	12	18
Extra crispy chicken, whole wing	1	150	10	60	6	1	5	11
Fiery buffalo dipping sauce	1 svg	25	0	0	6	0	6	0
Fiery buffalo hot wings	1	80	5	56	5	1	4	4
Fiery buffalo hot wings snack box	1	500	27	49	46	4	42	16
Fiery buffalo wings	1	80	5	56	4	1	3	4
Garlic parmesan dipping sauce	1 svg	130	13	90	2	0	2	0
Georgia Gold Hot Wings	25 g	90	7	70	4	0	4	4

	Serving Size	Calories	Fat (g)	Calories from Fat (%)	Total Carbs (g)	Fiber (g)	Net Carbs (g)	Protein (g)
Georgia Gold Kentucky grilled chicken, breast	1	250	10	36	1	0	1	38
Georgia Gold Kentucky grilled chicken, drumstick	1	90	6	60	0	0	0	11
Georgia Gold Kentucky grilled chicken, thigh	1	170	11	58	0	0	0	17
Georgia Gold Kentucky grilled chicken, whole wing	1	90	6	60	1	0	1	9
Green beans	1 svg	25	0	0	4	2	2	1
Grilled chicken, breast	1	180	4	20	0	0	0	35
Grilled chicken, drumstick	1	70	4	51	0	0	0	10
Grilled chicken, thigh	1	140	9	58	0	0	0	15
Grilled chicken, whole wing	1	80	4	45	0	0	0	10
HBBQ dipping sauce	1 svg	40	0	0	9	0	9	0
HBBQ hot wings	1	90	5	50	7	0	7	4
HBBQ hot wings snack box	1	520	27	47	53	4	49	16
BBQ wings	1	80	5	56	5	1	4	4
Heinz buttermilk dressing	1 oz	160	17	96	1	0	1	0
Heinz buttermilk ranch dressing	1 oz	160	17	96	1	0	1	0
Hidden Valley, The Original Ranch, fat free dressing	1.5 oz	35	0	0	8	0	8	1
Honey BBQ sandwich	1	310	4	12	42	1	41	23
Honey mustard dipping sauce	1 svg	120	10	75	6	0	6	0
Hot honey Kentucky grilled chicken, breast	1	260	11	38	3	0	3	38
Hot honey Kentucky grilled chicken, drumstick	1	90	5	50	1	0	1	11
Hot honey Kentucky grilled chicken, thigh	1	180	12	60	2	0	2	17
Hot honey Kentucky grilled chicken, whole wing	1	80	4.5	51	1	0	1	9
Hot & spicy, breast	1	470	28	54	15	4	11	38
Hot & spicy, drumstick	1	160	10	56	5	1	4	12
Hot & spicy, thigh	1	380	28	66	11	2	9	22
Hot & spicy, whole wing	1	160	8	45	10	1	9	12
Hot wings	1	70	5	64	3	0	3	4

	Serving Size	Calories	Fat (g)	Calories from Fat (%)	Total Carbs (g)	Fiber (g)	Net Carbs (g)	Protein (g)
Kentucky Fried Chicken *(cont.)*	***	***	*	*	*	*	*	*
Hot wings snack box	1	470	27	52	41	4	37	16
House side salad	1	15	0	0	3	2	1	1
Jalapeno peppers	1 svg	20	Tr	0	1	1	0	0
Kentucky grilled chicken, breast	1	210	7	30	0	0	0	38
Kentucky grilled chicken, drumstick	1	90	4	40	0	0	0	11
Kentucky grilled chicken, thigh	1	150	9	54	0	0	0	17
Kentucky grilled chicken, whole wing	1	70	3	39	0	0	0	9
KFC cornbread muffin	1	210	9	39	28	1	27	3
KFC creamy parmesan Caesar dressing	2 oz	260	26	90	4	0	4	2
KFC famous bowls, mashed potato w/ gravy	1	700	32	41	77	6	71	26
KFC famous bowls, rice & gravy	1	790	28	32	106	5	101	29
KFC gizzards	1 svg	200	11	50	15	1	14	11
KFC Kentucky nuggets	1	45	3	60	2	0	2	3
KFC livers	1 svg	180	10	50	11	0	11	11
KFC mean greens	1 svg	30	0	0	4	2	2	3
KFC red beans w/ sausage & rice	1 svg	160	3	17	26	4	22	24
KFC snacker w/ crispy strip	1	300	14	42	28	2	26	15
KFC snacker w/ crispy strip, buffalo	1	260	9	31	30	2	28	15
KFC snacker w/ crispy strip, ultimate cheese	1	280	11	35	29	2	27	16
KFC snacker w/ original recipe strip	1	300	14	42	28	2	26	15
KFC snacker w/ original recipe strip, buffalo	1	240	7	26	29	2	27	15
KFC snacker w/ original recipe strip, ultimate cheese	1	260	9	31	29	2	27	15
KFC snacker, fish	1	320	14	39	31	2	29	16
KFC snacker, honey BBQ	1	210	3	13	32	2	30	13
Macaroni & cheese	1 svg	180	9	45	20	2	18	6

	Serving Size	Calories	Fat (g)	Calories from Fat (%)	Total Carbs (g)	Fiber (g)	Net Carbs (g)	Protein (g)
Macaroni salad	1 svg	180	9	45	20	1	19	3
Marzetti Lite Italian dressing	1 oz	15	0.5	30	2	0	2	0
Mashed potatoes w/ gravy	1 svg	130	5	35	20	2	18	2
Mashed potatoes w/o gravy	1 svg	100	3	27	16	1	15	2
Original recipe chicken BLT salad	1	300	15	45	13	4	9	29
Original recipe chicken Caesar salad	1	280	14	45	11	4	7	28
Original recipe chicken, breast	1	370	21	51	7	0	7	38
Original recipe chicken, breast, w/o skin or breading	1	140	2	13	1	0	1	29
Original recipe chicken, drumstick	1	110	7	57	2	0	2	10
Original recipe chicken, thigh	1	260	19	66	6	0	6	16
Original recipe chicken, whole wing	1	110	7	57	3	0	3	9
Original recipe filet sandwich	1	480	23	43	38	2	36	25
Original recipe strips	2	200	10	45	7	1	6	21
Original recipe strips	3	310	15	44	11	2	9	32
Parmesan garlic croutons, 1 pouch	1	70	3	39	8	1	7	2
Popcorn chicken, snack box	1	660	38	52	55	5	50	25
Popcorn chicken, individual size	1	400	26	59	22	3	19	21
Potato salad	1 svg	200	10	45	24	3	21	2
Potato wedges	1 svg	260	13	45	33	3	30	4
Roasted chicken BLT salad	1	200	7	32	7	3	4	30
Roasted chicken Caesar salad	1	190	6	28	5	2	3	29
Seasoned rice	1 svg	140	Tr	0	31	1	30	3
Smokey Mountain BBQ Kentucky grilled chicken, breast	1	260	11	38	2	0	2	38
Smokey Mountain BBQ Kentucky grilled chicken, drumstick	1	100	5	45	1	0	1	11
Smokey Mountain BBQ Kentucky grilled chicken, thigh	1	180	11	55	1	0	1	17

	Serving Size	Calories	Fat (g)	Calories from Fat (%)	Total Carbs (g)	Fiber (g)	Net Carbs (g)	Protein (g)
Kentucky Fried Chicken *(cont.)*	***	***	*	*	*	*	*	*
Smokey Mountain BBQ Kentucky grilled chicken, whole wing	1	90	5	50	1	0	1	9
Snack bowl	1	320	15	42	34	3	31	12
Sweet & sour dipping sauce	1 svg	45	0	0	12	0	12	0
Sweet kernel corn	1 svg	110	Tr	0	23	2	21	4
Tender roast sandwich	1	400	15	34	29	1	28	34
Tender roast twister	1	440	18	37	42	2	40	29
Three bean salad	1 svg	70	0	0	14	3	11	3
Toasted wrap w/ crispy strip	1	360	20	50	27	2	25	17
Toasted wrap w/ original recipe strip	1	340	18	48	27	2	25	17
Toasted wrap w/ tender roast filet	1	310	14	41	24	1	23	22
Krispy Kreme Doughnuts	***	***	*	*	*	*	*	*
Apple fritter	1	380	20	47	47	2	45	4
Caramel kreme crunch	1	380	19	45	49	Tr	49	4
Chocolate glazed cruller	1	290	15	47	37	Tr	37	2
Chocolate iced cake	1	280	14	45	36	Tr	36	3
Chocolate iced custard filled	1	300	17	51	35	Tr	35	3
Chocolate iced glazed	1	250	12	43	33	Tr	33	3
Chocolate iced kreme filled	1	300	17	51	35	Tr	35	3
Chocolate iced w/ sprinkles	1	270	12	40	38	Tr	38	3
Cinnamon apple filled	1	290	16	50	32	Tr	32	3
Cinnamon bun	1	260	16	55	28	Tr	28	3
Cinnamon twist	1	240	15	56	23	Tr	23	3
Doughnut holes, glazed blueberry	4	220	12	49	27	Tr	27	3
Doughnut holes, glazed cake	4	210	10	43	29	Tr	29	2
Doughnut holes, glazed chocolate cake	4	210	10	43	29	Tr	29	2
Doughnut holes, glazed pumpkin spice	4	210	10	43	29	Tr	29	2
Doughnut holes, original glazed	4	200	11	50	25	Tr	25	2
Dulce de leche	1	300	18	54	31	Tr	31	3

	Serving Size	Calories	Fat (g)	Calories from Fat (%)	Total Carbs (g)	Fiber (g)	Net Carbs (g)	Protein (g)
Glazed chocolate cake	1	300	15	45	42	2	40	3
Glazed cinnamon	1	210	12	51	24	Tr	24	2
Glazed cruller	1	240	14	53	26	Tr	26	2
Glazed kreme filled	1	340	20	53	39	Tr	39	3
Glazed lemon filled	1	290	16	50	35	Tr	35	3
Glazed pumpkin spice	1	300	14	42	42	Tr	42	2
Glazed raspberry filled	1	300	16	48	36	Tr	36	3
Glazed sour cream	1	300	13	39	43	Tr	43	2
Maple iced glazed	1	240	12	45	32	Tr	32	2
New York cheesecake	1	340	20	53	34	Tr	34	4
Original glazed	1	200	12	54	22	Tr	22	2
Powdered cake	1	290	14	43	37	Tr	37	3
Powdered strawberry filled	1	290	16	50	33	Tr	33	3
Sugar	1	200	12	54	21	Tr	21	2
Traditional Cake	1	230	13	51	25	Tr	25	3
Little caesars	***	***	*	*	*	*	*	*
Antipasto Salad	1 svg	220	14	57	10	4	6	15
Buffalo Ranch Dip	1 svg	230	24	94	3	0	3	2
Cheezy Jalapeno Dip	1 svg	220	22	90	3	0	3	1
Hot-N-Ready Caesar Wings (oven roasted)	1	64	4.4	62	Tr	0	Tr	6
Hot-N-Ready Buffalo Wings	1	64	4.4	62	0	0	0	6
Ranch Dip	1 svg	240	24	90	4	0	4	2
Long John Silver's	***	***	*	*	*	*	*	*
Alaskan flounder	1	250	11	40	26	2	24	12
Baja fish taco	1	350	22	57	29	1	28	9
Baked cod	1	120	5	38	1	0	1	22
Breaded clam strips, snack box	1	320	19	53	29	2	27	9
Breadstick	1	170	4	21	29	1	28	6
Broccoli cheese soup, bowl	1	220	18	74	8	1	7	5
Buttered lobster bites, snack box	1	230	9	35	24	2	22	13
Chicken plank	1	140	8	51	9	0	9	8
Chicken sandwich	1	360	15	38	40	3	37	14

	Serving Size	Calories	Fat (g)	Calories from Fat (%)	Total Carbs (g)	Fiber (g)	Net Carbs (g)	Protein (g)
Long John Silver's (cont.)	***	***	*	*	*	*	*	*
Chocolate cream pie	1 slice	310	22	64	24	1	23	5
Cocktail sauce	1 oz	25	0	0	6	0	6	0
Cole slaw	4 oz	200	15	68	15	3	12	1
Corn cobbette w/ butter oil	1	150	10	60	14	3	11	3
Corn cobbette w/o butter oil	1	90	3	30	14	3	11	3
Crumblies	1 oz	170	12	64	14	1	13	1
Fish sandwich	1	470	23	44	48	3	45	18
Fish sandwich, ultimate	1	530	28	48	49	3	46	21
Fish, battered	1	260	16	55	17	0	17	12
Fries, basket portion	1	310	14	41	45	4	41	3
Fries, platter portion	1	230	10	39	34	3	31	3
Ginger teriyaki sauce	1 pkt	80	0	0	18	0	18	1
Grilled Pacific salmon, 2 filets	1	150	5	30	2	0	2	24
Grilled tilapia, 1 filet	1	110	3	25	1	0	1	22
Hushpuppy	1	60	3	45	9	1	8	1
Ketchup	1 pkt	10	0	0	2	0	2	0
Lobster stuffed crab cake	1	170	9	48	16	1	15	6
Louisiana hot sauce	1 tsp	0	0	0	0	0	0	0
Malt vinegar	0.5 oz	0	0	0	0	0	0	0
Pecan pie	1 slice	370	15	36	55	2	53	4
Pineapple cream pie	1 slice	290	13	40	39	1	38	4
Popcorn shrimp, snack box	1	270	16	53	23	1	22	9
Rice	5 oz	180	1	5	37	2	35	4
Salmon bowl, w/ sauce	1	460	8	16	65	4	61	30
Salmon, Freshside Grille Smart Choice	1	280	7	23	27	3	24	27
Shrimp bowl, w/ sauce	1	380	5	12	64	4	60	21
Shrimp scampi (8 pc)	1	110	5	41	1	0	1	16
Shrimp scampi, Freshside Grille Smart Choice	1	250	7	25	27	3	24	19
Shrimp, battered	3 pc	130	9	62	8	0	8	5
Tartar sauce	1 oz	100	9	81	4	0	4	0
Tilapia, Freshside Grille Smart Choice	1	250	5	18	27	3	24	25

	Serving Size	Calories	Fat (g)	Calories from Fat (%)	Total Carbs (g)	Fiber (g)	Net Carbs (g)	Protein (g)
Vegetable medley	4 oz	50	2	36	8	3	5	1
McDonald's	***	***	*	*	*	*	*	*
Americano, sm	12 fl oz	0	0	0	0	0	0	0
Americano, med	16 fl oz	0	0	0	0	0	0	0
Americano, lg	20 fl oz	0	0	0	1	0	1	0
Angus Bacon & Cheese	1	790	39	44	63	4	59	45
Angus Deluxe	1	750	39	47	31	4	27	40
Angus Mushroom & Swiss	1	770	40	47	59	4	55	44
Apple Dippers	1 pkg	35	0	0	8	0	8	0
Artificial Sweetener (*Splenda* or *Equal*)	1 pkt	0	0	0	1	0	1	0
Artisan Grilled Chicken Sandwich - no bun	1	160	4	23	2	0	2	29
Bacon, Egg & Cheese Bagel - no bagel	1	300	23	69	6	1	5	17
Bacon, Egg & Cheese Bagel - no bagel, sauce	1	270	20	67	5	1	4	16
Bacon, Egg & Cheese Biscuit, lg size biscuit	1	480	27	51	43	3	40	15
Bacon, Egg & Cheese Biscuit, lg - no biscuit	1	450	24	48	40	2	38	18
Bacon, Egg & Cheese Biscuit, reg size biscuit	1	420	23	49	37	2	35	15
Bacon, Egg & Cheese Biscuit, reg - no biscuit	1	190	13	62	4	1	3	14
Bacon, Egg & Cheese McGriddles	1	420	18	39	48	2	46	15
Bacon McDouble - no bun, ketchup	1	290	21	65	4	0	4	23
Bacon Smokehouse Artisan Grilled Chicken - no bun, sauces, onion strings	1	300	14	42	3	0	3	41
Bacon Smokehouse Burger, double - no bun, sauces, onion strings	1	690	50	65	4	0	4	56
Bacon Smokehouse Burger, regular - no bun, sauces, onion strings	1	390	28	65	3	0	3	32

	Serving Size	Calories	Fat (g)	Calories from Fat (%)	Total Carbs (g)	Fiber (g)	Net Carbs (g)	Protein (g)
McDonald's (cont.)	***	***	*	*	*	*	*	*
Bacon Ranch Grilled Chicken Salad	1	320	14	39	8	3	5	42
Baked Hot Apple Pie	1	250	13	47	32	4	28	2
Barbecue sauce	1 pkt	50	0	0	12	0	12	0
Big Breakfast, lg size biscuit	1	800	52	59	56	4	52	28
Big Breakfast, reg size biscuit	1	740	48	58	51	3	48	28
Big Breakfast - no biscuit, hash browns	1	340	29	77	2	0	2	19
Big Mac	1	540	29	48	45	3	42	25
Big Mac - no bun	1	330	25	68	7	1	6	18
Big Mac - no bun, sauce	1	240	16	60	5	1	4	18
Big N' Tasty	1	460	24	47	37	3	34	24
Big N' Tasty w/ cheese	1	510	28	49	38	3	35	27
Biscuit, lg	1	320	16	45	39	3	36	5
Biscuit, reg	1	260	12	42	33	2	31	5
Butter garlic croutons	½ oz	60	2	30	10	1	9	2
Cheeseburger	1	300	12	36	33	2	31	15
Cheeseburger, no bun, ketchup	1	140	10	64	3	0	3	10
Cheeseburger, triple - no bun, ketchup	1	370	26	63	5	1	4	27
Cheeseburger, double - no bun, ketchup	1	280	20	64	4	1	3	20
Chicken McNuggets	10 pc	460	29	57	27	0	27	24
Chicken McNuggets	6 pc	280	17	55	16	0	16	14
Chicken McNuggets	4 pc	190	12	57	11	0	11	10
Chicken Selects Premium Breast Strips	3 pc	400	24	54	23	0	23	23
Chicken Selects Premium Breast Strips	5 pc	660	40	55	39	0	39	38
Chipotle BBQ Snack Wrap (crispy)	1	330	15	41	35	1	34	14
Chipotle BBQ Snack Wrap (grilled)	1	260	9	31	28	1	27	18
Chocolate Chip Cookie	1	160	8	45	21	1	20	2
Chocolate Triple Thick Shake, sm	12 fl oz	440	10	20	76	1	75	10

	Serving Size	Calories	Fat (g)	Calories from Fat (%)	Total Carbs (g)	Fiber (g)	Net Carbs (g)	Protein (g)
Cinnamon Melts	1 svg	460	19	37	66	3	63	6
Coffee, black (add *Splenda* or *Equal* if desired), sm	12 fl oz	0	0	0	1	0	1	2
Coffee, w/ *Splenda* or *Equal*, sm	12 fl oz	0	0	0	2	0	2	2
Coffee, black (add *Splenda* or *Equal* if desired), med	16 fl oz	0	0	0	2	0	2	2
Coffee, black (add *Splenda* or *Equal* if desired), lg	20 fl oz	0	0	0	2	0	2	2
Coffee w/ coffee cream (add *Splenda* or *Equal* if desired), sm	12 fl oz	20	1.5	0	2	0	2	2
Coffee w/ coffee cream & *Splenda* or *Equal*, sm	12 fl oz	25	1.5	0	3	0	3	2
Coffee creamer, individual	1	20	1.5	68	1	0	1	0
Creamy Ranch sauce	1.5 oz	200	22	99	2	0	2	0
Deluxe Breakfast, lg size biscuit, w/o syrup & margarine	1	1090	60	50	111	6	105	36
Double Cheeseburger	1	440	23	47	34	2	32	25
Double Quarter Pounder w/ cheese	1	380	42	99	40	3	37	48
Egg McMuffin	1	300	12	36	30	2	28	18
Egg McMuffin - no muffin	1	160	11	62	3	0	3	12
Egg White Delight McMuffin - no muffin	1	140	9	58	2	0	2	13
English muffin	1	160	3	17	27	2	25	5
Filet-O-Fish	1	380	18	43	38	2	36	15
French fries, lg	1	500	25	45	63	6	57	6
French fries, med	1	380	19	45	48	5	43	4
French fries, sm	1	230	11	43	29	3	26	3
Fruit 'n Yogurt Parfait	1	160	2	11	31	1	30	4
Fruit 'n Yogurt Parfait, w/o granola	1	130	2	14	25	0	25	4
Grape jam	½ oz	9	0	0	9	0	9	0
Hamburger	1	250	8	29	31	1	30	13
Hamburger - no bun, ketchup	1	90	6	60	1	0	1	7
Hash brown	2 oz	150	9	54	15	2	13	1

	Serving Size	Calories	Fat (g)	Calories from Fat (%)	Total Carbs (g)	Fiber (g)	Net Carbs (g)	Protein (g)
McDonald's (cont.)	***	***	*	*	*	*	*	*
Honey	1 pkt	50	0	0	12	0	12	0
Honey dressing	1 svg	45	0	0	12	0	12	0
Honey Mustard Snack Wrap (crispy)	1	330	16	44	34	1	33	14
Honey Mustard Snack Wrap (grilled)	1	260	9	31	27	1	26	18
Hot caramel sundae	1	340	8	21	60	1	59	7
Hot fudge sundae	1	330	10	27	54	2	52	8
Hotcake syrup	1 pkg	180	0	0	45	0	45	0
Hotcakes	1 svg	350	9	23	60	3	57	8
Hotcakes & Sausage	1 svg	520	24	42	10	3	7	15
Iced Tea (unsweetened)	30 fl oz	5	0	0	0	0	0	1
Ketchup	1 pkt	15	0	0	3	0	3	0
Kiddie cone	1	45	1	20	8	0	8	1
Low fat caramel dip	1 pkg	70	1	13	15	0	15	0
McChicken	1	360	16	40	40	2	38	14
McDonaldland cookies	1 svg	260	8	28	43	1	42	4
McDouble	1	390	19	44	33	2	31	22
McDouble - no bun, ketchup	1	230	16	63	3	0	3	17
McFlurry w/ *M&M's* Candies	12 fl oz	620	20	29	96	1	95	14
McFlurry w/ *Oreo* Cookies	12 fl oz	550	17	28	88	1	87	13
McRib	1	500	26	47	44	3	41	22
McSkillet Burrito w/ sausage	1	610	36	53	44	3	41	27
McSkillet Burrito w/ steak	1	570	30	47	44	3	41	32
Newman's Own Creamy Caesar Dressing	2 fl oz	190	18	85	4	0	4	2
Newman's Own Creamy Ranch Dressing	2 fl oz	170	15	79	9	0	9	1
Newman's Own Creamy Southwestern Dressing	1.5 fl oz	100	6	54	11	0	11	1
Newman's Own Low Fat Balsamic Vinaigrette	1.5 fl oz	40	3	68	4	0	4	0
Newman's Own Low Fat Family Recipe Italian Dressing	1.5 fl oz	60	3	45	8	0	8	1
Oatmeal raisin cookie	1	150	6	36	22	1	21	2

	Serving Size	Calories	Fat (g)	Calories from Fat (%)	Total Carbs (g)	Fiber (g)	Net Carbs (g)	Protein (g)
Peanuts, for sundaes	1 svg	45	4	80	2	1	1	2
Premium Bacon Ranch Salad	1	140	7	45	10	3	7	9
Premium Bacon Ranch Salad w/ crispy chicken	1	370	20	49	20	3	17	29
Premium Bacon Ranch Salad w/ grilled chicken	1	260	9	31	12	3	9	33
Premium Caesar Salad	1	90	4	40	9	3	6	7
Premium Caesar Salad w/ crispy chicken	1	330	17	46	20	3	17	26
Premium Caesar Salad w/ grilled chicken	1	220	6	25	12	3	9	30
Premium Crispy Chicken Classic Sandwich	1	530	20	34	59	3	56	28
Premium Crispy Chicken Club Sandwich	1	630	28	40	60	4	56	35
Premium Crispy Chicken Ranch BLT Sandwich	1	580	23	36	62	3	59	31
Premium Grilled Chicken Classic Sandwich	1	420	20	43	51	3	48	32
Premium Grilled Chicken Club Sandwich	1	530	17	29	52	4	48	39
Premium Grilled Chicken Ranch BLT Sandwich	1	470	12	23	54	3	51	36
Premium Southwest Salad	1	140	5	32	20	6	14	6
Premium Southwest Salad w/ crispy chicken	1	430	20	42	38	6	32	26
Premium Southwest Salad w/ grilled chicken	1	320	9	25	30	6	24	30
Quarter Pounder	1	410	19	42	37	2	35	24
Quarter Pounder w/ cheese	1	510	26	46	40	3	37	29
Quarter Pounder w/ cheese, double - no bun, ketchup	1	590	43	66	5	1	4	45
Quarter Pounder w/ cheese, regular - no bun, ketchup	1	340	25	66	4	1	3	25
Ranch Snack Wrap (crispy)	1	340	17	45	33	4	29	14
Ranch Snack Wrap (grilled)	1	270	10	33	26	1	25	18
Sausage Biscuit, lg size biscuit	1	480	31	58	39	3	36	11
Sausage Biscuit, reg size biscuit	1	430	27	57	34	2	32	11

	Serving Size	Calories	Fat (g)	Calories from Fat (%)	Total Carbs (g)	Fiber (g)	Net Carbs (g)	Protein (g)
McDonald's (cont.)	***	***	*	*	*	*	*	*
Sausage Biscuit - no biscuit	1	200	19	86	1	0	1	7
Sausage Biscuit w/ egg, lg size biscuit	1	570	37	58	42	3	39	18
Sausage Biscuit w/ egg, lg - no biscuit	1	260	23	80	2	0	2	12
Sausage Biscuit w/ egg, reg size biscuit	1	510	33	58	36	2	34	18
Sausage Biscuit w/ egg, reg - no biscuit	1	270	23	77	2	0	2	12
Sausage Burrito	1	430	27	57	34	2	32	11
Sausage McGriddles	1	420	22	47	44	2	42	11
Sausage McMuffin	1	370	22	54	29	2	27	14
Sausage McMuffin - no muffin	1	260	24	83	2	0	2	9
Sausage McMuffin w/ egg	1	450	27	54	30	2	28	21
Sausage McMuffin with egg - no muffin	1	340	29	77	3	0	3	16
Sausage patty	1	170	15	79	1	0	1	7
Sausage, Egg & Cheese McGriddles	1	560	32	51	48	2	46	20
Scrambled eggs	2	170	11	58	1	0	1	15
Side salad	1	20	0	0	4	1	3	1
Side Salad, no dressing	1	15	0	0	3	1	2	1
Snack Size Fruit & Walnut Salad	1 pkg	210	8	34	31	2	29	4
Southern Style Chicken Biscuit, lg size biscuit	1	470	24	46	46	3	43	17
Southern Style Chicken Biscuit, reg size biscuit	1	410	20	44	41	2	39	17
Southern Style Crispy Chicken Sandwich	1	400	17	38	39	1	38	24
Southwestern chipotle barbeque sauce	1.5 oz	70	0	0	18	1	17	0
Spicy buffalo sauce	1.5 oz	70	7	90	1	1	0	0
Steak, Egg & Cheese Biscuit - no biscuit	1	270	19	63	4	1	3	20

	Serving Size	Calories	Fat (g)	Calories from Fat (%)	Total Carbs (g)	Fiber (g)	Net Carbs (g)	Protein (g)
Steak, Egg & Cheese Biscuit - no biscuit, onion sauce	1	260	18	62	3	1	2	20
Strawberry preserves	½ oz	35	0	0	9	0	9	0
Strawberry sundae	1	280	6	19	49	1	48	6
Strawberry Triple Thick Shake, sm	12 fl oz	420	10	21	73	0	73	10
Sugar cookie	1	160	7	39	21	0	21	2
Sweet & sour sauce	1 pkt	50	0	0	12	0	12	0
Tangy honey mustard sauce	1.5 oz	70	3	39	13	0	13	1
Triple Breakfast Stacks Biscuits - no biscuits	1	620	53	77	6	1	5	30
Triple Breakfast Stacks McGriddles - no pancakes	1	620	53	77	6	1	5	29
Triple Breakfast Stacks McMuffin - no muffin	1	640	56	79	5	0	5	30
Vanilla reduced fat ice cream cone	1	150	4	24	24	0	24	4
Vanilla Triple Thick Shake, sm	12 fl oz	420	10	21	72	0	72	9
Whipped margarine	1 pat	40	5	100	0	0	0	0
Olive Garden	***	***	*	*	*	*	*	*
Insufficient information	***	***	*	*	*	*	*	*
Alfredo Sauce (appetizer size)	1 svg	440	43	88	5	0	5	8
Alfredo Sauce (kids' size)	1 svg	330	32	87	4	0	4	6
Chicken Piccata (lunch)	1	370	22	54	12	3	9	32
Chicken Piccata (dinner)	1	530	27	46	12	3	9	60
Chicken Margherita (lunch)	1	400	25	56	11	2	9	36
Chicken Margherita (dinner)	1	570	30	47	13	4	9	64
Fresh Brewed Unsweetened Iced Tea	***	0	0	0	1	0	1	0
Gorgonzola Sauce (appetizer size)	1 svg	170	17	90	2	0	2	2
Gorgonzola Sauce (entree size)	1 svg	500	50	90	5	0	5	7
Herb-Grilled Salmon	1	460	29	57	9	5	4	45
Italian Bottled Water	1 bottle	0	0	0	0	0	0	0
Italian Sausage	2 links	360	14	35	2	Tr	2	27
Salmon Piccata	1	580	40	62	12	3	9	45

	Serving Size	Calories	Fat (g)	Calories from Fat (%)	Total Carbs (g)	Fiber (g)	Net Carbs (g)	Protein (g)
Outback Steakhouse	***	***	*	*	*	*	*	*
Apps and Sides	***	***	*	*	*	*	*	*
Grilled Asparagus	1 svg	60	4	60	4	2	2	2
Kookaburra Wings, hot, small	1 svg	950	87	82	8	1	7	35
Kookaburra Wings, mild, small	1 svg	960	87	82	8	1	7	35
Pork	***	***	*	*	*	*	*	*
Pork Porterhouse	1	510	26	46	0	0	0	69
Seafood	***	***	***	*	*	*	*	*
Bacon bourbon salmon	10 oz	650	42	58	6	0	6	61
Bacon bourbon salmon	7 oz	480	32	60	3	0	3	45
Lobster tails entrée, 5 oz, grilled	2 tails	650	45	62	2	Tr	2	53
Lobster tails entrée, 5 oz, steamed	3 tails	630	30	43	2	Tr	2	80
Lobster tails entrée, 5 oz, steamed	2 tails	480	27	51	1	Tr	1	53
King crab	1 ¼ lb	500	34	61	1	0	1	43
King crab	½ lb	370	32	78	1	0	1	17
Side Salad, House	***	***	***	*	*	*	*	*
w/ Caesar dressing	1	190	19	90	2	0	2	2
w/ creamy blue cheese dressing	1	240	25	94	Tr	0	Tr	2
w/ mustard vinaigrette	1	220	22	90	4	0	4	0
w/ ranch dressing	1	210	23	99	1	0	1	Tr
w/ Thousand Island dressing	1	250	25	90	6	0	6	0
Steaks	***	***	***	*	*	*	*	*
Bone-in ribeye	22 oz	1080	74	62	0	0	0	104
Filet, 6 oz, and grilled lobster tail	1	660	42	57	2	0	2	66
Filet, 9 oz, and lobster tail	1	780	47	54	2	0	2	86
Filet, 8 oz, and lobster tail	1	740	45	55	2	0	2	80
Filet, 6 oz, and lobster tail	1	660	42	57	2	0	2	66
Melbourne/Porterhouse	32 oz	1610	114	64	7	0	7	140
Melbourne/Porterhouse	24 oz	1230	87	64	5	0	5	107

	Serving Size	Calories	Fat (g)	Calories from Fat (%)	Total Carbs (g)	Fiber (g)	Net Carbs (g)	Protein (g)
Melbourne/Porterhouse	22 oz	1110	78	63	5	0	5	96
Melbourne/Porterhouse	20 oz	1010	71	63	4	0	4	88
Melbourne/Porterhouse	18 oz	910	64	63	4	0	4	79
New York strip	14 oz	940	72	69	0	0	0	73
New York strip	13 oz	880	67	69	0	0	0	68
New York strip	12 oz	810	62	69	0	0	0	63
Outback center-cut sirloin	12 oz	420	13	28	Tr	0	Tr	76
Outback center-cut sirloin	11 oz	390	12	28	Tr	0	Tr	70
Outback center-cut sirloin	10 oz	350	11	28	Tr	0	Tr	63
Outback center-cut sirloin	9 oz	320	10	28	Tr	0	Tr	57
Outback center-cut sirloin	8 oz	280	9	29	0	0	0	51
Outback center-cut sirloin	6 oz	210	7	30	0	0	0	38
Prime center-cut filet	11 oz	440	17	35	Tr	0	Tr	73
Prime New York strip	16 oz	1100	84	69	0	0	0	85
Prime ribeye	16 oz	1400	114	73	0	0	0	92
Prime ribeye	14 oz	750	48	58	0	0	0	79
Prime ribeye	13 oz	710	45	57	0	0	0	75
Prime ribeye	12 oz	650	42	58	0	0	0	69
Prime ribeye	10 oz	540	35	58	0	0	0	58
Sirloin, 12 oz, and grilled shrimp on the barbie	1	580	22	34	5	Tr	5	90
Sirloin, 11 oz, and grilled shrimp on the barbie	1	540	21	35	5	Tr	5	84
Sirloin, 10 oz, and grilled shrimp on the barbie	1	510	20	35	4	Tr	4	77
Sirloin, 9 oz, and grilled shrimp on the barbie	1	470	19	36	4	Tr	4	71
Sirloin, 8 oz, and grilled shrimp on the barbie	1	440	18	37	4	Tr	4	65
Sirloin, 6 oz, and grilled shrimp on the barbie	1	370	15	36	4	Tr	4	52
Sirloin, 5 oz, and grilled shrimp on the barbie	1	330	14	38	4	Tr	4	46
Slow-roasted prime rib	24 oz	1230	87	64	5	0	5	107
Slow-roasted prime rib	16 oz	1400	114	73	0	0	0	92
Slow-roasted prime rib	12 oz	1050	86	74	0	0	0	69

	Serving Size	Calories	Fat (g)	Calories from Fat (%)	Total Carbs (g)	Fiber (g)	Net Carbs (g)	Protein (g)
Outback Steakhouse (cont.)	***	***	*	*	*	*	*	*
Slow-roasted prime rib	8 oz	700	57	73	0	0	0	46
Victoria's Filet Mignon	10 oz	400	15	34	Tr	0	Tr	66
Victoria's Filet Mignon	9 oz	360	14	35	Tr	0	Tr	60
Victoria's Filet Mignon	8 oz	320	12	34	Tr	0	Tr	53
Victoria's Filet Mignon	6 oz	240	9	34	0	0	0	40
Steak Mates	***	***	***	*	*	*	*	*
Five grilled shrimp	1 svg	170	9	48	4	Tr	4	17
Lobster and mushroom topping	1 svg	190	13	62	8	1	7	12
Lobster tail, 5 oz, grilled	1	420	33	71	1	0	1	27
Lobster tail, 5 oz, steamed	1	340	24	64	1	0	1	27
Roasted garlic butter topping	1 svg	170	18	95	2	0	2	Tr
Sautéed 'shrooms	1 svg	130	6	42	10	3	7	7
Smokey bacon bourbon topping	1 svg	110	6	49	6	0	6	7
Panda Express Chinese Food	***	***	*	*	*	*	*	*
Beef Dishes	***	***	*	*	*	*	*	*
Beijing beef	1 svg	660	41	56	52	4	48	24
Broccoli beef	1 svg	150	6	36	12	3	9	11
Mongolian beef	1 svg	200	9	41	16	3	13	15
Beverages	***	***	*	*	*	*	*	*
Lipton No Calorie Brisk Peach Tea, all sizes	***	0	0	0	0	0	0	0
Chicken Dishes	***	***	*	*	*	*	*	*
Black pepper chicken	1 svg	200	11	50	11	2	9	14
Broccoli chicken	1 svg	180	9	45	11	3	8	13
Grilled Asian Chicken (kid's menu)	1 svg	180	8	40	5	0	5	22
Grilled Teriyaki Chicken (kid's menu)	1 svg	180	8	40	5	0	5	22
Kung Pao chicken	1 svg	300	20	60	13	2	11	20
Mandarin chicken	1 svg	310	16	46	8	0	8	34
Mushroom chicken	1 svg	180	10	50	10	2	8	14
Orange chicken	1 svg	400	20	45	42	0	42	15

	Serving Size	Calories	Fat (g)	Calories from Fat (%)	Total Carbs (g)	Fiber (g)	Net Carbs (g)	Protein (g)
Pineapple chicken	1 svg	230	10	39	21	2	19	13
Pineapple chicken breast	1 svg	230	12	47	19	1	18	11
Potato chicken	1 svg	220	11	45	18	3	15	11
String bean chicken	1 svg	190	9	43	13	3	10	12
String bean chicken breast	1 svg	200	12	54	12	2	10	10
Sweet & sour chicken	1 svg	400	17	38	46	1	45	15
Thai cashew chicken breast	1 svg	330	22	60	17	2	15	15
Pork Dishes	***	***	*	*	*	*	*	*
BBQ pork	1 svg	360	19	48	13	1	12	34
Sweet & sour pork	1 svg	400	23	52	36	2	34	13
Vegetable Dishes	***	***	*	*	*	*	*	*
Eggplant & tofu	1 svg	310	24	70	19	3	16	7
Hot Szechuan Tofu	1 svg	140	8	51	10	2	8	6
Mixed vegetables, side	1 svg	100	6	54	7	3	4	3
Mixed vegetables, entrée	1 svg	190	13	62	14	5	9	5
Rice & Noodles	***	***	*	*	*	*	*	*
Chow mein	1 svg	400	12	27	61	8	53	12
Fried rice	1 svg	570	18	28	85	8	77	16
Steamed rice	1 svg	420	0	0	93	0	93	8
Appetizers & Sides	***	***	*	*	*	*	*	*
Chicken egg roll	1	200	12	54	16	2	14	8
Chicken potstickers	3 pc	220	11	45	23	1	22	7
Cream cheese rangoon	3 pc	190	8	38	24	2	22	5
Super Greens, side	7 oz	90	2.5	25	10	5	5	6
Super Greens, entrée	3.5 oz	45	1.5	30	5	3	2	3
Vegetable spring rolls	2	160	7	39	22	4	18	4
Sauces & Cookies	***	***	*	*	*	*	*	*
Mandarin sauce	1 svg	160	0	0	40	0	40	0
Potsticker sauce	1 svg	45	0	0	10	0	10	1
Sweet & sour sauce	1 svg	80	0	0	21	0	21	0
Fortune cookie	1	30	0	0	7	0	7	1
Seafood	***	***	*	*	*	*	*	*
Crispy shrimp	6 pc	260	13	45	26	1	25	9
Kung Pao shrimp	1 svg	230	14	55	13	2	11	13

	Serving Size	Calories	Fat (g)	Calories from Fat (%)	Total Carbs (g)	Fiber (g)	Net Carbs (g)	Protein (g)
Panda Express Chinese Food (cont.)	***	***	*	*	*	*	*	*
Steamed ginger fish (kid's menu)	1 svg	70	4	51	3	0	3	5
Tangy shrimp	1 svg	140	5	32	16	1	15	8
Soup	***	***	*	*	*	*	*	*
Egg flower soup	1	90	2	20	15	1	14	3
Hot & sour soup	1	90	4	40	12	1	11	4
Panera Bread								
(all sandwiches & salads are full size; "light" dressing refers to portion size)	***	***	*	*	*	*	*	*
Asiago cheese bagel	1	330	6	16	55	2	53	13
Asiago cheese demi	2 oz	160	4	23	22	1	21	7
Asiago cheese loaf	2 oz	160	4	23	22	1	21	7
Asiago roast beef sandwich, on asiago cheese bread	1	710	32	41	57	3	54	47
Asian sesame chicken salad	1	410	19	42	31	5	26	32
Asian sesame salad w/ chicken - "light" reduced-sugar Asian sesame dressing, no wonton strips	1	280	13	42	11	5	6	30
Bacon turkey bravo sandwich, on tomato basil bread	1	840	32	34	87	4	83	51
Bacon, egg & cheese sandwich	1	510	24	42	44	2	42	28
Baked potato soup	12 oz	370	22	54	33	3	30	8
Bear claw	1	460	24	47	54	2	52	9
Blueberry bagel	1	330	2	5	67	2	65	10
Broccoli cheddar soup	12 oz	290	16	50	24	7	17	12
Caesar dressing	1.5 oz	150	16	96	2	0	2	1
Caesar salad	1	390	27	62	25	3	22	12
Caesar salad w/ chicken - no croutons	1	380	25	59	7	2	5	32
Caramel pecan brownie	1	490	25	46	64	2	62	5
Carrot walnut muffin	1	430	19	40	61	2	59	8
Challah bread	2 oz	180	3	15	34	1	33	6
Cheese pastry	1	400	23	52	41	1	40	8

	Serving Size	Calories	Fat (g)	Calories from Fat (%)	Total Carbs (g)	Fiber (g)	Net Carbs (g)	Protein (g)
Cherry balsamic vinaigrette	1.5 oz	130	12	83	7	0	7	0
Cherry pastry	1	450	22	44	55	2	53	8
Chicken bacon Dijon panini, on country bread	1	940	36	34	96	4	92	59
Chicken bacon Dijon panini, on French bread	1	780	36	42	63	2	61	53
Chicken Caesar sandwich, on focaccia	1	860	39	41	82	4	78	43
Chicken Caesar sandwich, on three cheese bread	1	800	33	37	83	4	79	45
Chicken salad sandwich, on sesame semolina bread	1	710	25	32	101	13	88	31
Chicken salad sandwich, on whole grain bread	1	620	26	38	77	16	61	31
Chipotle chicken sandwich, on artisan French bread	1	1070	55	46	87	4	83	54
Chipotle chicken sandwich, on French bread	1	900	56	56	53	3	50	49
Chocolate chip bagel	1	370	6	15	69	2	67	10
Chocolate chip muffie	1	270	12	40	40	1	39	4
Chocolate chipper cookie	1	440	23	47	59	2	57	5
Chocolate duet w/ walnuts cookie	1	450	24	48	55	3	52	6
Chocolate pastry	1	340	20	53	37	2	35	6
Chopped chicken cobb salad	1	490	35	64	9	3	6	36
Ciabatta	6.25 oz	460	5	10	84	3	81	16
Cinnamon chip scone	1	530	27	46	67	2	65	8
Cinnamon crunch bagel	1	430	8	17	81	3	78	9
Cinnamon raisin loaf	2 oz	180	3	15	34	1	33	5
Cinnamon roll	1	620	24	35	89	3	86	13
Cinnamon swirl bagel	1	320	3	8	65	3	62	10
Classic café salad	1	170	11	58	19	4	15	3
Cobblestone roll	1	650	13	18	123	3	120	12
Coffee, dark roast	12 fl oz	15	0	0	3	0	3	1
Coffee, dark roast	16 fl oz	20	0	0	4	0	4	1
Coffee, dark roast	20 fl oz	25	0	0	5	0	5	2
Coffee, decaf	12 fl oz	10	0	0	2	0	2	1

	Serving Size	Calories	Fat (g)	Calories from Fat (%)	Total Carbs (g)	Fiber (g)	Net Carbs (g)	Protein (g)
Panera Bread (cont.)	***	***	*	*	*	*	*	*
Coffee, decaf	16 fl oz	15	0	0	2	0	2	1
Coffee, decaf	20 fl oz	20	0	0	3	0	3	2
Country loaf	2 oz	140	Tr	0	27	1	26	5
Country miche	2 oz	140	Tr	0	28	1	27	5
Cream of chicken & wild rice soup	12 oz	300	17	51	29	1	28	7
Creamy tomato soup	12 oz	290	20	62	28	3	25	4
Creamy tomato soup w/ croutons	12.75 oz	370	23	56	39	5	34	4
Dutch apple & raisin bagel	1	360	3	8	77	2	75	8
Egg & cheese sandwich	1	380	14	33	43	2	41	18
Espresso	1 shot	5	0	0	0	0	0	0
Everything bagel	1	300	3	9	59	2	57	10
Fat free raspberry dressing	1.5 oz	30	0	0	8	0	8	0
Fat free reduced sugar poppyseed dressing	1.5 oz	15	0	0	4	1	3	0
Focaccia	2 oz	160	2	11	29	1	28	5
Focaccia w/ asiago cheese	2 oz	160	5	28	23	1	22	5
Forest mushroom soup	12 oz	250	18	65	21	2	19	4
Four cheese soufflé	1	480	31	58	34	2	32	16
French baguette	2 oz	150	Tr	0	30	1	29	5
French croissant	1	290	17	53	31	1	30	6
French loaf	2 oz	150	2	12	29	1	28	5
French miche	2 oz	140	Tr	0	28	1	27	5
French onion soup w/ cheese & croutons	13.25 oz	250	11	40	30	3	27	10
French onion soup w/o cheese & croutons	12 oz	130	5	35	20	2	18	3
French roll	2.25 oz	180	2	10	35	1	34	6
French toast bagel	1	350	5	13	67	2	65	9
Fresh apple pastry	1	380	19	45	44	1	43	7
Fresh fruit cup, lg	1	70	0	0	19	1	18	1
Fresh fruit cup, sm	1	150	0	0	37	2	35	2
Frontega chicken panini, on focaccia	1	860	39	41	80	4	76	46

	Serving Size	Calories	Fat (g)	Calories from Fat (%)	Total Carbs (g)	Fiber (g)	Net Carbs (g)	Protein (g)
Frozen caramel drink	16 fl oz	580	25	39	83	1	82	6
Frozen lemonade	16 fl oz	90	0	0	21	0	21	0
Frozen mocha drink	16 fl oz	550	25	41	78	2	76	7
Fuji apple salad	1	410	29	64	33	5	28	8
Fuji apple salad w/ chicken	1	520	30	52	34	6	28	32
Gooey butter pastry	1	350	19	49	39	1	38	7
Greek dressing/herb vinaigrette	1.5 oz	220	24	98	1	0	1	0
Greek salad	1	440	39	80	15	6	9	10
Green goddess cobb salad w/ chicken - "light" green goddess dressing, no wedge tomatoes, pickled red onions	1	460	28	55	14	5	9	42
Grilled chicken Caesar salad	1	500	28	50	26	3	23	35
Honey wheat loaf	2 oz	160	3	17	30	2	28	5
Hot tea	8 fl oz	0	0	0	0	0	0	0
Iced coffee	16/20 oz	10	0	0	2	0	2	1
Iced coffee	32 fl oz	20	0	0	4	0	4	1
Iced tea, unsweetened	20 fl oz	0	0	0	2	0	2	0
Iced tea, unsweetened	32 fl oz	0	0	0	3	0	3	0
Italian combo sandwich, on ciabatta	1	1040	45	39	94	5	89	61
Lemon poppyseed mini bundt cake	1	460	20	39	63	0	63	6
Light buttermilk ranch	1.5 oz	80	4	45	9	1	8	1
Low fat chicken noodle soup	12 oz	140	3	19	20	1	19	9
Low fat vegetarian black bean soup	12 oz	170	4	21	29	5	24	10
Low fat vegetarian garden soup	12 oz	120	1	8	24	7	17	4
Mango smoothie	18 fl oz	330	10	27	61	3	58	2
Mediterranean veggie sandwich, on tomato basil bread	1	610	13	19	102	9	93	22
New England clam chowder	12 oz	450	34	68	29	3	26	8
Nutty chocolate chipper cookie	1	460	27	53	54	3	51	5
Oatmeal raisin cookie	1	370	14	34	57	2	55	5
Orange scone	1	460	20	39	65	1	64	8

	Serving Size	Calories	Fat (g)	Calories from Fat (%)	Total Carbs (g)	Fiber (g)	Net Carbs (g)	Protein (g)
Panera Bread (cont.)	***	***	*	*	*	*	*	*
Pastry ring, cherry cheese	1	220	10	41	27	1	26	3
Pecan braid	1	440	25	51	46	2	44	8
Pecan roll	1	720	38	48	88	2	86	11
Pineapple upside-down mini bundt cake	1	510	22	39	75	3	72	5
Plain bagel	1	290	2	6	59	2	57	10
Plain cream cheese spread	1 oz	100	10	90	1	0	1	2
Pumpkin muffie	1	250	10	36	39	1	38	3
Pumpkin muffin	1	530	20	34	81	2	79	6
Reduced-fat balsamic vinaigrette	1.5 oz	130	10	69	9	0	9	0
Reduced-fat hazelnut cream cheese spread	1 oz	80	6	68	3	0	3	2
Reduced-fat honey walnut cheese spread	1 oz	80	6	68	4	0	4	2
Reduced-fat plain cheese spread	1 oz	70	6	77	1	0	1	3
Reduced-fat raspberry cheese spread	1 oz	70	5	64	4	1	3	2
Reduced-fat sundried tomato cheese spread	1 oz	70	6	77	2	1	1	3
Reduced-fat veggie cheese spread	1 oz	60	5	75	1	1	0	2
Reduced-fat wild blueberry muffin	1	360	10	25	61	1	60	6
Reduced-sugar Asian sesame vinaigrette	1.5 oz	90	8	80	6	0	6	0
Salt bagel	1	290	2	6	58	2	56	10
Sausage, egg & cheese sandwich	1	550	30	49	44	2	42	25
Sesame bagel	1	310	3	9	59	2	57	10
Sesame semolina loaf	2 oz	140	Tr	0	29	1	28	4
Sesame semolina miche	2 oz	140	1	6	30	1	29	5
Shortbread	1	350	21	54	36	1	35	3
Sierra turkey sandwich, on focaccia w/ asiago cheese	1	970	54	50	80	4	76	39

	Serving Size	Calories	Fat (g)	Calories from Fat (%)	Total Carbs (g)	Fiber (g)	Net Carbs (g)	Protein (g)
Smoked ham & swiss sandwich, on rye bread	1	700	35	45	55	4	51	40
Smoked ham & swiss sandwich, on stone-milled rye bread	1	780	29	33	82	7	75	49
Smoked turkey breast sandwich, on country bread	1	730	23	28	92	7	85	36
Smoked turkey breast sandwich, on sourdough bread	1	470	17	33	49	3	46	30
Smokehouse turkey panini, on focaccia	1	860	36	38	82	4	78	52
Smokehouse turkey panini, on three cheese bread	1	810	30	33	83	5	78	54
Sourdough baguette	2 oz	160	Tr	0	31	1	30	6
Sourdough loaf	2 oz	140	Tr	0	28	1	27	5
Sourdough roll	2.5 oz	200	1	5	39	1	38	7
Sourdough soup bowl	8 oz	590	3	5	117	4	113	22
Southwest chili lime ranch salad w/ chicken - no quinoa/tomato/sofrito blend, adobo corn blend, tortilla strips	1	350	20	51	14	6	8	32
Spicy Thai salad w/ chicken - "light" Thai style peanut sauce, "light" Thai chili vinaigrette, no wonton strips, edamame blend	1	290	13	40	15	3	12	32
Spinach & artichoke soufflé	1	500	32	58	35	2	33	19
Spinach & bacon soufflé	1	570	37	58	36	2	34	21
Spindrift Lemon Seltzer	1 can	0	0	0	1	0	1	0
Spindrift Orange Mango Seltzer	1 can	10	0	0	3	0	3	0
Spindrift Raspberry Lime Seltzer	1 can	10	0	0	2	0	2	0
Stone-milled rye loaf	2 oz	140	Tr	0	28	2	26	5
Stone-milled rye miche	2 oz	140	Tr	0	27	2	25	5
Strawberry granola parfait	1	310	12	35	41	4	37	3
Strawberry poppyseed salad	1	170	6	32	27	5	22	3

	Serving Size	Calories	Fat (g)	Calories from Fat (%)	Total Carbs (g)	Fiber (g)	Net Carbs (g)	Protein (g)
Panera Bread *(cont.)*	***	***	*	*	*	*	*	*
Strawberry poppyseed salad w/ chicken	1	290	9	28	29	5	24	26
Strawberry smoothie	18 fl oz	240	2	8	51	3	48	5
Summer corn chowder	12 oz	260	14	48	28	6	22	5
Three cheese demi	2 oz	140	2	13	26	1	25	6
Three cheese loaf	2 oz	140	2	13	26	1	25	6
Three cheese miche	2 oz	150	2	12	27	1	26	6
Three seed demi	2 oz	160	4	23	27	2	25	6
Toffee nut cookie	2 oz	460	19	37	59	1	58	5
Tomato & mozzarella panini, on ciabatta	1	770	29	34	96	6	90	30
Tomato & mozzarella salad	1	890	47	48	83	6	77	36
Tomato basil loaf	2 oz	140	Tr	0	27	1	26	5
Tuna salad sandwich, on honey wheat bread	1	750	47	56	65	6	59	20
Turkey artichoke panini, on focaccia	1	750	27	32	89	7	82	40
Turkey sausage & potato soufflé	1	460	28	55	35	2	33	15
Very chocolate brownie	1	460	22	43	61	2	59	5
White balsamic apple vinaigrette	1.5 oz	150	12	72	11	0	11	0
White whole grain loaf	2 oz	140	3	19	27	2	25	5
Whole grain bagel	1	370	4	10	70	6	64	13
Whole grain baguette	2 oz	140	1	6	28	3	25	6
Whole grain loaf	2 oz	130	1	7	26	3	23	6
Whole grain miche	2 oz	130	1	7	25	3	22	5
Wild blueberry muffin	1	390	15	35	58	1	57	5
Wild blueberry scone	1	390	16	37	56	2	54	6
Papa John's Pizza	***	***	*	*	*	*	*	*
Specialty Pizzas	***	***	*	*	*	*	*	*
BBQ Chicken & Bacon	***	***	*	*	*	*	*	*
Original crust, 10"	1 slice	220	8	33	30	1	29	10
Original crust, 12"	1 slice	240	8	30	32	1	31	11
Original crust, 14"	1 slice	340	11	29	44	2	42	15

	Serving Size	Calories	Fat (g)	Calories from Fat (%)	Total Carbs (g)	Fiber (g)	Net Carbs (g)	Protein (g)
Original crust, 16"	1 slice	350	12	31	47	2	45	16
Thin crust, 14"	1 slice	270	13	43	27	Tr	27	12
Pan crust, 12"	1 slice	430	22	46	43	1	42	15
Cheese	***	***	*	*	*	*	*	*
Original crust, 10"	1 slice	180	6	30	25	1	24	7
Original crust, 12"	1 slice	210	8	34	27	1	26	9
Original crust, 14"	1 slice	280	10	32	38	2	36	12
Original crust, 16"	1 slice	200	10	45	41	2	39	12
Thin crust, 14"	1 slice	220	12	49	21	1	20	9
Pan crust, 12"	1 slice	410	23	50	28	1	27	13
Garden Fresh	***	***	*	*	*	*	*	*
Original crust, 10"	1 slice	190	6	28	26	2	24	8
Original crust, 12"	1 slice	200	7	32	28	2	26	8
Original crust, 14"	1 slice	280	9	29	39	2	37	11
Original crust, 16"	1 slice	290	9	28	42	3	39	12
Thin crust, 14"	1 slice	210	11	47	23	2	21	8
Pan crust, 12"	1 slice	370	19	46	39	2	37	11
Hawaiian BBQ Chicken	***	***	*	*	*	*	*	*
Original crust, 10"	1 slice	230	8	31	31	1	30	10
Original crust, 12"	1 slice	240	8	30	33	1	32	11
Original crust, 14"	1 slice	340	11	29	46	2	44	16
Original crust, 16"	1 slice	360	12	30	49	2	47	16
Thin crust, 14"	1 slice	290	14	43	31	1	30	13
Pan crust, 12"	1 slice	440	22	45	45	1	44	15
Pepperoni	***	***	*	*	*	*	*	*
Original crust, 10"	1 slice	210	9	39	25	1	24	9
Original crust, 12"	1 slice	220	9	37	26	1	25	9
Original crust, 14"	1 slice	310	13	38	38	2	36	13
Original crust, 16"	1 slice	330	13	35	40	2	38	13
Thin crust, 14"	1 slice	250	15	54	21	1	20	10
Pan crust, 12"	1 slice	410	24	53	37	1	36	13
Sausage	***	***	*	*	*	*	*	*
Original crust, 10"	1 slice	220	10	41	25	2	23	8
Original crust, 12"	1 slice	240	11	41	26	2	24	9

	Serving Size	Calories	Fat (g)	Calories from Fat (%)	Total Carbs (g)	Fiber (g)	Net Carbs (g)	Protein (g)
Papa John's Pizza (cont.)	***	***	*	*	*	*	*	*
Original crust, 14"	1 slice	330	15	41	37	3	34	13
Original crust, 16"	1 slice	340	15	40	40	3	37	13
Thin crust, 14"	1 slice	270	16	53	21	2	19	9
Pan crust, 12"	1 slice	420	25	54	37	2	35	12
Spicy Italian	***	***	*	*	*	*	*	*
Original crust, 10"	1 slice	230	7	27	26	2	24	9
Original crust, 12"	1 slice	260	8	28	27	2	25	11
Original crust, 14"	1 slice	370	11	27	38	4	34	15
Original crust, 16"	1 slice	390	12	28	41	4	37	16
Thin crust, 14"	1 slice	310	13	38	22	3	19	12
Pan crust, 12"	1 slice	470	21	40	38	3	35	15
Spinach Alfredo	***	***	*	*	*	*	*	*
Original crust, 10"	1 slice	190	7	33	24	1	23	8
Original crust, 12"	1 slice	210	8	34	26	1	25	8
Original crust, 14"	1 slice	280	11	35	36	2	34	11
Original crust, 16"	1 slice	310	12	35	39	2	37	12
Thin crust, 14"	1 slice	220	13	53	19	1	18	8
Pan crust, 12"	1 slice	380	22	52	35	1	34	11
The Meats	***	***	*	*	*	*	*	*
Original crust, 10"	1 slice	230	11	43	25	1	24	10
Original crust, 12"	1 slice	240	11	41	26	1	25	11
Original crust, 14"	1 slice	350	16	41	38	2	36	15
Original crust, 16"	1 slice	370	17	41	40	2	38	16
Thin crust, 14"	1 slice	280	17	55	21	1	20	12
Pan crust, 12"	1 slice	440	26	53	37	1	36	15
The Works	***	***	*	*	*	*	*	*
Original crust, 10"	1 slice	220	7	29	26	2	24	9
Original crust, 12"	1 slice	230	8	31	27	2	25	10
Original crust, 14"	1 slice	330	11	30	39	3	36	14
Original crust, 16"	1 slice	350	11	28	42	3	39	15
Thin crust, 14"	1 slice	260	13	45	22	2	20	11
Pan crust, 12"	1 slice	420	21	45	37	2	35	14
Tuscan Six Cheese	***	***	*	*	*	*	*	*

	Serving Size	Calories	Fat (g)	Calories from Fat (%)	Total Carbs (g)	Fiber (g)	Net Carbs (g)	Protein (g)
Original crust, 10"	1 slice	210	8	34	26	1	25	10
Original crust, 12"	1 slice	230	9	35	27	1	26	11
Original crust, 14"	1 slice	320	13	37	38	2	36	15
Original crust, 16"	1 slice	330	13	35	41	2	39	15
Thin crust, 14"	1 slice	250	14	50	21	1	20	12
Pan crust, 12"	1 slice	410	23	50	37	1	36	15
Sides & Desserts	***	***	*	*	*	*	*	*
Breadsticks	2	290	5	16	53	2	51	9
Garlic parmesan breadsticks	2	330	10	27	54	2	52	10
Cheesesticks	4	370	16	39	42	2	40	15
Chickenstrips	2	160	8	45	10	0	10	10
Wings, BBQ	2	160	10	56	4	0	4	14
Wings, buffalo	2	160	11	62	1	1	0	14
Wings, honey chipotle	2	190	12	57	8	0	8	12
Cinnapie	4	560	19	31	89	3	86	9
Apple pie	4	480	10	19	89	3	86	9
Sweetsticks	4	570	15	24	98	3	95	12
Chocolate pastry delights	1	180	11	55	18	1	17	2
Sauces	***	***	*	*	*	*	*	*
Barbecue	1 svg	45	0	0	11	0	11	0
Blue cheese	1 svg	160	16	90	1	0	1	1
Buffalo	1 svg	15	Tr	0	2	0	2	0
Cheese	1 svg	40	4	90	2	0	2	1
Honey mustard	1 svg	150	15	90	5	0	5	0
Pizza	1 svg	20	1	45	3	0	3	0
Ranch	1 svg	100	10	90	1	0	1	1
Special garlic	1 svg	150	17	100	0	0	0	0
Pizza Hut	***	***	*	*	*	*	*	*
Apps & Bone-In Wings	***	***	*	*	*	*	*	*
Baked hot wings	2 ea	120	7	53	1	0	1	11
Baked mild wings	2 ea	110	7	57	1	0	1	11
Breadsticks	1 ea	140	6	39	18	1	17	4
Buffalo burnin' hot wings	1	100	4.5	41	5	0	5	9
Buffalo medium wings	1	100	4.5	41	5	0	5	9

	Serving Size	Calories	Fat (g)	Calories from Fat (%)	Total Carbs (g)	Fiber (g)	Net Carbs (g)	Protein (g)
Pizza Hut (cont.)	***	***	*	*	*	*	*	*
Buffalo mild wings	1	100	4.5	41	5	0	5	9
Cajun rub wings	1	80	4.5	51	Tr	0	Tr	9
Cheese breadsticks	1 ea	180	7	35	20	1	19	7
Garlic-parmesan wings	1	140	11	71	Tr	0	Tr	10
Hawaiian teriyaki wings	1	100	4.5	41	4	0	4	10
Lemon pepper rub wings	1	80	4.5	51	Tr	0	Tr	9
Marinara dipping sauce	3 oz	60	0	0	12	2	10	2
Naked wings	1	80	4.5	51	0	0	0	9
Ranch rub wings	1	80	4.5	51	Tr	0	Tr	9
Spicy garlic wings	1	120	8	60	3	0	3	9
Stuffed pizza rolls	1 ea	230	11	43	24	1	23	9
Wing blue cheese dipping sauce	1.5 oz	230	24	94	2	0	2	1
Wing ranch cheese dipping sauce	1.5 oz	220	23	94	3	0	3	1
Fit 'n Delicious Pizza (⅛ of 12" pizza)	***	***	*	*	*	*	*	*
All natural chicken, mushrooms & jalapeno	1 slice	180	5	25	22	1	21	12
All natural chicken, red onion & green pepper	1 slice	180	5	25	24	1	23	11
Diced red tomato, mushroom & jalapeno	1 slice	150	4	24	23	2	21	6
Green pepper, red onion & diced red tomato	1 slice	150	4	24	24	2	22	6
Ham, pineapple & diced tomato	1 slice	160	5	28	24	1	23	7
Ham, red onion & mushroom	1 slice	160	5	28	23	1	22	8
Hand-Tossed Style Pizza (⅛ of 12" pizza)	***	***	*	*	*	*	*	*
All natural Italian sausage & red onion	1 slice	240	10	38	26	2	24	10
All natural pepperoni	1 slice	230	10	39	25	1	24	10
All natural pepperoni & mushroom	1 slice	210	8	34	26	2	24	9
Cheese only	1 slice	220	8	33	26	1	25	10

	Serving Size	Calories	Fat (g)	Calories from Fat (%)	Total Carbs (g)	Fiber (g)	Net Carbs (g)	Protein (g)
Dan's original	1 slice	260	12	42	26	2	24	11
Ham & pineapple	1 slice	200	6	27	27	1	26	9
Hawaiian luau	1 slice	230	10	39	27	1	26	10
Meat lover's	1 slice	310	17	49	26	2	24	14
Spicy Sicilian	1 slice	250	11	40	26	2	24	11
Supreme	1 slice	260	12	42	26	2	24	11
Triple meat Italiano	1 slice	260	12	42	25	2	23	12
Veggie lover's	1 slice	200	7	32	27	2	25	8
Pan Pizza (⅛ of 12" pizza)	***	***	*	*	*	*	*	*
All natural Italian sausage & red onion	1 slice	260	11	38	28	2	26	11
All natural pepperoni	1 slice	250	11	40	26	1	25	10
All natural pepperoni & mushroom	1 slice	230	9	35	27	1	26	10
Cheese only	1 slice	230	9	35	27	1	26	10
Dan's original	1 slice	270	13	43	27	2	25	12
Ham & pineapple	1 slice	220	8	33	28	1	27	9
Hawaiian luau	1 slice	260	10	35	28	1	27	11
Meat lover's	1 slice	330	18	49	27	1	26	15
Spicy Sicilian	1 slice	270	12	40	27	2	25	11
Supreme	1 slice	280	13	42	27	2	25	12
Triple meat Italiano	1 slice	280	13	42	27	1	26	12
Veggie lover's	1 slice	220	8	33	28	2	26	9
Stuffed Crust Pizza (⅙ of 14" pizza)	***	***	*	*	*	*	*	*
All natural Italian sausage & red onion	1 slice	390	18	42	40	2	38	17
All natural pepperoni	1 slice	380	18	43	39	2	37	16
All natural pepperoni & mushroom	1 slice	350	15	39	39	2	37	15
Cheese only	1 slice	340	14	37	39	2	37	15
Dan's original	1 slice	440	22	45	40	2	38	20
Ham & pineapple	1 slice	330	13	35	41	2	39	15
Hawaiian luau	1 slice	360	14	35	41	2	39	16
Meat lover's	1 slice	480	26	49	39	2	37	22
Spicy Sicilian	1 slice	430	21	44	40	2	38	19

	Serving Size	Calories	Fat (g)	Calories from Fat (%)	Total Carbs (g)	Fiber (g)	Net Carbs (g)	Protein (g)
Pizza Hut (cont.)	***	***	*	*	*	*	*	*
Supreme	1 slice	410	20	44	40	3	37	18
Triple meat Italiano	1 slice	440	23	47	40	2	38	21
Veggie lover's	1 slice	330	13	35	40	3	37	14
Thin & Crispy Pizza (⅛ of 12" pizza)	***	***	*	*	*	*	*	*
All natural Italian sausage & red onion	1 slice	220	10	41	23	1	22	9
All natural pepperoni	1 slice	200	9	41	21	1	20	9
All natural pepperoni & mushroom	1 slice	190	7	33	22	1	21	8
Cheese only	1 slice	190	8	38	22	1	21	9
Dan's original	1 slice	230	11	43	2	1	1	10
Ham & pineapple	1 slice	180	6	30	23	1	22	8
Hawaiian luau	1 slice	220	10	41	23	1	22	10
Meat lover's	1 slice	290	16	50	22	1	21	13
Spicy Sicilian	1 slice	230	11	43	22	1	21	10
Supreme	1 slice	230	11	43	23	1	22	10
Triple meat Italiano	1 slice	230	12	47	22	1	21	11
Veggie lover's	1 slice	180	6	30	23	1	22	7
Popeyes Louisiana Kitchen	***	***	*	*	*	*	*	*
Biscuits	1 svg	240	13	49	26	1	25	4
Blackened ranch dipping sauce	1 svg	118	13	99	2	0	2	1
Butterfly shrimp	1 svg	310	19	55	22	2	20	13
Buttermilk ranch dipping sauce	1 svg	150	15	90	3	0	3	0
Cajun rice	1 svg	170	6	32	22	20	2	8
Cajun wing segments	6 pc	600	43	65	19	0	19	34
Chicken biscuit	1	350	20	51	30	Tr	30	13
Chicken bowl	1	570	29	46	44	8	36	35
Chicken étouffée	1 svg	160	10	56	6	2	4	12
Chicken sausage jambalaya	1 svg	220	11	45	20	1	19	10
Cinnamon apple turnover	1	250	12	43	34	2	32	3
Coffee	1	0	0	0	0	0	0	0
Coleslaw	1 svg	260	23	80	14	9	5	Tr
Corn on the cob	1	19	2	95	37	4	33	6

	Serving Size	Calories	Fat (g)	Calories from Fat (%)	Total Carbs (g)	Fiber (g)	Net Carbs (g)	Protein (g)
Crawfish étouffée	1 svg	180	5	25	25	2	23	7
Crispy chicken sandwich	1	560	23	37	56	3	53	33
Delta mini	1	300	13	39	30	1	29	15
French fries	1 svg	310	17	49	35	3	32	4
Green beans, reg size	1 svg	55	2	33	7	2	5	3
Grilled chicken sandwich	1	360	10	25	46	2	44	21
Handcrafted Tenders, blackened	5 pc	283	3	10	3	0	3	43
Handcrafted Tenders, blackened	3 pc	170	2	11	2	0	2	26
Loaded chicken wrap	1	400	17	38	44	4	40	19
Louisiana Travelers, mild tenders	3 pc	380	17	40	24	0	24	33
Louisiana Travelers, nuggets	6 pc	220	12	49	13	Tr	13	15
Louisiana Travelers, spicy tenders	3 pc	410	17	37	30	0	30	33
Mardi Gras mustard dipping sauce	1 svg	95	9	85	5	1	4	1
Mashed potatoes & gravy	1 svg	120	4	30	18	2	16	3
Mashed potatoes, no gravy	1 svg	100	3	27	17	Tr	17	1
Mild chicken, breast	1	350	20	51	8	0	8	33
Mild chicken, breast, no skin & breading	1	120	2	15	0	0	0	24
Mild chicken, leg	1	110	7	57	3	0	3	11
Mild chicken, leg, no skin & breading	1	50	2	36	0	0	0	9
Mild chicken, strips, no skin & breading	2 pc	130	3	21	3	0	3	25
Mild chicken, thigh	1	280	20	64	7	0	7	16
Mild chicken, thigh, no skin & breading	1	80	4	45	0	0	0	11
Mild chicken, wing	1	150	10	60	5	0	5	9
Mild chicken, wing, no skin & breading	1	40	2	45	0	0	0	7
Po boy sandwich		330	17	46	36	0	36	8
Popcorn shrimp		280	16	51	22	Tr	22	12
Red beans & rice		320	19	53	31	17	14	10

	Serving Size	Calories	Fat (g)	Calories from Fat (%)	Total Carbs (g)	Fiber (g)	Net Carbs (g)	Protein (g)
Popeyes Louisiana Kitchen (cont.)	***	***	*	*	*	*	*	*
Smothered chicken	210	8	34	24	1	23	10	
Spicy chicken, breast	1	360	22	55	8	1	7	31
Spicy chicken, breast, no skin & breading	1	120	2	15	Tr	Tr	Tr	25
Spicy chicken, leg	1	100	5	45	3	0	3	9
Spicy chicken, leg, no skin & breading	1	50	2	36	0	0	0	9
Spicy chicken, strips, no skin & breading	2 pc	150	4	24	5	0	5	23
Spicy chicken, thigh	1	300	24	72	7	0	7	15
Spicy chicken, thigh, no skin & breading	1	80	3	34	0	0	0	12
Spicy chicken, wing	1	140	9	58	5	0	5	8
Spicy chicken, wing, no skin & breading	1	40	2	45	0	0	0	6
Tartar dipping sauce	1 svg	140	15	96	1	0	1	0
Unsweetened Iced Tea	22 fl oz	0	0	0	0	0	0	0
Red Lobster	***	***	*	*	*	*	*	*
Beverages	***	***	*	*	*	*	*	*
Harbor Café Coffee	1 svg	0	0	0	0	0	0	0
Iced Tea	1 svg	0	0	0	1	0	1	0
Chicken and Beef	***	***	*	*	*	*	*	*
Buffalo Chicken Wings, starter	1 svg	660	48	0	5	1	4	52
7-oz Wood-Grilled Sirloin, entrée or CYO	1	290	13	0	2	1	1	41
Seafood	***	***	*	*	*	*	*	*
Arctic Char (Today's Catch), lunch or dinner	1	350	16	41	Tr	0	Tr	41
Catfish, Farm-Raised, blackened, lunch	1	210	10	43	2	0	2	26
Cod (Today's Catch), lunch or dinner	1	250	3	11	Tr	0	Tr	40
Crab	***	***	*	*	*	*	*	*

	Serving Size	Calories	Fat (g)	Calories from Fat (%)	Total Carbs (g)	Fiber (g)	Net Carbs (g)	Protein (g)
North Pacific King Crab Legs, 1.5 lb (Today's Catch)	1	480	35	66	Tr	0	Tr	41
King Crab Legs, add-on	1	360	34	85	0	0	0	14
Snow Crab Legs, entrée or add-on	1	370	34	83	0	0	0	16
Wild-Caught Snow Crab Legs	1	440	34	70	0	0	0	32
Flounder	***	***	*	*	*	*	*	*
Today's Catch, lunch or dinner	1	200	4.5	20	Tr	0	Tr	35
Wild-Caught (oven-broiled), classic or lunch	1	210	5	21	1	0	1	35
Wild-Caught Flounder/ Sole (oven-broiled), early dining	1	420	11	24	1	0	1	70
Grouper (Today's Catch), lunch or dinner	1	220	3.5	14	Tr	0	Tr	42
Gulf Snapper (Today's Catch), lunch or dinner	1	230	4.5	18	Tr	0	Tr	45
Haddock (Today's Catch), lunch or dinner	1	220	3.5	14	Tr	0	Tr	43
Halibut (Today's Catch), lunch or dinner	1	220	4	16	Tr	0	Tr	38
Lake Whitefish (Today's Catch), lunch or dinner	1	310	14	41	Tr	0	Tr	42
Lobster	***	***	*	*	*	*	*	*
Whole Steamed Maine Lobster	1.25 lb	440	34	70	0	0	0	33
Classic Maine Lobster Tail, entrée or add-on	1	370	36	88	Tr	0	Tr	12
Wood-Grilled Maine Lobster Tail, entrée or add-on	1	390	37	85	Tr	0	Tr	13
Ono/Wahoo (Today's Catch), lunch or dinner	1	300	18	54	Tr	0	Tr	33
Pacific Snapper (Today's Catch), lunch or dinner	1	170	4	21	Tr	0	Tr	33
Perch (Today's Catch), lunch or dinner	1	190	3	14	Tr	0	Tr	36

	Serving Size	Calories	Fat (g)	Calories from Fat (%)	Total Carbs (g)	Fiber (g)	Net Carbs (g)	Protein (g)
Red Lobster (cont.)	***	***	*	*	*	*	*	*
Rainbow Trout (Today's Catch), lunch	1	250	11	40	Tr	0	Tr	34
Rainbow Trout (Today's Catch), dinner	1	490	22	40	Tr	0	Tr	67
Red Rockfish (Today's Catch), lunch or dinner	1	170	4	21	Tr	0	Tr	33
Salmon (Today's Catch), lunch	1	310	19	55	Tr	0	Tr	32
Salmon (Today's Catch), dinner	1	630	39	56	Tr	0	Tr	64
Scallops	***	***	*	*	*	*	*	*
Bay Scallops (oven-broiled), CYO lunch	1	50	0.5	9	1	0	1	11
Wood-Grilled Sea Scallops, entrée or add-on	1	80	2.5	28	2	0	2	12
Wood-Grilled Sea Scallops, CYO	1	240	18	68	4	Tr	4	17
Shrimp	***	***	*	*	*	*	*	*
Garlic Grilled Red Shrimp, add-on	1	110	6	49	0	0	0	15
Garlic Grilled Shrimp Scampi (Endless Shrimp Monday initial order)	1	440	18	37	5	1	4	24
Garlic Shrimp Scampi (entrée, lunch, add-on, refill) or Shrimp Your Way Scampi	1	220	18	74	3	0	3	12
Garlic Shrimp Scampi, CYO	1	240	18	68	4	Tr	4	17
Garlic Shrimp Scampi, CYO lunch	1	120	9	68	2	0	2	8
Wood-Grilled Jumbo Shrimp Skewer	1	80	3	34	Tr	Tr	Tr	12
Wood-Grilled Shrimp Skewer, no rice (Endless Shrimp Monday refill)	1	60	3.5	53	0	0	0	7
Sole	***	***	*	*	*	*	*	*
Today's Catch, lunch or dinner	1	200	4.5	20	Tr	0	Tr	35

	Serving Size	Calories	Fat (g)	Calories from Fat (%)	Total Carbs (g)	Fiber (g)	Net Carbs (g)	Protein (g)
Wild-Caught Flounder/ Sole (oven-broiled), early dining	1	420	11	24	1	0	1	70
Tilapia	***	***	*	*	*	*	*	*
Today's Catch, dinner	1	430	11	23	Tr	0	Tr	82
Wood-Grilled Tilapia, CYO	1	220	6	25	Tr	0	Tr	41
Tuna (Today's Catch), lunch or dinner	1	250	2.5	9	Tr	0	Tr	52
Dressings and Condiments	***	***	*	*	*	*	*	*
Melted butter	1 svg	300	33	99	0	0	0	0
Blue cheese dressing	1 svg	230	24	94	2	0	2	2
Caesar dressing	1 svg	300	32	96	Tr	0	Tr	2
Marinara sauce	1 svg	35	2	51	4	0	4	0
Pico de Gallo	1 svg	10	0	0	2	0	2	0
Ranch dressing	1 svg	150	16	96	2	0	2	0
Tartar sauce	1 svg	210	21	90	4	0	4	0
TFF Toppings	***	***	*	*	*	*	*	*
Blackened Seasoning	1 svg	15	0	0	3	1	2	0
Broiled Fish Seasoning	1 svg	10	0	0	2	0	2	0
Langostino Lobster Beurre Blanc	1 svg	140	9	58	7	0	7	8
Olive Oil	1 svg	40	4.5	100	0	0	0	0
Pineapple Relish	1 svg	10	0	0	3	0	3	0
Yucatan Shrimp	1 svg	170	15	79	5	0	5	7
Sides & Additions	***	***	*	*	*	*	*	*
Fresh Seasonal Asparagus	1 svg	80	7	79	4	2	2	3
Grilled Shrimp added to salad	1 svg	60	4	60	0	0	0	5
Roasted Green Beans	1 svg	150	14	84	7	3	4	2
Seasoned Fresh Broccoli	1 svg	40	0	0	8	3	5	3
Ruby Tuesday	***	***	*	*	*	*	*	*
Appetizers	***	***	*	*	*	*	*	*
Chicken Wings, Hot	1 svg	490	24	44	1	0	1	55
Chicken Wings, Mild	1 svg	600	42	63	1	0	1	55
Dressings & Sauces	***	***	*	*	*	*	*	*
Buttermilk Blue Cheese	1 svg	180	19	95	1	0	1	1

	Serving Size	Calories	Fat (g)	Calories from Fat (%)	Total Carbs (g)	Fiber (g)	Net Carbs (g)	Protein (g)
Ruby Tuesday (cont.)	***	***	*	*	*	*	*	*
Cocktail Sauce	1 svg	22	0	0	5	0	5	0
Creamy Caesar	1 svg	170	19	100	1	0	1	1
Garden Herb Ranch	1 svg	113	12	96	0	0	0	0
Italian Herb Vinaigrette	1 svg	130	14	97	2	0	2	0
Mayonnaise	1 svg	220	24	98	0	0	0	0
Mustard	1 svg	2	0	0	0	0	0	0
Parmesan Cream Sauce	1 svg	58	4	62	2	0	2	1
Sour Cream	1 svg	18	1	50	1	0	1	0
Spicy Shrimp Sauce	1 svg	170	18	95	2	0	2	0
Tomato Basil Sauce	1 svg	22	1	41	3	0	3	0
Whipped Butter	1 svg	140	14	90	0	0	0	0
White Cheddar Sauce	1 svg	230	19	74	5	0	5	7
Garden Bar Add-Ons	***	***	*	*	*	*	*	*
Avocado	1 svg	180	14	70	8	6	2	1
Broiled Shrimp	1 svg	220	12	49	1	0	1	22
Chopped Garden Bar Mix	1 svg	10	0	0	2	1	1	1
Cilantro Lime Vinaigrette	1 svg	60	6	90	1	0	1	0
Crispy Cheese Crisps	1 svg	230	14	55	2	0	2	22
Crispy Onions	1 svg	25	2	72	2	0	2	0
Diced Grilled Chicken	1 svg	170	9	48	0	0	0	20
Diced Grilled Sirloin	1 svg	230	14	55	0	0	0	19
Garden Herb Ranch Dressing	1 svg	110	11	90	1	0	1	0
Italian Herb Vinaigrette	1 svg	130	14	97	2	0	2	0
Pico de Gallo	1 svg	80	0	0	17	2	15	2
Salmon	1 svg	70	3	39	1	0	1	6
Spicy Roasted Broccoli	1 svg	70	5	64	4	2	2	2
Lunch & Dinner	***	***	*	*	*	*	*	*
Asiago Peppercorn Sirloin	8 oz	354	16	41	7	0	7	43
Asiago Peppercorn Sirloin	6 oz	297	14	42	6	0	6	33
Asiago Peppercorn Strip	1 svg	604	39	58	5	0	5	55
Blackened Tilapia	1 svg	204	6	26	2	0	2	31
Cajun Rib Eye, 12 oz	1 svg	639	49	69	0	0	0	56
Chicken Bella	1 svg	288	10	31	4	1	3	34

	Serving Size	Calories	Fat (g)	Calories from Fat (%)	Total Carbs (g)	Fiber (g)	Net Carbs (g)	Protein (g)
Chicken Fresco	1 svg	368	22	54	2	0	2	32
Grilled Salmon	1 svg	491	30	55	0	0	0	53
New Orleans Seafood	1 svg	347	14	36	4	0	4	44
New York Strip, 10 oz	1 svg	563	40	64	0	0	0	48
Petite Sirloin, 6 oz	1 svg	310	17	49	1	0	1	32
Skewered Shrimp	1 svg	393	33	76	0	0	0	18
Top Sirloin, 8 oz	1 svg	317	11	31	2	0	2	50
Sides	***	***	*	*	*	*	*	*
Fresh Green Beans	1 svg	37	0	0	5	2	3	1
Fresh Grilled Asparagus	1 svg	70	2	26	7	2	5	3
Fresh Grilled Zucchini	1 svg	22	0	0	2	1	1	1
Seasoned Steamed Broccoli	1 svg	44	2	41	5	2	3	3
Schlotzsky's								
(all salads are listed w/ no dressing)	***	***	*	*	*	*	*	*
Albuquerque turkey sandwich	1 sm	700	37	48	57	4	53	34
Angus beef & provolone sandwich	1 sm	500	19	34	55	3	52	27
Angus corned beef Reuben sandwich	1 sm	620	27	39	54	4	50	40
Angus corned beef sandwich	1 sm	390	9	21	53	4	49	27
Angus pastrami & swiss sandwich	1 sm	610	24	35	56	4	52	43
Angus pastrami Reuben sandwich	1 sm	620	26	38	54	4	50	41
Angus roast beef & cheese sandwich	1 sm	530	22	37	50	2	48	33
Asian chicken wrap	1	540	12	20	80	5	75	56
Baby spinach & feta salad	1	110	7	57	6	3	3	8
Baby spinach salad pizza	1	450	7	14	80	4	76	18
Bacon, tomato & portobello pizza	1	620	23	33	75	4	71	28
Barbecue chips	1	220	12	49	25	1	24	3
BBQ chicken & jalapeno pizza	1	720	16	20	99	3	96	69
BLT	1 sm	370	14	34	49	2	47	14
Boston clam chowder	1 cup	180	11	55	20	0	20	4

	Serving Size	Calories	Fat (g)	Calories from Fat (%)	Total Carbs (g)	Fiber (g)	Net Carbs (g)	Protein (g)
Schlotzsky's (cont.)	***	***	*	*	*	*	*	*
Broccoli cheese soup	1 cup	170	14	74	12	1	11	4
Brownie	1	420	22	47	54	3	51	5
Caesar salad	1	100	5	45	10	3	7	6
Carrot cake	1	720	42	53	80	3	77	7
Cheese sandwich, original style	1 sm	560	27	43	51	3	48	28
Chicken & pesto sandwich	1 sm	380	9	21	49	3	46	27
Chicken breast sandwich	1 sm	340	4	11	52	3	49	26
Chicken salad	1	290	15	47	12	3	9	61
Chicken tortilla soup	1 cup	140	6	39	15	1	14	8
Chipotle chicken sandwich	1 sm	380	10	24	47	3	44	27
Chocolate chip cookie	1	160	8	45	22	1	21	2
Classic swiss & tomato panini	1	620	26	38	63	1	62	33
Combination special pizza	1	640	25	35	76	4	72	27
Cracked pepper chips	1	220	12	49	25	1	24	3
Deluxe sandwich, original style	1 sm	740	38	46	55	3	52	43
Dijon chicken sandwich	1 sm	380	7	17	52	5	47	29
Double cheese pizza	1	600	21	32	74	3	71	27
Feta & portobello wrap	1	620	39	57	55	4	51	14
Fresh tomato & pesto pizza	1	560	19	31	73	3	70	25
Fresh veggie sandwich	1 sm	340	10	26	50	4	46	14
Fudge chocolate chip cookie	1	160	8	45	22	1	21	2
Garden salad	1	50	1	18	12	4	8	3
Greek salad	1	140	8	51	13	4	9	7
Grilled chicken & guacamole wrap	1	690	36	47	60	8	52	63
Grilled chicken & pesto pizza	1	680	22	29	75	4	71	72
Grilled chicken Caesar salad	1	220	8	33	12	3	9	53
Grilled chicken Romano panini	1	570	16	25	62	1	61	70
Ham & cheese sandwich, original style	1 sm	510	19	34	54	3	51	31
Ham & turkey chef salad	1	250	13	47	14	4	10	22
Hearty vegetable beef soup	1 cup	60	3	45	7	1	6	3
Homestyle tuna sandwich	1 sm	380	11	26	48	3	45	22

	Serving Size	Calories	Fat (g)	Calories from Fat (%)	Total Carbs (g)	Fiber (g)	Net Carbs (g)	Protein (g)
Homestyle tuna wrap	1	460	17	33	55	4	51	23
Jalapeno chips	1	220	12	49	25	1	24	3
Mediterranean pizza	1	560	20	32	74	4	70	21
Mesquite BBQ baked crisps	1	140	4	26	24	2	22	2
Mozzarella & portobello panini	1	490	15	28	63	2	61	24
New York style cheesecake	1	350	23	59	30	1	29	6
Oatmeal raisin cookie	1	150	6	36	22	1	21	2
Old fashioned chicken noodle soup	1 cup	80	2	23	12	1	11	6
Original baked crisps	1	140	3	19	26	2	24	2
Original kettle chips	1	190	11	52	18	2	16	2
Panini Italiano	1	740	32	39	67	2	65	43
Parmesan chicken Caesar wrap	1	560	21	34	61	5	56	61
Pasta salad	1	70	3	39	12	1	11	0
Pepperoni & double cheese pizza	1	690	30	39	74	3	71	31
Plain chips	1	220	12	49	25	1	24	3
Potato salad	1	240	13	49	29	3	26	3
Potato w/ bacon soup	1 cup	180	10	50	22	1	21	4
Salt & vinegar chips	1	220	12	49	25	1	24	3
Santa Fe chicken sandwich	1 sm	430	10	21	53	3	50	31
Side salad	1	25	1	36	7	2	5	1
Smoked ham crostini panini	1	640	23	32	67	2	65	39
Smoked turkey & guacamole panini	1	600	21	32	69	5	64	32
Smoked turkey & jalapeno pizza	1	650	21	29	78	4	74	36
Smoked turkey breast sandwich	1 sm	350	6	15	52	2	50	20
Smoked turkey Reuben sandwich	1 sm	610	26	38	57	4	53	34
Sour cream & onion chips	1	220	12	49	25	1	24	3
Sugar cookie	1	160	7	39	22	0	22	2
Texas Schlotzsky's sandwich	1 sm	540	23	38	51	2	49	32
Thai chicken pizza	1	720	23	29	85	4	81	71
The original sandwich	1 sm	560	26	42	52	3	49	28

	Serving Size	Calories	Fat (g)	Calories from Fat (%)	Total Carbs (g)	Fiber (g)	Net Carbs (g)	Protein (g)
Schlotzsky's (cont.)	***	***	*	*	*	*	*	*
Timberline chile	1 cup	280	9	29	31	7	24	18
Tomato basil soup	1 cup	200	5	23	30	2	28	6
Turkey & guacamole sandwich	1 sm	370	7	17	54	4	50	21
Turkey bacon club sandwich	1 sm	560	25	40	51	3	48	32
Turkey chef salad	1	310	18	52	14	4	10	26
Turkey sandwich, original style	1 sm	600	27	41	54	3	51	34
Vegetarian special pizza	1	540	17	28	74	4	70	22
Vegetarian vegetable soup	1 cup	100	1	9	22	5	17	2
White chocolate macadamia nut cookie	1	170	9	48	21	1	20	2
Wisconsin cheese soup	1 cup	260	20	69	20	0	20	4
Sonic	***	***	*	*	*	*	*	*
Apple slices	1 svg	35	0	0	9	2	7	0
Apple slices, w/ fat free caramel dipping sauce	1 svg	120	0	0	27	2	25	0
Bacon cheeseburger toaster sandwich	1	670	39	52	52	3	49	29
Banana cream pie shake	14 oz	590	19	29	98	1	97	7
Banana fudge sundae	1	440	16	33	70	2	68	4
Banana malt	14 oz	490	17	31	78	1	77	7
Banana shake	14 oz	470	16	31	76	1	75	7
Banana split	1	420	9	19	80	2	78	4
Barq's Root Beer float	14 oz	300	8	24	56	0	56	3
BBQ sauce	1 oz	45	0	0	11	0	11	0
BLT toaster sandwich	1	500	29	52	45	2	43	17
Blue coconut Creamslush Treat	14 oz	430	13	27	76	0	76	5
Blue coconut slush	14 oz	190	0	0	52	0	52	0
Breakfast burrito, bacon, egg & cheese	1	450	27	54	38	1	37	19
Breakfast burrito, sausage, egg & cheese	1	480	31	58	38	1	37	18
Breakfast Toaster, bacon, egg & cheese	1	530	32	54	40	2	38	20
Breakfast Toaster, sausage, egg & cheese	1	620	42	61	40	2	38	20

	Serving Size	Calories	Fat (g)	Calories from Fat (%)	Total Carbs (g)	Fiber (g)	Net Carbs (g)	Protein (g)
Bubble gum slush	14 oz	190	0	0	52	0	52	0
Burrito	1	370	18	44	40	6	34	10
Burrito deluxe	1	420	22	47	43	6	37	13
Butterfinger Sonic Blast	14 oz	580	22	34	88	0	88	8
California cheeseburger	1	690	39	51	57	5	52	29
Caramel malt	14 oz	550	18	29	90	0	90	7
Caramel shake	14 oz	530	17	29	88	0	88	6
Caramel sundae	1	390	13	30	64	0	64	4
Ched "r" bites	12 pc	280	15	48	22	1	21	13
Ched "r" bites	4 pc	330	17	46	36	2	34	8
Cherry Creamslush Treat	14 oz	440	13	27	77	0	77	5
Cherry slush	14 oz	200	0	0	53	0	53	0
Chicken club toaster sandwich	1	740	46	56	55	4	51	29
Chicken strip dinner	4 pc	930	43	42	100	7	93	36
Chili cheeseburger	1	660	35	48	56	5	51	31
Chocolate cream pie shake	14 oz	660	19	26	114	0	114	7
Chocolate malt	14 oz	550	17	28	91	0	91	7
Chocolate shake	14 oz	540	16	27	89	0	89	6
Chocolate sundae	1	410	13	29	67	0	67	4
Coca-Cola float	14 oz	290	8	25	54	0	54	3
Coconut cream pie shake	14 oz	580	20	31	93	0	93	7
Corn dog	1	210	11	47	23	2	21	6
Country fried steak toaster sandwich	1	670	37	50	71	4	67	14
Crispy chicken bacon ranch sandwich	1	610	34	50	48	4	44	30
Crispy chicken sandwich	1	550	32	52	46	4	42	22
Crispy chicken wrap	1	480	21	39	54	3	51	20
CroissSonic breakfast sandwich, w/ bacon, egg & cheese	1	510	36	64	29	0	29	18
CroissSonic breakfast sandwich, w/ sausage, egg & cheese	1	600	46	69	29	0	29	19
Diet Coke float	14 oz	220	8	33	33	0	33	3
Diet Dr Pepper float	14 oz	220	8	33	33	0	33	3

	Serving Size	Calories	Fat (g)	Calories from Fat (%)	Total Carbs (g)	Fiber (g)	Net Carbs (g)	Protein (g)
Sonic (cont.)	***	***	*	*	*	*	*	*
Dr Pepper float	14 oz	310	8	23	58	0	58	3
Ex-long chili cheese coney	1	660	39	53	55	4	51	28
Ex-long slaw dog	1	670	38	51	60	4	56	24
French fries, w/ cheese, lg	1	580	28	43	70	5	65	11
French fries, w/ cheese, med	1	420	21	45	51	4	47	8
French fries, w/ cheese, sm	1	270	13	43	32	2	30	5
French fries, w/ chili & cheese, lg	1	690	37	48	75	7	68	19
French fries, w/ chili & cheese, med	1	490	27	50	54	5	49	14
French fries, w/ chili & cheese, sm	1	300	16	48	33	3	30	8
French fries, lg	1	450	18	36	67	5	62	5
French fries, med	1	330	13	35	48	4	44	4
French fries, sm	1	200	8	36	30	2	28	2
French toast sticks	4 pc	500	31	56	49	2	47	7
Fritos chili cheese pie, lg	1	940	64	61	72	6	66	25
Fritos chili cheese pie, med	1	470	32	61	36	3	33	13
Fritos chili cheese wrap	1	670	39	52	66	4	62	21
Grape Creamslush Treat	14 oz	430	13	27	76	0	76	5
Grape slush	14 oz	190	0	0	52	0	52	0
Green apple slush	14 oz	200	0	0	52	0	52	0
Green chili cheeseburger	1	630	31	44	46	5	41	29
Grilled chicken bacon ranch sandwich	1	470	22	42	35	3	32	35
Grilled chicken salad	1	250	10	36	12	3	9	29
Grilled chicken sandwich	1	400	19	43	32	3	29	28
Grilled chicken wrap	1	400	14	32	39	2	37	28
Hickory burger	1	580	26	40	60	5	55	25
Hickory cheeseburger	1	640	31	44	61	5	56	28
Hidden Valley fat free Italian dressing	1.5 oz	40	0	0	10	0	10	0
Hidden Valley honey mustard dressing	1.5 oz	180	16	80	10	0	10	1

	Serving Size	Calories	Fat (g)	Calories from Fat (%)	Total Carbs (g)	Fiber (g)	Net Carbs (g)	Protein (g)
Hidden Valley original light Ranch dressing	1.5 oz	110	5	41	14	0	14	3
Hidden Valley original Ranch dressing	1.5 oz	190	20	95	2	0	2	1
Hidden Valley Thousand Island dressing	1.5 oz	190	19	90	7	0	7	1
Honey mustard sauce	1 oz	90	7	70	7	0	7	0
Hot fudge cake sundae	1	500	20	36	73	2	71	5
Hot fudge malt	14 oz	580	22	34	87	1	86	7
Hot fudge shake	14 oz	570	21	33	75	1	74	6
Hot fudge sundae	1	440	18	37	63	1	62	4
Jalapeno burger	1	550	26	43	53	5	48	25
Jalapeno cheeseburger	1	620	31	45	54	5	49	28
Jr. bacon cheeseburger	1	410	23	50	31	3	28	20
Jr. breakfast burrito	1	320	21	59	25	0	25	12
Jr. burger	1	310	15	44	30	3	27	15
Jr. *Butterfinger* sundae	1	170	6	32	26	0	26	2
Jr. deluxe burger	1	350	20	51	28	3	25	15
Jr. double cheeseburger	1	570	35	55	33	3	30	30
Jr. *Fritos* chili cheese wrap	1	330	17	46	34	3	31	12
Jr. *M&M's* sundae	1	180	7	35	26	0	26	2
Jr. Oreo sundae	1	150	5	30	22	0	22	2
Jr. *Reese's* sundae	1	160	5	28	27	0	27	3
Jumbo popcorn chicken salad	1	420	25	54	32	5	27	21
Jumbo popcorn chicken, lg	6 oz	560	32	51	41	5	36	27
Jumbo popcorn chicken, sm	4 oz	380	22	52	27	3	24	18
Lemon Creamslush Treat	14 oz	430	13	27	77	0	77	5
Lemon real fruit slush	14 oz	200	0	0	53	0	53	0
Lemon-berry Creamslush Treat	14 oz	460	12	23	85	1	84	5
Lemon-berry real fruit slush	14 oz	210	0	0	55	0	55	0
Lime Creamslush Treat	14 oz	430	13	27	77	0	77	5
Lime real fruit slush	14 oz	200	0	0	52	0	52	0
M&M's Sonic Blast	14 oz	600	24	36	88	1	87	8
Mozzarella sticks	1 svg	440	22	45	40	2	38	19
Nuts, add-on for sundaes	3.5 oz	20	2	90	1	0	1	1

	Serving Size	Calories	Fat (g)	Calories from Fat (%)	Total Carbs (g)	Fiber (g)	Net Carbs (g)	Protein (g)
Sonic (cont.)	***	***	*	*	*	*	*	*
Onion rings, lg	1	640	31	44	80	4	76	9
Onion rings, med	1	440	21	43	55	3	52	6
Orange Creamslush Treat	14 oz	430	13	27	77	0	77	5
Orange slush	14 oz	200	0	0	52	0	52	0
Oreo Sonic Blast	14 oz	540	21	35	80	1	79	7
Peanut butter fudge malt	14 oz	620	29	42	83	1	82	9
Peanut butter fudge shake	14 oz	610	28	41	81	1	80	8
Peanut butter fudge sundae	1	470	25	48	58	1	57	6
Peanut butter malt	14 oz	670	36	48	78	0	78	11
Peanut butter shake	14 oz	640	34	48	75	0	75	10
Peanut butter sundae	1	510	31	55	53	0	53	8
Pickle-O's	1 svg	310	16	46	36	2	34	5
Pineapple malt	14 oz	510	17	30	82	0	82	7
Pineapple shake	14 oz	500	16	29	80	0	80	6
Pineapple sundae	1	370	13	32	58	0	58	4
Ranch sauce	1 oz	150	16	96	1	0	1	0
Reese's Peanut Butter Cups Sonic Blast	14 oz	560	19	31	89	1	88	9
Regular coney	1	390	23	53	32	2	30	17
Santa Fe grilled chicken salad	1	310	12	35	22	6	16	31
Sausage biscuit dippers w/ gravy	3 pc	690	44	57	57	0	57	16
Sonic bacon cheeseburger, w/ mayo	1	780	48	55	57	5	52	33
Sonic burger, w/ ketchup	1	560	26	42	57	5	52	26
Sonic burger, w/ mayo	1	650	37	51	55	5	50	26
Sonic burger, w/ mustard	1	560	26	42	54	5	49	26
Sonic cheeseburger, w/ ketchup	1	630	31	44	59	5	54	29
Sonic cheeseburger, w/ mayo	1	720	42	53	56	5	51	29
Sonic cheeseburger, w/ mustard	1	620	31	45	55	5	50	29
Sprite float	14 oz	290	8	25	53	0	53	3
Sprite Zero float	14 oz	220	8	33	33	0	33	3
Steak & egg breakfast burrito	1	590	34	52	47	5	42	28

	Serving Size	Calories	Fat (g)	Calories from Fat (%)	Total Carbs (g)	Fiber (g)	Net Carbs (g)	Protein (g)
Strawberry cream pie shake	14 oz	620	19	28	106	1	105	7
Strawberry Creamslush Treat	14 oz	4150	12	3	84	1	83	5
Strawberry malt	14 oz	520	17	29	85	1	84	7
Strawberry real fruit slush	14 oz	210	0	0	55	0	55	0
Strawberry shake	14 oz	510	16	28	83	1	82	7
Strawberry sundae	1	380	13	31	61	1	60	4
SuperSonic breakfast burrito	1	570	36	57	48	3	45	19
SuperSonic cheeseburger w/ ketchup	1	900	53	53	60	5	55	46
SuperSonic cheeseburger w/ mayo	1	980	64	59	58	5	53	46
SuperSonic cheeseburger w/ mustard	1	890	53	54	57	5	52	46
SuperSonic jalapeno cheeseburger	1	890	53	54	56	5	51	46
Syrup	1 oz	80	0	0	21	0	21	0
Tacos	2	340	20	53	35	4	31	8
Tater tots, w/ cheese, lg	1	660	44	60	55	6	49	10
Tater tots, w/ cheese, med	1	420	28	60	35	3	32	7
Tater tots, w/ cheese, sm	1	270	18	60	22	2	20	5
Tater tots, w/ chili cheese, lg	1	760	53	63	61	7	54	18
Tater tots, w/ chili cheese, med	1	490	34	62	38	5	33	13
Tater tots, w/ chili cheese, sm	1	290	21	65	23	3	20	7
Tater tots, lg	1	530	34	58	52	6	46	4
Tater tots, med	1	320	21	59	32	3	29	2
Tater tots, sm	1	200	13	59	20	2	18	2
Thousand Island burger	1	610	32	47	56	5	51	26
Vanilla cone	1	180	6	30	30	0	30	2
Vanilla dish	1	240	9	34	36	0	36	3
Vanilla malt	14 oz	480	18	34	72	0	72	7
Vanilla shake	14 oz	470	17	33	71	0	71	7
Watermelon Creamslush Treat	14 oz	440	13	27	77	0	77	5
Watermelon slush	14 oz	200	0	0	53	0	53	0
Starbucks	***	***	*	*	*	*	*	*
Avocado Spread	57 g	90	8	80	5	4	1	1

	Serving Size	Calories	Fat (g)	Calories from Fat (%)	Total Carbs (g)	Fiber (g)	Net Carbs (g)	Protein (g)
Starbucks (cont.)	***	***	*	*	*	*	*	*
Blonde Roast, plain	***	***	*	*	*	*	*	*
Short	8 fl oz	5	0	0	0	0	0	0
Tall	12 fl oz	5	0	0	0	0	0	0
Grande	16 fl oz	5	0	0	0	0	0	1
Venti	20 fl oz	5	0	0	0	0	0	1
Bottled Cold Brew, black, unsweetened	11 fl oz	15	0	0	0	0	0	1
Clover Brewed Coffee, plain	***	***	*	*	*	*	*	*
Short	8 fl oz	10	0	0	0	0	0	0
Tall	12 fl oz	10	0	0	0	0	0	0
Grande	16 fl oz	10	0	0	0	0	0	1
Venti	20 fl oz	10	0	0	0	0	0	1
Comfort Wellness Brewed Tea, all sizes	***	0	0	0	0	0	0	0
Defense Wellness Brewed Tea	***	***	*	*	*	*	*	*
Short	8 fl oz	5	0	0	2	0	2	0
Tall	12 fl oz	5	0	0	2	0	2	0
Grande	16 fl oz	10	0	0	3	0	3	0
Venti	20 fl oz	10	0	0	3	0	3	0
Emperor's Cloud and Mist Green Tea, all sizes	***	0	0	0	0	0	0	0
Featured Dark Roast	***	***	*	*	*	*	*	*
Short	8 fl oz	5	0	0	0	0	0	0
Tall	12 fl oz	5	0	0	0	0	0	0
Grande	16 fl oz	5	0	0	0	0	0	1
Venti	20 fl oz	5	0	0	0	0	0	1
Galvanina Sparkling Water, plain and lime	1 bottle	0	0	0	0	0	0	0
Half & Half - see Creamer	***	***	*	*	*	*	*	*
Heavy Cream	1 Tbsp	51	5	88	Tr	0	Tr	Tr
Iced Coffee, unsweetened	***	***	*	*	*	*	*	*
Tall	12 fl oz	0	0	0	0	0	0	0
Grande	16 fl oz	5	0	0	0	0	0	0
Venti	24 fl oz	5	0	0	0	0	0	0
Trenta	30 fl oz	5	0	0	0	0	0	1

	Serving Size	Calories	Fat (g)	Calories from Fat (%)	Total Carbs (g)	Fiber (g)	Net Carbs (g)	Protein (g)
Jade Citrus Mint Green Tea, all sizes	***	0	0	0	0	0	0	0
Justin's Classic Almond Butter	32 g (1 pkt)	190	18	85	6	3	3	7
Mint Majesty Herbal Tea, all sizes	***	0	0	0	0	0	0	0
Organic Jade Citrus Mint Brewed Tea, all sizes	***	0	0	0	0	0	0	0
Passion Tango Herbal Tea, all sizes	***	0	0	0	0	0	0	0
Peach Tranquility Herbal Tea, all sizes	***	0	0	0	0	0	0	0
Pike Place Roast, regular or decaf	***	***	*	*	*	*	*	*
Short	8 fl oz	5	0	0	0	0	0	0
Tall	12 fl oz	5	0	0	0	0	0	0
Grande	16 fl oz	5	0	0	0	0	0	1
Venti	20 fl oz	5	0	0	0	0	0	1
Rev Up Wellness Brewed Tea, all sizes	***	0	0	0	0	0	0	0
Royal English Breakfast Tea, all sizes	***	0	0	0	0	0	0	0
Sous Vide Egg Bites, Bacon and Gruyere	130 g	310	22	64	9	0	9	19
Sugar-Free Syrup (all flavors)	1 pump	0	0	0	0	0	0	0
Teavana Earl Grey Brewed Tea, all sizes	***	0	0	0	0	0	0	0
Teavana Organic Chai Tea, all sizes	***	0	0	0	0	0	0	0
Youthberry White Tea, all sizes	***	0	0	0	0	0	0	0
Subway	***	***	*	*	*	*	*	*
Breakfast Flatbread Sandwiches	***	***	*	*	*	*	*	*
Black forest ham & cheese	1	480	22	41	46	3	43	27
Cheese	1	460	21	41	45	3	42	23
Double bacon & cheese	1	560	28	45	46	3	43	30
Mega	1	750	48	58	46	3	43	34
Sausage & cheese	1	700	44	57	46	3	43	30

	Serving Size	Calories	Fat (g)	Calories from Fat (%)	Total Carbs (g)	Fiber (g)	Net Carbs (g)	Protein (g)
Subway (cont.)	***	***	*	*	*	*	*	*
Steak & cheese	1	520	23	40	48	3	45	32
Western & cheese	1	490	22	40	47	3	44	28
Breakfast Sandwiches, on 6" Bread	***	***	*	*	*	*	*	*
Black forest ham & cheese	1	450	19	38	47	5	42	27
Cheese	1	420	18	39	46	5	41	22
Double bacon & cheese	1	520	25	43	47	5	42	29
Mega	1	720	45	56	47	5	42	33
Sausage & cheese	1	670	41	55	46	5	41	30
Steak & cheese	1	490	20	37	48	5	43	31
Western & cheese	1	450	19	38	48	5	43	27
Cheese	***	***	*	*	*	*	*	*
American	11 g	40	3.5	79	1	0	1	2
Cheddar	14 g	60	4.5	68	0	0	0	4
Monterey Cheddar	14 g	50	4.5	81	0	0	0	3
Parmesan	0 g	5	0	0	0	0	0	1
Pepper Jack	11 g	50	4	72	0	0	0	2
Provolone	14 g	50	4	72	0	0	0	4
Shredded mozzarella	14 g	40	3	68	0	0	0	3
Swiss	14 g	50	4.5	81	0	0	0	4
Cookies & Desserts	***	***	*	*	*	*	*	*
Apple pie	1 svg	250	10	36	37	1	36	0
Apple slices	1 pkg	35	0	0	9	2	7	0
Chocolate chip cookie	1	220	10	41	30	1	29	2
Chocolate chunk cookie	1	220	10	41	30	Tr	30	2
Double chocolate chip	1	210	10	43	30	1	29	2
M&M's cookie	1	210	10	43	32	Tr	32	2
Oatmeal raisin cookie	1	200	8	36	30	1	29	3
Peanut butter cookie	1	220	12	49	26	1	25	4
Sugar cookie	1	220	12	49	28	Tr	28	2
White chip macadamia nut cookie	1	220	11	45	29	Tr	29	2
Yogurt, *Dannon* Light & Fit	1	80	0	0	16	0	16	5
Flatbread Sandwiches	***	***	*	*	*	*	*	*
Black forest ham	1	320	7	20	47	3	44	18

	Serving Size	Calories	Fat (g)	Calories from Fat (%)	Total Carbs (g)	Fiber (g)	Net Carbs (g)	Protein (g)
Oven roasted chicken breast	1	350	7	18	48	3	45	24
Roast beef	1	340	8	21	45	3	42	27
Subway club	1	350	8	21	47	3	44	26
Sweet onion chicken teriyaki	1	410	7	15	59	3	56	26
Turkey breast	1	310	6	17	47	3	44	18
Turkey breast & black forest ham	1	330	7	19	47	3	44	20
Veggie Delite	1	260	5	17	44	3	41	9
Hash browns	4 pc	150	9	54	17	2	15	1
Pizza, 8"	***	***	*	*	*	*	*	*
Cheese	1	680	0	0	7	0	7	1
Cheese & veggie	1	740	3	4	12	4	8	12
Pepperoni	1	790	3	3	10	4	6	20
Sausage	1	820	30	33	3	0	3	1
Salads (w/o dressing)	***	***	*	*	*	*	*	*
Black forest ham	1	120	3	23	12	4	8	13
Chicken and bacon ranch	1	460	32	63	15	4	11	27
Cold cut combo	1	180	11	55	13	4	9	12
Ham	1	110	3	25	12	4	8	12
Italian BMT	1	240	15	56	13	4	9	14
Oven roasted chicken	1	130	2.5	17	12	4	8	17
Roast beef	1	140	3.5	23	12	4	8	19
Rotisserie-style chicken	1	170	5	26	11	4	7	23
Spicy Italian	1	310	23	67	13	4	9	14
Subway club	1	140	3	19	12	4	8	18
Sweet onion chicken teriyaki	1	200	3	14	25	4	21	20
Tuna salad	1	310	24	70	11	4	7	15
Turkey breast	1	110	2	16	12	4	8	12
Turkey breast & ham	1	120	3	23	12	4	8	14
Veggie Delite	1	50	1	18	10	4	6	3
Salad Dressings & Vinaigrettes	***	***	*	*	*	*	*	*
Fat free Italian dressing	2 oz	35	0	0	7	0	7	1
Ranch dressing	14 g	70	8	100	1	0	1	0

	Serving Size	Calories	Fat (g)	Calories from Fat (%)	Total Carbs (g)	Fiber (g)	Net Carbs (g)	Protein (g)
Subway (cont.)	***	***	*	*	*	*	*	*
Savory Caesar dressing	14 g	80	9	100	1	0	1	1
Subway vinaigrette	14 g	35	3.5	90	1	0	1	0
Six Inch Subs	***	***	*	*	*	*	*	*
Big Philly cheesesteak	1	520	18	31	53	6	47	39
Black forest ham	1	290	5	16	47	5	42	18
BLT	1	360	13	33	45	5	40	17
Chicken & bacon ranch	1	570	28	44	49	6	43	35
Cold cut combo	1	410	16	35	48	5	43	21
Italian BMT	1	450	20	40	48	5	43	22
Meatball marinara	1	580	23	36	70	9	61	24
Oven roasted chicken breast	1	320	5	14	49	5	44	23
Roast beef	1	310	5	15	46	5	41	26
Spicy Italian	1	520	28	48	47	5	42	22
Subway club	1	320	5	14	47	5	42	26
Subway melt	1	380	11	26	49	5	44	25
Sweet onion chicken teriyaki	1	380	5	12	60	5	55	26
The Feast	1	540	22	37	50	5	45	39
Tuna	1	530	30	51	46	5	41	21
Turkey breast	1	280	4	13	47	5	42	18
Turkey breast & black forest ham	1	300	4	12	47	5	42	19
Veggie Delite	1	230	3	12	45	5	40	8
Toppings & Extras	***	***	*	*	*	*	*	*
Bacon	15 g	70	6	77	1	0	1	5
Banana peppers	4 g	0	0	0	0	0	0	0
Black Olives	3 g	0	0	0	0	0	0	0
Chipotle Southwest sauce	14 g	80	7	79	1	0	1	0
Cucumbers	14 g	0	0	0	1	0	1	0
Green peppers	7 g	0	0	0	0	0	0	0
Guacamole	35 g	70	6	77	3	2	1	1
Jalapenos	4 g	0	0	0	0	0	0	0
Lettuce	21 g	0	0	0	1	0	1	0
Light mayonnaise	15 g	50	5	90	1	0	1	0

	Serving Size	Calories	Fat (g)	Calories from Fat (%)	Total Carbs (g)	Fiber (g)	Net Carbs (g)	Protein (g)
Oil	5 g	45	5	100	0	0	0	0
Pickles	9 g	0	0	0	0	0	0	0
Red onions	7 g	0	0	0	1	0	1	0
Spicy brown mustard	14 g	15	1	60	1	0	1	0
Spinach	7 g	0	0	0	0	0	0	0
Tomatoes	35 g	5	0	0	1	0	1	0
Yellow mustard	14 g	10	0.5	45	1	0	1	0
Taco Bell	***	***	*	*	*	*	*	*
Bean burrito	1	350	9	23	54	9	45	13
Brisk Unsweetened No Lemon Iced Tea	16 fl oz	0	0	0	0	0	0	0
Burrito supreme, beef	1	410	15	33	52	8	44	17
Burrito supreme, chicken	1	390	12	28	51	6	45	20
Burrito supreme, steak	1	380	12	28	50	6	44	17
Caramel apple empanada	1	310	15	44	39	2	37	2
Chalupa Baja, beef	1	410	26	57	31	4	27	13
Chalupa Baja, chicken	1	390	23	53	29	2	27	17
Chalupa Baja, steak	1	380	23	54	29	2	27	14
Chalupa nacho cheese, beef	1	370	21	51	32	3	29	12
Chalupa nacho cheese, chicken	1	350	18	46	30	2	28	16
Chalupa nacho cheese, steak	1	340	18	48	30	2	28	13
Chalupa supreme, beef	1	370	21	51	31	3	28	14
Chalupa supreme, chicken	1	350	18	46	30	2	28	17
Chalupa supreme, steak	1	340	18	48	29	2	27	15
Cheese roll-up	1	200	10	45	19	2	17	9
Cheesy double beef burrito	1	470	20	38	54	6	48	18
Cheesy fiesta potatoes	1 svg	270	16	53	28	3	25	4
Chicken grilled taquitos	1	320	11	31	37	2	35	18
Chicken quesadilla	1	520	27	47	41	4	37	28
Cinnamon twists	1	170	7	37	26	1	25	1
Crunchwrap supreme	1	540	21	35	71	6	65	16
Crunchy taco	1	170	10	53	12	3	9	8
Double decker taco	1	320	13	37	38	7	74	14
Double decker taco supreme	1	350	15	39	40	7	34	14
Enchirito, beef	1	360	17	43	35	7	28	18

	Serving Size	Calories	Fat (g)	Calories from Fat (%)	Total Carbs (g)	Fiber (g)	Net Carbs (g)	Protein (g)
Taco Bell (cont.)	***	***	*	*	*	*	*	*
Enchirito, chicken	1	340	13	34	33	6	27	22
Enchirito, steak	1	330	14	38	33	6	27	19
Fiesta burrito, beef	1	380	14	33	50	5	45	14
Fiesta burrito, chicken	1	360	10	25	49	3	46	17
Fiesta burrito, steak	1	350	18	46	48	3	45	14
Fresco burrito supreme, chicken	1	340	8	21	49	6	43	18
Fresco burrito supreme, steak	1	330	8	22	49	6	43	15
Fresco crunchy taco	1	150	7	42	13	3	10	7
Fresco bean burrito	1	330	7	19	55	9	46	11
Fresco fiesta burrito, chicken	1	340	8	21	50	4	46	16
Fresco grilled steak soft taco	1	160	5	28	21	2	19	9
Fresco ranchero chicken soft taco	1	170	4	21	22	2	20	12
Fresco soft taco, beef	1	180	7	35	22	3	19	8
Gordita Baja, beef	1	360	21	53	30	5	25	13
Gordita Baja, chicken	1	340	18	48	29	3	26	17
Gordita Baja, steak	1	330	18	49	28	3	25	14
Gordita nacho cheese, beef	1	320	16	45	31	4	27	12
Gordita nacho cheese, chicken	1	300	13	39	30	2	28	15
Gordita nacho cheese, steak	1	290	13	40	29	2	27	13
Gordita supreme, beef	1	320	16	45	30	4	26	13
Gordita supreme, chicken	1	300	13	39	29	3	26	17
Gordita supreme, steak	1	290	13	40	29	3	26	14
Grilled chicken burrito	1	440	20	41	48	3	45	16
Grilled chicken soft taco	1	200	8	36	19	1	18	12
Grilled Stuft burrito, beef	1	690	30	39	79	10	69	26
Grilled Stuft burrito, chicken	1	650	23	32	76	7	69	33
Grilled Stuft burrito, steak	1	630	24	34	75	7	68	28
Guacamole, side	1	35	3	77	2	1	1	0
Half pound beef combo burrito	1	450	17	34	51	9	42	21
Half pound beef & potato burrito	1	510	22	39	66	7	59	14
Half pound cheesy bean & rice burrito	1	470	21	40	60	6	54	12

	Serving Size	Calories	Fat (g)	Calories from Fat (%)	Total Carbs (g)	Fiber (g)	Net Carbs (g)	Protein (g)
Iced coffee	13 fl oz	10	0	0	0	0	0	2
Mexican pizza	1	530	30	51	46	7	39	20
Mexican rice	1 svg	130	4	28	21	1	20	2
MexiMelt	1	280	14	45	23	4	19	15
Nachos	1 svg	330	21	57	31	2	29	4
Nachos BellGrande	1 svg	760	42	50	77	12	65	19
Nachos supreme	1 svg	430	24	50	41	7	34	13
Pintos n' cheese	1 svg	170	6	32	18	7	11	9
Rainforest coffee, hot	13 fl oz	10	0	0	0	0	0	2
Salsa, side	1	5	0	0	1	0	1	0
Seven layer burrito	1	490	17	31	67	10	57	17
Soft taco, beef	1	210	9	39	21	3	18	10
Soft taco, grilled steak	1	250	14	50	20	2	18	11
Soft taco, ranchero chicken	1	270	14	47	21	2	19	14
Soft taco supreme, beef	1	240	11	41	24	3	21	11
Sour cream, side	1	30	2	60	2	0	2	1
Steak grilled taquitos	1	310	11	32	37	2	35	15
Steak quesadilla	1	510	28	49	41	4	37	25
Taco salad, chicken ranch, fully loaded	1	960	57	53	78	8	70	36
Taco salad, chipotle steak, fully loaded	1	950	59	56	96	8	88	29
Taco salad, express	1	600	30	45	57	15	42	25
Taco salad, fiesta	1	820	43	47	81	15	66	30
Taco salad, fiesta, w/o shell	1	400	22	50	41	13	28	24
Taco supreme, crunchy	1	200	12	54	15	3	12	9
Triple layer nachos	1 svg	340	18	48	38	6	32	7
Volcano burrito	1	800	42	47	81	8	73	24
Volcano taco	1	240	17	64	14	3	11	8
Taco del Mar	***	***	*	*	*	*	*	*
Beef baja bowl	1	830	35	38	81	10	71	44
Beef enchilada	1	1030	37	32	115	13	102	55
Beef mondito burrito	1	560	19	31	71	6	65	28
Beef mondo burrito	1	1070	36	30	134	12	122	54
Beef quesadilla	1	800	37	42	66	6	60	49

	Serving Size	Calories	Fat (g)	Calories from Fat (%)	Total Carbs (g)	Fiber (g)	Net Carbs (g)	Protein (g)
Taco del Mar (cont.)	***	***	*	*	*	*	*	*
Beef taco salad	1	930	49	47	75	12	63	47
Beef taco, hard	1	270	15	50	17	1	16	17
Beef taco, soft	1	280	11	35	28	4	24	18
Beef, side	1 svg	200	11	50	4	1	3	24
Black beans	1 svg	140	2	13	24	8	16	7
Breakfast taco, flour	1	260	15	52	18	1	17	13
Butter cookies	1	220	10	41	31	0	31	2
Cheese enchilada	1	820	27	30	112	12	100	31
Cheese mondito burrito	1	460	13	25	69	5	64	16
Cheese mondo burrito	1	870	24	25	130	10	120	30
Cheese quesadilla	1	710	35	44	63	4	59	32
Cheese, side	1 svg	110	9	74	1	0	1	7
Chicken baja bowl	1	790	31	35	79	9	70	44
Chicken enchilada	1	990	33	30	113	12	101	55
Chicken mondito burrito	1	550	17	28	70	6	64	28
Chicken mondo burrito	1	1030	32	28	131	11	120	54
Chicken quesadilla	1	770	33	39	64	5	59	49
Chicken taco salad	1	900	45	45	73	11	62	47
Chicken taco, hard	1	260	13	45	16	1	15	17
Chicken taco, soft	1	260	9	31	27	3	24	19
Chicken, side	1 svg	170	7	37	1	0	1	24
Chips & salsa	1	590	27	41	78	5	73	8
Chocolate chip & nut cookie	1	240	13	49	30	2	28	3
Chocolate chip cookie	1	240	12	45	34	1	33	2
Cod, side	2 pc	120	4	30	13	0	13	10
Corn tortillas	2	120	2	15	24	3	21	3
Diced potatoes	1 svg	60	1	15	11	1	10	2
Egg & cheese burrito	1	490	19	35	59	6	53	22
Egg & cheese taco, flour	1	200	10	45	17	1	16	9
Eggs	1 svg	90	7	70	1	0	1	7
Enchilada sauce	1 svg	35	0	0	7	0	7	1
Fish baja bowl	1	880	41	42	95	9	86	31
Fish mondito burrito	1	510	21	37	61	7	54	21
Fish mondo burrito	1	840	30	32	110	12	98	32

	Serving Size	Calories	Fat (g)	Calories from Fat (%)	Total Carbs (g)	Fiber (g)	Net Carbs (g)	Protein (g)
Fish taco salad	1	1040	61	53	89	11	78	34
Fish taco, hard	1	270	15	50	23	1	22	10
Fish taco, soft	1	270	11	37	34	3	31	12
Flour tortilla, 13"	1	350	9	23	57	3	54	11
Flour tortilla, 10"	1	210	5	21	33	2	31	7
Flour tortilla, 6"	1	100	3	27	15	0	15	3
Green sauce	2 Tbsp	5	0	0	1	0	1	0
Guacamole	1 svg	40	4	90	2	1	1	1
Habanero sauce	2 Tbsp	10	0	0	1	0	1	0
Hash browns	1	110	6	49	13	2	11	1
Milk chocolate cookie	1	240	12	45	31	0	31	3
Mondito breakfast burrito	1	640	31	44	62	7	55	29
Mondo breakfast burrito	1	1190	59	45	110	13	97	54
Nachos	1	1190	65	49	110	12	98	37
Oatmeal, raisin & walnut cookie	1	240	11	41	35	1	34	3
Oreo brownie	1	400	17	38	59	1	58	4
Peanut butter cookie	1	240	13	49	27	0	27	4
Pinto beans, whole	1 svg	90	0	0	20	6	14	6
Pork baja bowl	1	790	33	38	81	9	72	40
Pork enchilada	1	990	35	32	114	12	102	51
Pork mondito burrito	1	550	18	29	71	6	65	26
Pork mondo burrito	1	920	24	23	132	11	121	43
Pork quesadilla	1	770	35	41	65	5	60	45
Pork taco salad	1	900	46	46	74	11	63	43
Pork taco, hard	1	260	14	48	17	1	16	15
Pork taco, soft	1	260	10	35	28	3	25	16
Pork, side	1 svg	170	8	42	3	0	3	20
Queso	¼ cup	80	6	68	2	0	2	3
Red sauce	2 Tbsp	5	0	0	1	0	1	0
Refried beans	1 svg	160	4	23	24	5	19	7
Rice	1 svg	230	3	12	45	1	44	4
Rice & black beans	1 svg	370	5	12	69	9	60	12
Rice & pinto beans	1 svg	320	3	8	66	8	58	10
Rice & refried beans	1 svg	390	7	16	69	6	63	12

	Serving Size	Calories	Fat (g)	Calories from Fat (%)	Total Carbs (g)	Fiber (g)	Net Carbs (g)	Protein (g)
Taco del Mar (cont.)	***	***	*	*	*	*	*	*
Salsa, side	1 svg	15	0	0	4	1	3	1
Sausage	1 svg	100	8	72	1	0	1	6
Sour cream	1 svg	70	6	77	2	0	2	1
Spinach tortilla, 13"	1	350	10	26	56	5	51	10
Taco salad shell	1	280	16	51	29	1	28	4
Taco shell	1	110	5	41	14	0	14	2
Tomato tortilla, 13"	1	350	10	26	56	5	51	10
Triple chocolate cookie	1	230	12	47	31	1	30	3
Vegan mondito	1	430	11	23	70	6	64	13
Vegan mondo	1	800	19	21	133	12	121	24
Veggie taco, soft	1	310	8	23	49	5	44	11
White chocolate macadamia nut cookie	1	270	16	53	30	0	30	3
White sauce	2 Tbsp	120	13	98	1	0	1	0
Whole wheat tortilla, 13"	1	300	5	15	54	8	46	12
TGI Fridays	***	***	*	*	*	*	*	*
Insufficient information	***	***	*	*	*	*	*	*
Side of blue cheese	1 svg	200	21	95	1	0	1	2
Side of ranch	1 svg	130	14	97	1	0	1	1
Traditional wings, *Frank's RedHot* buffalo	1 svg	640	39	55	3	0	3	71
Tim Horton's	***	***	*	*	*	*	*	*
Angel cream donut	1	310	13	38	46	1	45	4
Apple fritter	1	300	11	33	49	2	47	4
Apple fritter Timbit	1	50	2	36	9	0	9	1
Bacon, egg & cheese sandwich	1	420	23	49	34	1	33	16
Bagel BLT	1	450	14	28	58	3	55	21
Banana cream filled Timbit	1	60	2	30	9	0	9	1
Beef stew	10 oz	240	8	30	25	3	22	17
BLT	1	450	18	36	53	2	51	18
Blueberry filled donut	1	230	8	31	36	1	35	4
Blueberry filled Timbit	1	60	2	30	10	0	10	1
Blueberry fritter	1	330	10	27	55	2	53	6
Boston cream donut	1	250	9	32	38	1	37	4

	Serving Size	Calories	Fat (g)	Calories from Fat (%)	Total Carbs (g)	Fiber (g)	Net Carbs (g)	Protein (g)
Café mocha	10 oz	160	7	39	25	1	24	1
Canadian maple filled donut	1	260	9	31	41	1	40	4
Caramel chocolate pecan cookie	1	230	11	43	32	1	31	3
Chicken noodle soup	10 oz	120	2	15	18	1	17	5
Chicken salad sandwich	1	380	9	21	55	3	52	21
Chili	10 oz	300	16	48	18	5	13	21
Chocolate chunk cookie	1	230	9	35	35	1	34	2
Chocolate dip donut	1	210	9	39	30	1	29	4
Chocolate glazed donut	1	260	10	35	39	2	37	4
Chocolate glazed Timbit	1	70	3	39	10	0	10	1
Coffee w/ cream & sugar	10 oz	75	4	48	9	0	9	1
Cream of broccoli soup	10 oz	160	9	51	16	1	15	6
Creamy field mushroom soup	10 oz	150	3	18	28	1	27	3
Egg & cheese sandwich	1	370	19	46	34	1	33	13
Egg salad sandwich	1	390	13	30	52	2	50	17
English toffee beverage	10 oz	220	6	25	40	0	40	3
Flavor shot	1 ml	5	0	0	1	0	1	0
French vanilla beverage	10 oz	240	7	26	39	0	39	4
Ham & swiss sandwich	1	440	12	25	56	3	53	28
Hash brown	1	100	5	45	12	1	11	1
Hearty potato bacon soup	10 oz	250	13	47	23	1	22	6
Hearty vegetable soup	10 oz	70	0	0	14	3	11	4
Honey cruller donut	1	320	19	53	37	0	37	1
Honey dip donut	1	210	8	34	33	1	32	4
Honey dip Timbit	1	60	2	30	9	0	9	1
Hot chocolate	10 oz	240	6	23	45	2	43	2
Hot smoothee	10 oz	260	10	35	39	2	37	5
Iced cappuccino	12 oz	300	15	45	41	0	41	0
Iced cappuccino, w/ milk	12 oz	180	2	10	39	0	39	3
Lemon filled Timbit	1	60	2	30	9	0	9	1
Maple dip donut	1	210	8	34	31	1	30	4
Minestrone	10 oz	120	4	30	24	2	22	3
Oatmeal raisin spice cookie	1	220	8	33	35	1	34	3
Old fashion glazed donut	1	320	19	53	35	1	34	3
Old fashion plain donut	1	260	19	66	20	1	19	3

	Serving Size	Calories	Fat (g)	Calories from Fat (%)	Total Carbs (g)	Fiber (g)	Net Carbs (g)	Protein (g)
Tim Horton's (cont.)	***	***	*	*	*	*	*	*
Old fashion plain Timbit	1	70	5	64	5	0	5	1
Peanut butter cookie	1	280	16	51	27	2	25	6
Sausage, egg & cheese sandwich	1	540	35	58	35	1	34	19
Sour cream glazed Timbit	1	90	5	50	12	0	12	1
Sour cream plain donut	1	270	17	57	27	1	26	3
Split pea w/ ham soup	10 oz	150	3	18	27	5	22	8
Strawberry filled donut	1	230	8	31	36	1	35	4
Strawberry filled Timbit	1	60	2	30	10	0	10	1
Tea w/ cream & sugar	10 oz	50	1	18	10	0	10	1
Toasted chicken club sandwich	1	460	7	14	70	2	68	30
Triple chocolate cookie	1	250	13	47	31	2	29	3
Turkey & wild rice soup	10 oz	120	2	15	21	1	20	3
Turkey bacon club sandwich	1	440	8	16	63	2	61	30
Vegetable beef barley soup	10 oz	110	2	16	21	2	19	4
Walnut crunch donut	1	360	23	58	35	1	34	4
White chocolate macadamia nut cookie	1	240	12	45	31	1	30	3
White country bun	1	240	1	4	49	2	47	9
Whole wheat country bun	1	230	1	4	46	4	42	10
Togo's								
(all sandwiches regular size)	***	***	*	*	*	*	*	*
Albacore tuna sandwich	1	660	28	38	73	4	69	30
Asian chicken salad	1	200	9	41	17	3	14	21
Asian chicken salad wrap w/ Asian dressing	1	670	32	43	74	8	66	28
Asian dressing	2.5 oz	380	33	78	10	0	10	0
Avocado & cheese sandwich	1	740	40	49	73	9	64	25
Avocado & cucumber sandwich	1	560	25	40	75	9	66	13
BBQ beef sandwich, hot	1	670	19	26	85	3	82	40
BBQ chicken ranch salad	1	230	4	16	31	5	26	20
BBQ chicken ranch salad wrap w/ buttermilk dressing	1	630	26	37	77	8	69	27
BBQ ranch chicken sandwich	1	750	27	32	88	4	84	42

	Serving Size	Calories	Fat (g)	Calories from Fat (%)	Total Carbs (g)	Fiber (g)	Net Carbs (g)	Protein (g)
Black forest ham & cheese sandwich	1	670	31	42	67	4	63	35
Blue cheese dressing	2.5 oz	260	26	90	3	0	3	2
Broccoli cheddar soup	12 oz	350	22	57	28	2	26	10
Buttermilk ranch dressing	2.5 oz	250	26	94	3	0	3	2
Caesar dressing	2.5 oz	150	12	72	8	0	8	2
Capicola, dry salami & provolone sandwich	1	1080	59	49	69	4	65	73
Cheese sandwich	1	800	45	51	68	4	64	34
Chicken Caesar salad	1	210	6	26	17	3	14	24
Chicken Caesar salad wrap w/ Caesar dressing	1	550	20	33	67	8	59	31
Chicken salad sandwich	1	650	29	40	74	5	69	26
Chicken sandwich, hot	1	630	20	29	72	4	68	44
Chili	12 oz	310	6	17	45	10	35	17
Chipotle roast beef sandwich	1	990	49	45	66	3	63	66
Chocolate chunk brownie	1	430	22	46	57	3	54	6
Classic white bread	1"	50	0	0	10	0	10	2
Cobb salad	1	330	20	55	12	6	6	29
Cobb salad wrap w/ blue cheese dressing	1	680	36	48	63	11	52	32
Dark chocolate chunk cookie	1	390	19	44	51	1	50	4
Dutch crunch bread	1"	50	0	0	10	0	10	1
Egg salad & cheese sandwich	1	750	39	47	70	4	66	31
Farmer's market salad	1	160	6	34	20	5	15	7
Farmer's market salad wrap w/ balsamic vinaigrette	1	440	14	29	72	9	63	12
Fat free serrano grape vinaigrette	2.5 oz	90	0	0	23	0	23	1
French dip sandwich, hot	1	840	33	35	67	3	64	67
Fresh mushroom & brie soup	12 oz	310	21	61	24	2	22	8
Garden vegetable soup	12 oz	120	1	8	25	4	21	5
Honey wheat bread	1"	50	Tr	0	10	Tr	10	2
Hummus sandwich	1	650	27	37	90	9	81	18
Italian vinaigrette	2.5 oz	300	32	96	4	0	4	0
Low fat balsamic vinaigrette	2.5 oz	90	4	40	16	0	16	0
Meatball sandwich, hot	1	690	27	35	78	5	73	33

	Serving Size	Calories	Fat (g)	Calories from Fat (%)	Total Carbs (g)	Fiber (g)	Net Carbs (g)	Protein (g)
Togo's (cont.)	***	***	*	*	*	*	*	*
Moroccan lentil soup	12 oz	190	2	9	34	12	22	10
Mortadella, salami & provolone sandwich	1	870	41	42	71	4	67	58
New England clam chowder	12 oz	370	24	58	31	1	30	10
Oatmeal raisin cookie	1	360	13	33	57	3	54	6
Old fashioned chicken noodle soup	12 oz	170	4	21	27	1	26	10
Onion herb bread	1"	50	0	0	10	0	10	2
Pacific cobb sandwich	1	710	36	46	68	6	62	34
Parmesan bread	1"	60	2	30	9	0	9	3
Pastrami Reuben sandwich	1	990	55	50	67	3	64	52
Pastrami sandwich, hot	1	750	33	40	69	4	65	43
Peanut butter chip cookie	1	420	23	49	45	2	43	7
Roast beef & avocado sandwich	1	720	29	36	70	6	64	46
Roast beef sandwich, hot	1	730	25	31	67	4	63	58
Roasted Yukon baked potato soup	12 oz	460	31	61	28	2	26	14
Salami & cheese sandwich	1	1100	53	43	73	4	69	87
Santa Fe chicken salad	1	370	16	39	33	10	23	27
Santa Fe chicken salad wrap w/ spicy pepitas dressing	1	800	44	50	75	13	62	34
Sicilian chicken sandwich, hot	1	710	28	35	73	4	69	41
Southwestern chicken & green chile soup	12 oz	400	27	61	21	2	19	18
Spicy pepitas dressing	2.5 oz	340	35	93	3	0	3	3
Spinach tortilla, for wraps	12"	320	8	23	53	2	51	7
Sundried tomato basil tortilla, for wraps	12"	320	8	23	54	2	52	7
Taco salad	1	600	39	59	36	9	27	26
Taco salad wrap w/ taco sauce	1	670	26	35	90	13	77	24
Taco sauce	1 oz	30	2	60	7	0	7	0
The Italian sandwich	1	860	43	45	71	4	67	51
Turkey & avocado sandwich	1	640	26	37	74	9	65	36
Turkey & cheese sandwich	1	670	28	38	68	4	64	42
Turkey & cranberry sandwich	1	670	19	26	95	4	91	34
Turkey bacon club sandwich	1	680	32	42	68	4	64	35

	Serving Size	Calories	Fat (g)	Calories from Fat (%)	Total Carbs (g)	Fiber (g)	Net Carbs (g)	Protein (g)
Turkey, ham & cheese sandwich	1	690	29	38	68	4	64	42
Turkey, ham, salami & cheese sandwich	1	920	41	40	71	4	67	70
Turkey, roast beef & cheese sandwich	1	770	30	35	69	4	65	59
Turkey, salami & cheese sandwich	1	900	40	40	70	4	66	59
Whole wheat tortilla, for wraps	12"	300	8	24	52	6	46	8
Wendy's	***	***	*	*	*	*	*	*
Ancho chipotle ranch dressing	1 svg	90	8	80	3	0	3	1
Baconator	1	590	51	78	35	1	34	56
Baked potato, w/ bacon & cheese	1	460	13	25	67	7	60	19
Baked potato, w/ broccoli & cheese	1	340	4	11	70	8	62	10
Baked potato, plain	1	270	0	0	61	7	54	7
Baked potato, w/ sour cream & chives	1	320	3	8	63	7	56	8
Balsamic vinaigrette	1 svg	90	6	60	8	0	8	0
Barbecue sauce	1	45	0	0	11	0	11	1
Bold buffalo boneless wings	1	520	18	31	58	2	56	31
Caesar salad, side	1	70	4	51	4	2	2	6
Chicken BLT salad	1	470	27	52	23	3	20	35
Chicken Caesar salad	1	180	4	20	8	3	5	28
Chicken club sandwich	1	550	26	43	48	2	46	34
Chicken nuggets	5 pc	230	16	63	11	0	11	12
Chicken nuggets	10 pc	470	32	61	21	0	21	23
Chili, lg	1	280	9	29	29	7	22	21
Chili, sm	1	190	6	28	19	5	14	14
Chunky blue cheese dressing	1 svg	230	24	94	2	0	2	2
Classic ranch dressing	1 svg	200	20	90	3	0	3	1
Coffee, all sizes	***	0	0	0	0	0	0	0
Crispy chicken sandwich	1	360	18	45	36	2	34	15
Crispy noodles	1 svg	70	3	39	10	0	10	1
Double Stack	1	360	18	45	26	1	25	23
Double w/ everything & cheese	1	700	40	51	38	2	36	47

	Serving Size	Calories	Fat (g)	Calories from Fat (%)	Total Carbs (g)	Fiber (g)	Net Carbs (g)	Protein (g)
Wendy's (cont.)	***	***	*	*	*	*	*	*
Fat free French dressing	1 svg	70	0	0	17	1	16	0
Fish fillet sandwich, premium	1	470	24	46	47	1	46	17
French fries, lg	1	540	26	43	71	7	64	7
French fries, med	1	420	20	43	55	5	50	5
French fries, sm	1	330	16	44	44	4	40	4
Grilled chicken Go Wrap	1	250	10	36	24	1	23	17
Heartland ranch sauce	1	160	17	96	1	0	1	0
Homestyle chicken fillet sandwich	1	440	16	33	47	2	45	25
Homestyle chicken Go Wrap	1	310	15	44	30	1	29	15
Homestyle garlic croutons	1 svg	70	3	39	9	0	9	2
Honey BBQ boneless wings	1	580	18	28	75	2	73	32
Honey Dijon dressing	1 svg	250	24	86	9	0	9	1
Honey mustard sauce	1	130	12	83	6	0	6	0
Hot Tea	16 fl oz	0	0	0	1	0	1	0
Italian vinaigrette	1 svg	130	11	76	8	0	8	0
Junior bacon cheeseburger	1	310	16	46	25	1	24	17
Junior cheeseburger	1	270	11	37	26	1	25	15
Junior cheeseburger deluxe	1	300	14	42	28	2	26	15
Junior hamburger	1	230	8	31	26	1	25	13
Light classic ranch dressing	1 svg	90	8	80	4	0	4	1
Light honey Dijon dressing	1 svg	100	5	45	13	1	12	1
Mandarin chicken salad	1	180	2	10	16	2	14	24
Mandarin orange cup	1	80	0	0	19	1	18	1
Oriental sesame dressing	1 svg	170	10	53	19	0	19	1
Reduced fat acidified sour cream	1 svg	45	4	80	2	0	2	1
Roasted almonds	1 svg	130	11	76	4	2	2	5
Seasoned tortilla strips	1 svg	110	5	41	13	1	12	2
Side salad	1	35	0	0	8	2	6	1
Single w/ everything	1	430	20	42	38	2	36	25
Southwest taco salad	1	400	22	50	26	7	19	27
Spicy chicken fillet sandwich	1	440	16	33	49	2	47	26
Spicy chicken Go Wrap	1	320	15	42	30	1	29	16
Supreme Caesar dressing	1 svg	120	13	98	1	0	1	1

	Serving Size	Calories	Fat (g)	Calories from Fat (%)	Total Carbs (g)	Fiber (g)	Net Carbs (g)	Protein (g)
Sweet & sour sauce	1	50	0	0	12	0	12	0
Sweet & spicy Asian chicken boneless wings	1	550	18	29	67	3	64	31
Thousand Island dressing	1 svg	290	28	87	9	0	9	1
Triple w/ everything and cheese	1	970	60	56	39	2	37	69
Ultimate chicken grill sandwich	1	320	7	20	36	2	34	28
Unsweetened Iced Tea, sm	20 fl oz	0	0	0	1	0	1	0
Unsweetened Iced Tea, med	30 fl oz	0	0	0	1	0	1	0
Unsweetened Iced Tea, lg	40 fl oz	5	0	0	2	0	2	0
Whataburger	***	***	*	*	*	*	*	*
Biscuit	1	300	17	51	32	1	31	5
Biscuit & gravy	1	530	36	61	52	1	51	9
Biscuit sandwich w/ bacon, egg & cheese	1	500	32	58	33	1	32	16
Biscuit sandwich w/ egg & cheese	1	450	28	56	33	1	32	13
Biscuit sandwich w/ sausage, egg & cheese	1	690	49	64	33	1	32	26
Biscuit w/ bacon	1	350	20	51	32	1	31	8
Biscuit w/ sausage	1	540	37	62	32	1	31	18
Breakfast On a Bun, w/ bun	1	360	21	53	25	1	24	15
Breakfast On a Bun, w/ sausage	1	550	38	62	25	1	24	25
Breakfast platter w/ bacon	1	740	45	55	53	2	51	24
Breakfast platter w/ sausage	1	930	62	60	53	2	51	34
Chicken strip	1 pc	200	12	54	11	0	11	9
Chicken strips	2 pc	380	24	57	22	0	22	18
Chicken strips	3 pc	580	37	57	34	0	34	28
Chicken strips salad	1	430	25	52	33	4	29	19
Chicken strips w/ gravy	4 pc	840	54	58	53	0	53	37
Chocolate chunk cookie	1	230	11	43	33	1	32	2
Chocolate malt, med	1	1050	25	21	188	3	185	21
Chocolate shake, med	1	1000	26	23	171	3	168	22
Chop house cheddar burger	1	1170	76	58	56	2	54	55
Cinnamon roll	1	390	9	21	71	3	68	7
Egg sandwich	1	310	17	49	25	1	24	12

	Serving Size	Calories	Fat (g)	Calories from Fat (%)	Total Carbs (g)	Fiber (g)	Net Carbs (g)	Protein (g)
Whataburger (cont.)	***	***	*	*	*	*	*	*
French fries, lg	1	530	27	46	63	5	58	8
French fries, med	1	400	20	45	47	4	43	6
French fries, sm	1	260	13	45	31	2	29	4
Garden salad	1	50	1	18	11	4	7	1
Grilled chicken salad	1	220	8	33	18	4	14	21
Grilled chicken sandwich	1	470	19	36	49	3	46	27
Honey butter chicken biscuit	1	610	38	56	51	1	50	14
Hot apple pie	1	230	11	43	29	2	27	3
Hot lemon pie	1	230	12	47	35	1	34	3
Junior chop house burger	1	630	44	63	28	1	27	30
Justaburger	1	290	15	47	26	1	25	13
Onion rings, lg	1	630	42	60	55	4	51	8
Onion rings, med	1	420	28	60	36	3	33	5
Pancakes, w/ bacon	1	630	12	17	112	5	107	20
Pancakes, w/ sausage	1	820	29	32	112	5	107	30
Pancakes, plain	1	580	8	12	112	5	107	17
Ranch sauce	3 oz	480	51	96	4	0	4	1
Strawberry malt, med	1	1040	24	21	188	0	188	19
Strawberry shake, med	1	990	26	24	171	0	171	20
Taquito, w/ bacon & egg	1	380	21	50	27	3	24	17
Taquito, w/ bacon, egg & cheese	1	420	24	51	27	3	24	19
Taquito, w/ potato & egg	1	430	23	48	37	3	34	15
Taquito, w/ potato, egg & cheese	1	470	27	52	37	3	34	17
Taquito, w/ sausage & egg	1	410	24	53	27	3	24	17
Taquito, w/ sausage, egg & cheese	1	450	28	56	27	3	24	19
Texas toast	1 pc	150	7	42	20	1	19	3
Vanilla malt, med	1	940	27	26	155	0	155	21
Vanilla shake, med	1	890	28	28	139	0	139	22
Whataburger	1	620	30	44	58	2	56	26
Whataburger Jr	1	300	15	45	28	1	27	13
Whataburger, w/ bacon & cheese	1	780	43	50	59	2	57	36

	Serving Size	Calories	Fat (g)	Calories from Fat (%)	Total Carbs (g)	Fiber (g)	Net Carbs (g)	Protein (g)
Whataburger, double meat	1	870	49	51	58	2	56	43
Whataburger, triple meat	1	1120	68	55	58	2	56	61
Whatacatch dinner	1	1580	92	52	161	8	153	29
Whatacatch sandwich	1	460	29	57	38	2	36	15
Whatachick'n sandwich	1	550	20	33	65	4	61	26
White chocolate chunk macadamia nut cookie	1	250	14	50	30	0	30	3
White peppered gravy, for chicken strips	1 svg	60	5	75	8	0	8	0
White Castle	***	***	*	*	*	*	*	*
Sandwiches	***	***	*	*	*	*	*	*
Bacon cheeseburger	1	200	11	50	15	Tr	15	10
Bacon jalapeno cheeseburger	1	210	12	51	15	Tr	15	11
Cheeseburger	1	170	9	48	15	Tr	15	7
Chicken breast sandwich	1	170	5	26	21	Tr	21	11
Chicken breast sandwich, w/ cheese	1	200	7	32	21	Tr	21	12
Chicken ring sandwich	1	170	8	42	19	Tr	19	7
Chicken ring sandwich, w/ cheese	1	200	10	45	19	Tr	19	8
Double bacon cheeseburger	1	370	22	54	23	1	22	19
Double cheeseburger	1	300	17	51	23	1	22	14
Double fish, w/o cheese	1	290	11	34	32	1	31	15
Double fish, w/ cheese	1	310	13	38	32	1	31	16
Double jalapeno cheeseburger	1	320	19	53	23	1	22	15
Double White Castle	1	250	13	47	22	1	21	11
Fish sandwich	1	160	6	34	19	Tr	19	8
Fish sandwich, w/ cheese	1	190	8	38	19	Tr	19	9
Jalapeno cheeseburger	1	180	10	50	15	Tr	15	8
Pulled pork BBQ sandwich	1	170	5	26	24	1	23	9
Surf & turf	1	340	18	48	28	1	27	17
Surf & turf, w/ cheese	1	390	22	51	28	1	27	20
Traditional bun, w/ cheese	1	100	4	36	13	Tr	13	3
White Castle	1	140	7	45	14	Tr	14	6

	Serving Size	Calories	Fat (g)	Calories from Fat (%)	Total Carbs (g)	Fiber (g)	Net Carbs (g)	Protein (g)
White Castle (cont.)	***	***	*	*	*	*	*	*
Breakfast Sandwiches	***	***	*	*	*	*	*	*
Bacon	1	90	3	30	12	1	11	3
Bacon & cheese	1	120	5	38	12	1	11	5
Bacon & egg	1	160	8	45	12	1	11	10
Bacon, egg & cheese	1	190	10	47	12	1	11	11
Egg	1	140	6	39	12	1	11	8
Egg & cheese	1	160	8	45	12	1	11	10
Hamburger & cheese	1	150	9	54	12	1	11	7
Hamburger & egg	1	200	11	50	12	1	11	12
Hamburger, egg & cheese	1	120	13	98	12	1	11	13
Sausage	1	210	15	64	12	1	11	7
Sausage & cheese	1	230	17	67	12	1	11	8
Sausage & egg	1	280	20	64	12	1	11	13
Sausage, egg & cheese	1	310	22	64	12	1	11	15
Sides & Sauces	***	***	*	*	*	*	*	*
BBQ sauce	1 oz	35	Tr	0	8	0	8	0
Chicken rings	3 pc	150	10	60	8	0	8	8
Chicken rings	6 pc	310	20	58	17	0	17	15
Chicken rings	9 pc	460	30	59	25	0	25	23
Clam strips, reg	1	250	22	79	5	0	5	8
Fat free honey mustard sauce	1 oz	50	0	0	13	0	13	0
Fish nibblers, reg	1	280	16	51	24	5	19	19
French fries, reg	1	400	29	65	25	3	22	3
Homestyle onion ring, reg	1	400	21	47	49	1	48	4
Marinara sauce	1 oz	15	0	0	3	0	3	1
Mozzarella cheese sticks	3 pc	250	14	50	22	1	21	10
Mozzarella cheese sticks	5 pc	420	23	49	37	2	35	17
Onion chips, reg	1	480	23	43	62	2	60	7
Onion rings, reg	1	200	9	41	28	1	27	2
Ranch dressing	1 oz	150	17	100	1	0	1	0
Seafood sauce	1 oz	30	0	0	7	0	7	0
White Castle Zesty Zing sauce	1 oz	120	11	83	4	0.	4	0